THE POWERHOUSE DIET

THE POWERHOUSE DIET

The High-raw, Low-grain Miracle for
Radiant Health, Good Looks and a
Great Body

LESLIE KENTON

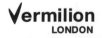
Vermilion
LONDON

First published in the United Kingdom in 2004 by
Vermilion, an imprint of Ebury Press
Random House UK Ltd.
Random House
20 Vauxhall Bridge Road,
London SW1V 2SA

Random House Australia (Pty) Limited
20 Alfred Street, Milsons Point, Sydney,
New South Wales 2061, Australia

Random House New Zealand Limited
18 Poland Road, Glenfield,
Auckland 10, New Zealand

Random House (Pty) Limited
Endulini, 5a Jubilee Road, Parktown 2193, South Africa

Random House UK Limited Reg. No. 954009
www.randomhouse.co.uk

Papers used by Vermilion are natural, recyclable products made from wood grown in sustainable forests.

ISBN: 0091891639

Typeset by Palimpsest Book Production Limited,
Polmont, Stirlingshire

Printed and bound in Australia by
Griffin Press

For Jo Jordan
whose courage and spirit inspires me

AUTHOR'S NOTE

This book explores a life-enhancing way of eating for high-level energy, good looks and emotional balance. *The Powerhouse Diet* offers protection from premature ageing and degenerative diseases, as well as rejuvenating mind and body. I will reveal how a high-raw, low-grain diet can be used to help strengthen the immune system, expand awareness and de-age the body. Light, nutrient-rich Powerhouse eating enhances life energy, naturally reversing the ageing process and assuring us of protection against illness and degeneration.

Recent research into the power of plant chemicals is creating a whole new approach to preventative and life-nurturing nutrition and is making a huge contribution to natural health and holistic medicine. A high-raw, low-grain diet based on foods rich in these plant compounds, essential fatty acids and other nutrients can actually bring about age reversal. This can be measured by orthodox medical parameters, such as lowered cholesterol and blood pressure, improved insulin resistance as well as the loss of many symptoms normally associated with degeneration. It also enhances our mental clarity, improves our emotional balance and heightens vitality.

And the power of foods for life enhancement cannot be quantified in chemical terms alone. It also depends on the way in which the foods have been grown and handled, and on the quality of life energy they carry. Raw vegetables and fruits contain enzymes and life energy that is lost when they are cooked. Even protein foods such as fish and game are higher quality when eaten raw or undercooked, as heat denatures the protein. So *The Powerhouse Diet* explores the life energy of fresh foods as well and contains many recipes – from sashimi to raw energy salads – specially designed to preserve it.

The information in this book is in no way intended to be prescriptive, to replace medical advice or be a substitute for a good doctor or a well-trained health-care practitioner – especially one knowledgeable in nutrition and natural healing. If you are ill or suspect you are ill, it is important that you see a physician. If you have been taking prescription medication, don't change your diet drastically without consulting your doctor. Neither the publisher nor the author can accept responsibility for injuries or illnesses arising out of a failure by a reader to take medical advice. I want to make clear that I have no commercial interest in any product, treatment or organisation mentioned in this book. I do, however, have a profound interest in helping myself and others to maximise their potential for positive health, awareness and creativity. For it is my belief that the more each one of us is able to re-establish harmony within ourselves and with our environment, the better equipped we will be to wrestle with the challenges now facing us in the world.

CONTENTS

ONE

REACH FOR THE TOP

If someone told you you could be healthy, lean for life and free from premature ageing, as well as remain highly protected against degenerative diseases, what would you say? And what if you could also look and feel 10 or more years younger than your chronological age – all by making simple changes to what you eat? Would you believe them? Sound too good to be true? Read on.

QUANTUM HEALTH

Let's take things further. What if you learned of a way of eating that brought you ongoing vitality, year after year, that improved athletic performance, helped clear cellulite and PMS, and offered emotional balance, enhanced mental clarity and virtually endless energy? Such things are not only possible, they are the experience of a growing number of men and women throughout the world who now choose to eat the way our Paleolithic ancestors did.

High Power Health

These savvy people – among them some of Hollywood's top stars and some of the world's best endurance athletes – know stuff that most of us have yet to discover. I call them the health élitists. Their goal is to live life at the peaks. They need an ongoing ability to access high levels of energy, creativity and freedom, stamina and good looks. These are but a few of the gifts that accompany eating foods on which we as human beings have been genetically programmed to thrive for over a million years of our evolution. When you supply a body with everything it needs to function optimally, it is not only often capable of healing itself, it can also reach heights of vitality, clarity and functioning that most of us would not believe possible. How to make such experiences possible for you is what this book is all about.

DOUBLE YOUR ENERGY

Scientific discoveries with the potential to fundamentally transform human health are rare. Few of them see the light of day; still fewer get translated into the kind of information and practices you or I can use to change our lives for the better. This book is about some such discoveries and how to apply them to your life. It shows you how you can shed excess weight while becoming fitter, healthier and brimming with energy. The information, tools, techniques and recipes it provides can also help you stay that way.

I am fully aware of what a huge statement this is. Yet it is true. The major discoveries come from three separate but closely related areas of nutrition which as yet few know about:

1. The discovery that returning to an approximation of what our Paleolithic ancestors ate – fresh raw foods plus top-quality proteins – stops swings in energy and mood, realigns the body to a high level of health, and curbs Syndrome X (more about this later).
2. The findings that by eliminating wheat and maize from your diet, along with sugars, starches and sweets, and reducing or even cutting out other cooked grains, you can transform the bio-chemistry of your body, trigger fat loss, restore energy, wipe out cravings for alcohol, drugs and sweets, and help your body grow lean naturally.
3. The mounting scientific evidence that human beings thrive on a high-raw diet thanks to the high level of life order and support it imparts to a living system, both physically and energetically.

Discoveries and clinical experience in all these areas feed into each other and form the foundation on which *The Powerhouse Diet* is built.

Quantum Health

I have long believed that few of us reach our potentials for radiant health, energy, clarity, emotional balance and creative power. This is what I call life at the peaks – quantum health. By this I mean a real leap into a totally different way of living – which most people don't think is possible. I mean a way of living where you wake in the morning feeling fresh and good about yourself and your life, in which your physical and mental potential has the best chance of being used to full effect – that realm of consciousness in which your capacity for fun, passion and excitement just about being alive can be like that of a joyous child. For real health is not just the absence of disease. It is a dynamic state of mind, body and spirit which makes it possible for us to participate fully and spontaneously in life, whatever it throws at us.

EXCITING NEW PARADIGM

People at the further reaches of human health do not face the future with fears about getting old and falling prey to degenerative disease. They live in anticipation that the best is yet to come. They know they are capable of moving towards an even more positive state of health and fulfilment as the years pass. They are no longer ruled by outdated ideas about ageing which teach that getting older includes illness as a 'natural' part of life. They know different. Their paradigms of ageing are closer to that of world-famous age researcher Johan Bjorksten who speaks of giving 'as many people as possible as many more healthy vigorous years of life as possible'.

The Missing Pieces

Twenty years ago my daughter and I wrote a ground-breaking book about the wonders of high-raw eating called *Raw Energy*. I am not a scientist, I am merely a reporter. I make no claims for 'healing' with raw foods. Yet, ever since the publication of *Raw Energy*, letters have flooded in from around the world. People have written to tell me about their experiments with high-raw eating and all the payoffs they have had. Together with new information from many scientific disciplines, they have added missing pieces to the original *Raw Energy* puzzle. They have expanded exponentially the understanding of how to use diet to encourage healing and enhance health. Here are some of the things I have learned from them:

❏ An *all-raw* diet is useful *temporarily* for deep detoxification and encouraging the body to heal both acute and chronic diseases.

❏ It is *not* advisable for *most* people to eat nothing but raw foods for long periods. An all-raw diet is great for short-term healing. People who carry on with it for years may continue to feel energetic and well, yet they seem to lose power and stamina, both physically and mentally, and sometimes even find it hard to live in the 'real' world. This is often because they do not get enough top-quality protein foods which give good architecture to body and psyche.

❏ In addition to fresh raw vegetables and fruits, seeds and nuts, we also need plenty of high-quality protein to keep our feet on the ground and give us the ability to function effectively in the world.

❑ Adequate protein is far healthier for bones than a low-protein diet. Organic and free-range meat, fish, game and eggs can contribute enormously to your power and vitality and help protect from premature ageing and degenerative disease (something I, like many others, for years did not know to be true).

❑ Too many concentrated fruit products, too many sweeteners like honey, raw sugar, rice syrup and malt extract which all-raw foodies often get, are not good. They can disturb insulin balance and in the long term predispose us to Syndrome X (*see below*) and all the degeneration that brings with it.

❑ The majority of people living on a Western diet show signs of Syndrome X or *insulin resistance syndrome.* This epidemic of abnormalities includes high blood pressure, distorted blood fats or triglycerides, high cholesterol and blood sugar disorders. It carries with it an increased risk of just about every age-related disorder you can name: from eye problems, heart disease, nervous system disorders, obesity, diabetes and Alzheimer's to chronic fatigue, exhaustion, anxiety, depression and poor sense of self-worth. Why? Because the way we are eating and living now is so far removed from what our bodies are genetically programmed to thrive on.

❑ Raw foods carry light energy – photons – gathered by plants and animals from the sun's own energy. These *biophotons* interact with our body's own light-based, energy-based cellular control and communication systems – *the living matrix* – to heal, to energise, to bring mental and emotional clarity and to help keep our bodies strong and resistant to the build-up of toxic waste which invites disease and degeneration.

❑ Eating a no-grain – or a low-grain – diet together with good-quality protein foods and lots of raw non-starchy vegetables and fruits reduces fatigue for virtually everyone while eliminating weight problems, banishing inflammation and further enhancing health, energy and good looks.

❑ Today's fruits and vegetables too often lack yesterday's nutrition, so a few well-chosen natural nutritional supplements can further enhance well-being. We need if at all possible to go for organic foods and so help avoid the toxic build-ups that can occur from foods grown using conventional farming methods.

❑ Finally – and most important of all – high-raw, low-grain eating helps rebalance metabolism, allowing the body's own remarkable inner power for healing to regenerate and rejuvenate the whole person. Why? Because the high-raw, low-grain diet with adequate protein foods is as close as you can get to eating as our ancestors have done for more than a million years of human evolution. It is the kind of diet we are genetically predisposed to thrive on. When we eat this way we provide our body with everything it needs to raise itself to even higher levels of health, energy and clarity of mind.

In this book I make available the research and opinions of scientists – many of them Nobel laureates – working in studies related to the actions of uncooked food on health. I also wish to share with you the benefits I and others have found using a high-raw diet.

This information is in no way intended to be prescriptive. No book can replace adequate medical care. If you are seriously unwell, it is important you seek the attention and care of a nutritionally aware physician. Everyone is biochemically and energetically unique. It is good to find a professional savvy enough to work well with you in the light of your own individuality.

I believe that all of us have far more resources for happiness, health and creativity than we use. *The Powerhouse Diet* is bringing more and more people to an experience of high energy and health which delights them, and which has them looking towards the future with enthusiasm. May you be blessed with its gifts.

MOVE INTO POWER

Twenty-five years ago I became fascinated by a high-raw diet. I had been chronically ill as a child – one 'infection' after another, nightmares, anxiety – but no one seemed able to help me. Then a wonderful break came my way. I met some truly remarkable doctors.

These were men and women who had been highly trained in orthodox medicine where drugs are the primary means of treating symptoms. Yet lucky for me, these were *doctors with a difference*. Disillusioned with the symptomatic approach, they had decided to look deeper and to ask questions like 'What can be done to help a living body heal itself from inside without the negative side-effects of toxic chemicals in drugs?' These physicians in Britain, the United States and Europe were enormously generous with their time and their knowledge. They taught me things they had spent decades learning: how to detoxify my body using a high-raw or all-raw diet, how to enhance my energy and – most important of all – how to trust my body's ability to heal itself.

I practised what they taught and experimented with countless natural techniques. My discoveries turned my life around. I learned that my tendency to 'infection' was in fact food allergies. I learned that my body had become toxic from years of eating convenience foods. I watched and marvelled as high-raw eating cleared the toxicity, the illness and the depression. I lost fat from my body spontaneously. I felt great. I had so much energy that my children suggested I start smoking to put a damper on it. (There is nothing worse than waking up to an ultra-dynamic, hypercheerful mother.) I never looked back. It was these changes that threw me into a career in health: TV programmes, articles, books, seminars, workshops, creating teaching modules for universities – the lot. I saw clearly that few of us ever live out our potentials for dynamism, creativity, good looks and radiant health. I felt passionate about sharing what I had been taught and had experienced for myself with others.

My children also became intrigued by the changes they saw happening to me on a high-raw diet. They loved the delicious foods and natural sweet treats I prepared for them. One day, my daughter Susannah, who has always been fascinated by health and energy, suggested we write a book about the transformation high-raw eating could bring about. Gail Rebuck, my first editor – now CEO of Random House UK – loved the idea. And so we began our research.

UNANSWERED QUESTIONS

I discovered that a diet which is 50–75 per cent raw makes most people look and feel their best, gives high levels of energy and stamina to cope with day-to-day living and protects from minor illnesses like flu and colds, as well as from premature ageing and degeneration. So profound were the energising effects that a high-raw diet had on myself and others, I was determined to learn as much as possible about why (having grown up in the 20th century with its passion for scientific explanations of phenomena). What is so special about uncooked foods, I wanted to know? What gives them the power to heal even long-standing illnesses? What is it about a diet of raw foods and juices – the typical regime of the world's most exclusive health spas – that has men and women looking 10 years younger after a fortnight?

Gathering Facts

My aim was simple: to gather together all the facts I could find about the effects of raw food. I delved through hundreds of books and research papers on the biochemistry and clinical uses of uncooked foods. I discovered a vast quantity of evidence showing how a way of eating in which 50–75 per cent of your foods are taken raw can reverse bodily degeneration and short-and long-term illness, can slow the rate at which a body ages, bring you boundless energy and help restore emotional balance. I found out that there is far more to the health-giving properties of uncooked foods than merely their high vitamin and mineral content. I came to understand that the body is a highly complex tapestry of energy, physical matter and biochemistry. In the past 20 years, this interconnected web of life has been identified, and named by scientists *the living matrix*. Many of the implications of these findings are beginning to alter our whole way of looking at health and life.

FROM PERSONAL TO UNIVERSAL

I discovered that the Germans, the Austrians, the Swedes and the Swiss have for generations catalogued the health-promoting effects of a diet high in raw fresh vegetables and fruits. I found that such a diet had been credited with the healing of long-term crippling diseases like arthritis and cancer, gastric ulcers, diabetes and heart disease. I uncovered reports of how athletes, taken off their usual diet high in cooked foods and put on a raw regime, not only lost none of their physical prowess but also improved their performances.

But my research into the benefits of high-raw eating did not end with the publication of *Raw Energy*. I knew that this was not the whole story. Since then I have worked with people all over the world to answer the question 'what are the fundamental principles that allow the finest expression of health and vitality, protection from degeneration, and let people live their life at the peaks?' With the help of doctors and scientists, including exciting new research which has only emerged in the last five to 10 years and is still little known to the public, I have finally put together the protocols for *The Powerhouse Diet*.

The Transformative Triad

The Powerhouse Diet is based on the discoveries of leading-edge science, facts which even 20 years ago were completely unknown. Now we understand that an optimal experience of human health and vitality is only possible when what we eat and the way we live is in line with what we have been genetically predisposed to thrive on. Such a simple idea. Yet what dazzling payoffs it brings. In practical terms this means three things:

1. A high-raw diet like that of our hunter-gatherer ancestors.

2. Adequate top-quality protein foods.

3. A low- or no-grain and low- or no-sugar way of eating.

There is an epidemic overtaking the Western world, and you need to know about it. Known as *insulin resistance syndrome* or *Syndrome X*, it's a serious condition based on your body's inability to handle the kinds of foods you eat. Syndrome X is not one condition but a collection of abnormalities which tend to occur together including high blood pressure, distorted cholesterol measurements and many other things your doctor worries about. They include, among others, a loss of muscle and an increase in fat in the body, furred arteries, and blood sugar disorders that screw up our energy. Together, these abnormalities make us vulnerable to overweight and obesity and put us at increased risk of getting just about every age-related disorder you can name: eye problems, diabetes, heart disease, cancer and Alzheimer's, to mention only a few. Syndrome X can be responsible for all sorts of other miseries too – from chronic fatigue and anxiety to obesity and irritability, depression and a poor sense of personal worth. Most frightening of all, people still consider these things to be a 'normal' part of growing older. They are not.

Beware Syndrome X

Syndrome X is not caused by a virus or accident of nature. It's a result of a sedentary lifestyle coupled with the high-grain, high-carbohydrate way of eating which we have followed for a very long time, believing – as government directives still tell us we should – that such a diet constitutes nutrition for health.

TOO MUCH GRAIN CAN BREED DESTRUCTION

In the so-called civilised world, people are fatter than ever. What's worse, we grow fatter still with each year that passes. Food manufacturers, government bodies and well-meaning doctors urge us to eat more low-fat, high-carb foods: masses of bread and cereals, rice and pasta. Fats, not carbohydrates, are supposed to be the villains of the piece. Only they're not. Extensive research into the effects of a low-fat, high-carbs diet on insulin resistance, obesity and the development of degenerative diseases shows quite clearly that these are precisely the foods which make us fat in the first place.

Impeccable scientific research indicates that these directives are wrong. Eating this way messes up the human metabolism. It is contrary to what our bodies throughout the whole of evolution have been programmed to thrive on – so contrary that it actually causes degeneration.

Here's the Gen

It happens like this: the hormone insulin delicately controls how your body turns the carbohydrates you eat into energy. But eating too much high-carbohydrate, grain-based and sugar-based food *floods* cells with insulin. This leads to a cascade of problems. The cells in your body lose their sensitivity to insulin, which means even more of it has to be produced to have any effect. Too much insulin circulating in the blood causes your body to convert food into fat, yet prevents it from releasing the fat to use as fuel. Instead it stores more fat in your cells, creates plaque in your arteries, distorts brain chemistry causing mood swings, and makes your energy unstable so you reach for another cup of coffee at 11 a.m. just to keep going. It's not hard to see that the high-carb diet based on too many grains and sugars (not to mention chemicals which the human body does not handle) can lead both directly and indirectly to degeneration, obesity and the rest of Syndrome X's grim tally.

So much for the bad news. The goods news is actually the magnificent news. Begin to eat in a way that is as close as possible to what your body has been genetically accustomed to – the Powerhouse eating you will find in this book – and you can turn your life around. What's more, these kinds of foods are absolutely delicious – a far cry from the health-food fodder and the high-carbs, low-fat stuff that is still too often foisted upon us.

High-Raw, No-Grain, Delicious

What is slowly beginning to replace all the high-carbs stuff in people's minds is 'high-protein, low-carbs' eating. That's good. At least it's a step in the right direction. But it does not go far enough. Of course the human body *needs* carbohydrates, but it needs the *right kind* of carbohydrates – the carbs friendly to our genes, not masses of manufactured foods riddled with junk fats, wheat, other refined grains, sugars and chemicals. It also needs *adequate*, not 'high', amounts of protein.

The kind of carbohydrates we thrive on are found in fresh, raw, non-starchy vegetables like broccoli, herbs, cauliflower, salad greens, carrots, celery and fresh fruits. Why? Because these are the kinds of carbohydrates our ancestors ate and therefore the foods our bodies need.

TOO MUCH, TOO SOON

Our genes change slowly. It takes 100,000 years to make even one significant evolutionary change to genes. The forces of natural selection have acted on us for millions of years, shaping and moulding our genetic makeup and biochemical functioning. Our bodies have only been subjected to high-density carbohydrate foods like bread and sugar for the last 4,000 years, since the advent of widespread agriculture. Before that we were always hunter-gatherers who ate raw foods primarily throughout the whole of evolution. We have eaten raw foods for more than a million years. Our bodies have come to need and to expect them. Most important of all, they thrive on a wide variety of fresh raw vegetable foods plus good proteins and essential fats.

Express Your Genes with Excellence

The Powerhouse high-raw, no-grain way of eating – complete with fish, game, herbs and seeds, eggs and meat (preferably organic) or vegan proteins like tofu – makes it possible for the human body to experience élite levels of *genetic expression.* What few people yet know is that more important than the genes we inherit are the ways in which those genes are *expressed.* This is the scientific term for how your genetic inheritance is lived out in day-to-day life. Do your genes express themselves by creating massive vitality for you? Clarity of mind? Creativity and freedom from illness? Or do they express themselves in negative ways by creating obesity, chronic fatigue, sagging skin and spirit, early ageing and degeneration? The quality of genetic expression depends primarily on how you eat and live, since it is this which determines the quality of the fluids in which your genes bathe within your cells.

Slow to Change

Although it takes about 100,000 years for a single significant genetic change to evolve in a human being, we have only had cooked foods and grains for a few thousand years. We have only had convenience foods, sugar and all this high-carbs stuff for the last 100 years. And guess what? It is during this period that the epidemics which now plague the Western world – from obesity to heart disease, diabetes, arthritis and other inflammatory conditions – have developed.

Powerhouse eating, which honours our genetic inheritance, can not only protect you from the fatigue and low-level experience of health which most people struggle with, it may even reverse existing disorders in medically measurable ways, bringing your body an experience of élitist vitality and optimal health at any age. For your body has a remarkable ability to heal itself when you clear it of stuff that does not belong in it and bathe your genes in what they need to make you super healthy and full of life. For most people, Powerhouse eating knocks on the head all signs of Syndrome X with high cholesterol and lack of energy, and brings them to new heights of vitality.

WHAT IS RAW POWER EATING?

It is a way of eating that makes use of cutting-edge scientific discoveries and natural medicine principles about what our bodies have been genetically programmed to thrive on for over a million years of evolution.

- ❑ High in raw foods
- ❑ Contains good-quality protein
- ❑ Low in grains

The Powerhouse Experience

How does this transformation come about? Powerhouse eating alters both the *kind* and *ratio* of the three fundamental nutrients – proteins, carbohydrates and fats – in your diet as well as their *quality*. You'll only eat the best: slow-release, low-density carbohydrates – as many as possible in their raw state, rich in vital plant nutrients and life itself – which do not distort blood sugar, upset insulin balance and contribute to Syndrome X. You also get plenty of top-quality proteins, omega-3 essential fatty acids and delicious and nutritious oils and fats – from coconut oil to creamy butter. Together, such foods can bring about a total and permanent physical metamorphosis as well as an end to fatigue and food cravings. The best news yet? Powerhouse meals are a far cry from what you have come to think of as 'health foods'. You know – the kind of things you are 'supposed' to eat even though they taste revolting. The foods are absolutely delicious – splendid herb salads with shavings of the best Parmesan, fish or chicken cooked in a rich coconut sauce – even desserts and sweet treats if you have a sweet tooth. Eat them and enjoy, while your body gets busy making itself healthier, more radiant and more beautiful with each week that passes.

ESCAPE FROM THE TWILIGHT ZONE

Do you live in the full radiance of vitality, energy and well-being? Do you wake each morning the way a healthy child does, excited by what lies ahead in the day? Or do you find it difficult to extract yourself from the twilight zone of survival – coping with life instead of living it to the full?

Working with animals at the University of Rostock just before World War II, Professor Werner Kollath discovered an extraordinary phenomenon he called *meso-health* – middle-nourishment. He discovered that a diet which did not produce high-level health nonetheless would sustain so-called normal health. Kollath took animals and reared them on a diet of purified, processed foodstuffs devoid of all minerals except potassium, phosphate and zinc, and virtually empty of vitamins except a little thiamine. Despite their poorly nourished condition, his animals grew and showed no clinical signs of disease, not even vitamin deficiencies.

Degeneration Starts Here

By the time they reached adulthood, however, like the rest of us, Kollath's animals showed serious signs of degeneration – dental caries, constipation, large populations of harmful bacteria in their colon, furred arteries, loss of calcium from their bones. No amount of vitamin supplements was able to reverse unpleasant changes in Kollath's animals. The only thing that did, provided it was given early enough, was an abundance of fresh raw food containing green leaves and vegetables. Kollath's findings were later confirmed by researchers working in Stockholm and Munich and applied to human health in European clinics with similar success.

HONOUR THE ANCESTORS

When an animal, human or otherwise, is not provided with a diet akin to what its genetic inheritance thrives on, degeneration sets in. This awareness of the importance that our genetic inheritance has in determining the kind of diet we need to eat to prevent degeneration, and fully *thrive* instead of merely survive, is taking off in scientific circles. Our ancestors were hunter-gatherers. They lived on weeds and vegetables, grubs, small and large animals, fish and fruit plus a few seeds and nuts. Virtually all of these foods were eaten raw for more than a million years of human evolution.

Scientists estimate that 60–90 per cent of the calories our Paleolithic ancestors took in came in the form of large and small game animals, eggs, birds, reptiles and insects. Vegetables and seeds were still in their raw wild form and had not been cultivated to create the starchy potatoes, wheat and other crops we know today.

Superb Bodies
The physiology of the body has changed little over the millennia. We are still genetically adapted to wild foods, not to the refined and processed foods we now consume. A hard look at the skeletons of those early hunter-gatherers reveals that pre-agricultural people were not just robust, but about the same size as us. Their diet was three times higher in protein than ours and usually – although not always – lower in fat. Not only was their protein intake higher than ours, their fibre intake was much higher – around 100 grams a day – thanks to all the raw plant foods they consumed. The foods they were eating were of course raw, fibre-rich, unprocessed and unrefined. Their calcium intake was also higher than ours, even though dairy products as we know them did not exist. They also managed to consume more potassium than we do, and their vitamin C intake, estimated at 400mg, was several times higher than our government-recommended daily requirement. And their intake of phytonutrients – the amazing plant factors, from flavonoids to carotenoids, that sport powerful antioxidant and immune-enhancing properties – was a whopping 300 times greater than ours. Even their ratio of polyunsaturated to saturated fat was different from ours. For the beasts they hunted, including small animals, birds, fish and insects, were themselves high in polyunsaturated fats – in marked contrast to the meat from grain-fed animals we eat now, which is full of saturated fat.

When we return to such a way of eating, our body tends to rediscover what it's like to function in the highest possible ways. Our energy soars, healing happens and we look and feel our best.

Why Return to High-raw, Low-grain Eating?

- ❏ You have more energy and vitality and look better.
- ❏ You lose weight easily and keep it off without counting calories.
- ❏ You benefit from the 'information' whole live foods carry to your cells in the form of electrochemical light energy and complex nutritional information, enhancing health and radiance.
- ❏ You get the best possible complements of vitamins, minerals and trace elements as well as essential enzymes which are destroyed when foods are cooked.
- ❏ Eating raw foods strengthens immunity, making you more resistant to disease, degeneration and allergies.
- ❏ Many chronic conditions disappear when people switch to a high-raw, low-grain diet and, the best news yet, they often don't return.

HOW HEALTHY ARE YOU?

Scientists involved in raw-food research and the treatment of illness using high- or all-raw diets believe that most of us in the industrialised world are like Kollath's animals. Most of us live in a state of 'meso-health' – a condition of half-hearted health induced by years of eating devitalised and processed foods. They say that by increasing the quantity of fresh raw food we eat, and cutting out cooked, processed and junk-fat foods, it is not only possible to improve the health of people already suffering from degenerative illness, but also to dramatically improve the health of all of us.

Downhill All the Way

Despite our sophisticated medical system based on potent drugs, dramatic life-saving techniques and high-technology procedures such as coronary bypass surgery, kidney dialysis and prosthetic joints, the state of health of most people in Britain and the United States is poor.

The diseases from which we suffer – cancer, cardiovascular troubles, diabetes, arthritis, respiratory disorders such as emphysema and bronchitis, and depression – have shown little decline in their incidence since the beginning of the 20th century. Indeed most of them, like cancer and mental illness, are steadily increasing.

Until HIV and SARS came along, many viruses and bacteria had been tamed thanks to widespread vaccination, improved public hygiene and the discovery of antibiotics. The diseases our early 21st-century society is heir to are of two sorts: *degenerative* and *immunosuppressant*. Both are fundamentally lifestyle related. They develop out of the way we live, eat and the way our polluted environment compromises our immune system and undermines the body's health-supporting processes. Hospitals and doctors' surgeries are full of people suffering from degenerative diseases: heart disease, hypertension, circulatory ailments, cancer, diabetes, arthritis, obesity, hypoglycaemia, mental disorders. They are the result of stress, overeating, under-exercising and pollution of our environment, whether it be from radiation, airborne chemicals or chemicals in our foods.

VOLKSWAGEN ATTITUDE

High-technology medicine and 11th-hour intervention can do little to prevent or cure such illness. This is why we need to stop treating our bodies with what Kenneth Pelletier, author of *Holistic Medicine*, has dubbed 'the Volkswagen attitude'. He means we must give up the notion that we can run ourselves as long and as hard as we like and then expect the doctor to pick up the pieces or supply us with new parts when we break down. It is high time we took control of how we live and eat, and change things.

All Change
Ecology is the catchword of all the life sciences. It is finally being applied to the human body. Our body, like the earth itself, has finite resources, and the condition we find ourselves in after two, three, four or five decades of living depends primarily on how we have lived. Specifically, it depends on a number of variables over which, ultimately,

only *we* can exercise control. These variables include such things as how we cope with stress, how often and to what degree we subject our bodies to drugs, alcohol and cigarettes, how much physical exercise we take, and what levels of environmental pollution we allow our governments to pass as 'safe'. The single most important variable of all is nutrition.

EAT YOUR WAY TO RADIANCE

Numerous studies now show that when nutrition improves – as we eat more fresh foods and good-quality proteins and less convenience fare for instance – so does health. Even small changes, such as cutting down on processed foods, sugar, alcohol and fat, improve health relatively quickly. And these can be measured too. They show up as lower levels of cholesterol and triglycerides in the blood, lower blood pressure, and more effective functioning of the immune system which protects the body from infection, malignant growths and early ageing. More important, even minor improvements in diet profoundly affect how we look and feel – to me this is the most important 'proof' that what one is doing is right for one's body.

Old Hat Science

The notion most people still have of nutrition is naïve and incomplete. Based on 19th-century scientific thinking, it assumes that Disease A is caused by Nutritional Deficit B. It is known as the single cause/single effect model of disease. Even most standard texts on nutritional diseases still confine themselves to 'deficiency diseases' – scurvy, beriberi, pellagra, rickets and kwashiorkor. The list is short. The diseases it lists are those caused by a shortage of one specific nutrient in the diet. Yet gross manifestations of single-element deficiency are rare in developed countries today. By contrast, sub-clinical nutritional deficiencies which cause slow but inexorable physical decline are not. It is also still common for the average doctor to insist that, provided your diet is 'well-balanced' – and for most people the balance is between one highly processed food and another – it will offer adequate nutritional support for health. This is simply untrue.

COMPLEX SYNERGY

Between 50,000 and 100,000 different chemicals go into the making and running of the human body. They interact with each other in ways so complex that they make the world's most advanced computer look like an abacus. Nutritional science has so far isolated and identified some 17 vitamins and co-factors, 24 minerals, and eight to 10 amino acids as being 'essential' to the health and reproductive abilities of the human body. In truth, there are many more we need in good supply. New vital substances are discovered often – trace elements, fats, phyto-nutrients and enzymes – which are part of the synergy that creates radiant health and freedom from degenerative ageing. High-level well-being depends greatly on the quality and variety of the nutrients we take in. Without them we cannot build and maintain the elaborate machinery and perform the complex chemical transformations on which life depends.

The Whole is Greater

Far from being isolated in their workings, essential nutrients are syner-gistic. They *need* each other. They also enhance each other in their actions on the body. It is only by working together that they are able to enact the complicated routines that make our bodies function well. The human body has evolved to make use of the myriad co-operative and complementary substances which occur in foods in their natural state. There are many similarities between human blood and substances and fluids found in nature; for instance, blood serum has a compos-ition not unlike that of sea water, which is a veritable consommé of minerals. The blood pigment haemoglobin has a molecular structure that closely resembles the plant pigment chlorophyll. Life feeds on life. When we feed on living foods, the life they carry is imparted to us.

Biological Complexity

Foods in nature are highly complex; as the Soviet biochemist Professor I.I. Brekhman says, they are rich in *'structural information* for health' (*see Energy Raw and Free*). Cooking and other forms of processing interfere with this complexity and destroy much of this structural infor-mation on which health depends. To quote Dr Michael Colgan, sports expert, biochemist and former nutritional advisor to the US Olympics Committee, 'The multiple integration of these essential substances is the basis of their biological function. The adequacy of that function depends on the substances being supplied to the body in the same mixtures and concentrations that occur in raw, unprocessed foods. It was by use of these foods that genesis, over millions of years of evolution, developed the precise mechanisms to deal with them. It is not surprising that a diet which deviates too far from what our bodies have been genetically programmed to expect leads to progressive malnutrition. First, our body experiences deprivation at a cellular level, then gradual failure of the body's immune system, then illness.'

BEWARE CELLULAR MALNUTRITION

Another of the 20th century's most highly respected authorities on nutrition, the late American biochemist Roger Williams, said that cellular malnutrition is at the root of 10 times the number of disease conditions as clinically defined deficiencies. The diseases Williams refers to include allergies, arthritis, atherosclerosis (hardening of the arteries), coronary heart disease, emotional disorders, insomnia, periodontal (gum-related) diseases, infections, skeletal deformities, mental retardation and disorders of the immune system. If we are to overcome the current crisis in Western medicine, he always insisted, we must find ways of tackling malnutrition at the cellular level. That means altering the focus of our effort away from treating the symptoms of illness and looking for outside causes. Instead we must concentrate on the overall health and vitality and strengthening of the immune system. The easiest, most effective way of doing this in the long term is by changing our way of eating to one in keeping with what our genes have been designed to thrive on.

The All-important Immune System

The immune system is the Number One suspect in degenerative disease and premature ageing. It is really split into two interdependent parts – the thymus with its T-lymphocytes or T-cells, which is the main system of cellular immunity, and the thymic-independent B-lymphocytes or B-cells, which protect us from most viral and bacterial infections.

BOOST IMMUNITY

Numerous studies have shown that the nutrients which occur in optimal proportions and quantities in fresh uncooked vegetable foods, particularly in home-grown sprouts and vegetable juices – boost lymphocyte production and so increase resistance to illness. The nutrients that most favourably influence the immune system are vitamins E, C and A, many of the B-vitamins, and also zinc. Without a full complement of these fresh food nutrients (and probably others not yet tested and some perhaps not even discovered), immunity cannot be maintained, and we condemn ourselves to a state of mesotrophy. The body has quite extraordinary powers of compensation of course. For many years one can eat the wrong foods and show no clinical sign of illness. But the insidious degenerative process is at work within. Sooner or later, depending on one's constitution and how badly the body is abused, hidden degeneration turns into serious illness.

Self-regulating System

From my own investigations into the clinical effects of diets high in raw foods for healing – as well as from my own personal experience – I have discovered that a high-raw diet offers two precious things:

❏ A promise of greater resistance to illness and ageing.
❏ A key to greater 'aliveness' and vitality.

High-level health can only come from a finely tuned, self-regulating, self-enjoying system. Once you become aware enough of your own needs and your body's own responses to what you eat and don't eat by exploring what Powerhouse eating can do for you, you become the 'authority' on what is best for you. Then you can tap into new levels of energy, good looks and emotional balance and well-being.

LIFE IN THE TWILIGHT ZONE

No one living in what the great Swiss physician Max Bircher-Benner called 'the twilight zone of ill health' – mesotrophy by another name – has such a possibility. When an organism's vitality is lowered, or when its biochemical balance is disturbed, messages from the systems of the body become garbled. How can self-monitoring and self-correcting mechanisms be expected to work if both physical and mental perceptions are distorted? Perhaps the greatest satisfaction a high-raw, low-grain way of eating has to offer is the experience of finely tuned self-regulation day after day, year after year. 'Spiritual' is not a fashionable word with some people. Nevertheless, the benefits of a high-raw diet accrue as much on a spiritual level as they do on a physical one.

Kick the Habit

The American physician Dr John Douglass, who has for many years used a high-raw or all-raw diet in his treatments for countless conditions, discovered a strange pattern when talking to patients at the Kaiser-Permanente Medical Center in Los Angeles. A significant number of his patients report to him that after a few weeks on a high-raw diet they find themselves becoming 'declimatised to Western life'. Old habits such as cigarettes and alcohol often become distasteful and get left behind. This suggests that a high-raw diet tends to make the body more sensitive to whatever it is exposed to. Sexually and aesthetically, that can be enormously rewarding. Higher sensitivity to all kinds of stimuli make it easier to judge 'instinctively' what does you good and what does you harm. If you receive and heed those signals, you intuitively do what is best for you. This is just the beginning of the Powerhouse story.

ENDLESS PAYOFFS

Powerhouse eating creates what I call 'rhinoceros energy'. This is the kind of stamina that keeps you going when others have given up. Thanks to the way in which high-raw, low-grain eating continuously detoxifies the body of energy-depleting chemicals and by-products of stress, it also provides a high level of mental energy and clarity. It is an effective method of rejuvenating body and mind, sorting out female problems including cellulite, making you look great and lifting your spirits, better than anything I have ever found.

The harder you work, the greater the percentage of raw food you need to eat to function at your peak and still have energy left over for play. I belong to a family of amateur runners. Unless we have been out for a run along the cliffs of Pembrokeshire or around the Outer Circle of Regent's Park or on the shores of New Zealand, we feel that something is wrong somewhere. Many years ago when we began to eat a lot of our food raw, we noticed we could run far longer without fatigue. We also had a feeling of lightness on the road – a feeling which, by the way, disappeared when we had been to a party the night before and, in an attempt to be polite, eaten more 'normal' food.

Life Enhancement
It is not only physical energy that soars when you change to a high-raw diet. I also find I can work better for much longer periods – seven or eight hours at top efficiency, rather than three or four – provided I stick to my sprouted salads, eggs, fish, chicken, game and organic meat. I even need less sleep. When I do sleep, my sleep is deeper and more restful.

This experience of increased stamina and energy levels is not unique to me. I have had hundreds, maybe thousands, of letters from people all over the world who report the same experience. Some of them were super-fit even before making the switch to a high-raw diet. When I asked physicians, biochemists and other raw-food experts why raw foods have such an energising effect, they told me it was many things:

❑ A high-raw diet brings the body, in perfect and complementary combination, all the nutrients essential for maximum vitality, both as a whole and at a cellular level.

❑ Raw foods cleanse your body of stored wastes and toxins which interfere with the proper functioning of cells and organs and lower energy levels.

❑ Raw foods increase the micro-electric potential of cells, improving your body's use of oxygen so that both muscles and brain are energised.

❑ Raw foods carry a high level of biochemical and energetic order to the body, enabling it to eliminate illnesses and reach its optimal level of healthy functioning.

OXYGEN TO SPARE

Athletic performance is largely determined by how efficiently the body uses oxygen. This in turn depends on how good your heart is at delivering oxygenated blood to your muscles and how good your muscles are at extracting the oxygen once it arrives. Regular training helps a lot. It strengthens your heart so that it pumps more blood with each beat. It increases the number of oxygen-carrying red cells in your blood. In addition, it enlarges the smaller blood vessels so that more blood can flow through them. It also speeds up the rate at which the enzymes in muscle cells use the oxygen offered to them.

Oxygen is Premium

A high-raw diet greatly improves the last part of the process, the absorption and use of oxygen in muscle cells. In 1938, Professor Hans Eppinger, chief doctor at the First Medical Clinic of the University of Vienna, showed that raw foods increase cellular respiration. A high-raw diet also stimulates muscle cells to absorb nutrients and excrete wastes efficiently. In time it flushes away the noxious 'marsh' that develops between cells when too many starchy and sugary foods are being eaten: once the marsh has been cleared, speedy oxygen, nutrient and waste exchange can be resumed. Such a diet gradually detoxifies the whole body, giving the muscle cells ideal conditions in which to produce energy. A high-raw or all-raw diet also happens to be an excellent way for athletes to eat in the 48 hours leading up to a major event.

The high potassium content of raw vegetables and fruits enhances good muscle tone and stamina. Potassium deficiency is a common hazard encountered by long-distance runners; the mineral is rapidly depleted during hours of sustained exertion. If not replaced, even a trained athlete becomes chronically fatigued. Marathon runner and co-author of *The Sportsmedicine Book*, Dr Gabe Mirkin, says: 'When you lack potassium, you feel tired, weak and irritable.' Many athletes, amateur and professional alike, are not using their full potentials in performance because they, like the majority of people living on the average Western diet, are deficient in potassium.

THE MIND LIFT

Even more important than the way the high-raw diet makes you feel physically – how it increases stamina and energy, clears aches and pains and makes you highly resistant to fatigue and illness – is the way it makes you feel 'in yourself'. In a single word: terrific. Thinking processes become clearer. Instead of getting caught up in the emotional hassles when differences arise with other people, you can stand back and see what is happening. You no longer identify so much with what they think – you feel less threatened by someone who doesn't agree.

Dynamic Balance
High-raw, low-grain eating brings a sense of physical–psychic balance so life is not an endless seesaw of ups and downs. This experience makes you wonder if many of the negative feelings we all get from time to time are not so much psychological in origin as physiological, a sign that body chemistry is out of balance and toxins are building up. In my experience – and that of many others who have chosen to go high-raw, low-grain – the longer you eat this way, the more positive you feel about yourself and life in general.

Out with Fatigue
Chronic fatigue, marked by irritability, lethargy and the feeling that

almost everything is too much bother, has been called 'the plague of modern civilisation'. A certain wit once observed that 99 per cent of the world's work is done by people who feel under the weather. However, only 30 per cent of people who go to their doctor complaining of tiredness are diagnosed as suffering from something detectable. Anaemia is one of the commonest detectable causes of tiredness. Other causes include the under-production of certain hormones (as in diabetes, hypothyroidism and hypopituitarism), chronic infections and occasionally heart disease, especially if there is valve damage which prevents the heart from pumping enough oxygenated blood around the body. The rest of those who feel chronically tired are told there is nothing wrong with them according to laboratory tests and X-rays. They go home as tired as they came.

A deficit of the minerals potassium and magnesium is known to be a major cause of fatigue. Because Powerhouse eating is rich in fresh green vegetables and sprouts, it is also rich in chlorophyll, and therefore in magnesium, for chlorophyll is built around a core of magnesium. It is also, in contrast to the average Western diet, very high in potassium. Any long-term physical effort requires large reserves of potassium.

BIG CALMERS

In the 1960s, an American physician, Dr Palma Formica, was curious to know what effect magnesium and potassium supplements would have on fatigue. Her volunteers for the experiment were 100 chronically tired people, 84 women and 16 men. For five or six weeks she gave them extra potassium and magnesium. Then she recorded her findings: 'The change was startling. They (became) alert, cheerful, animated and energetic, and walked with a lively step. Their sleep became refreshing as it had not been for months. Some said they could get along on six hours a night. Formerly they had not felt rested on 12 or more. Morning exhaustion vanished.' Eighty-seven of Dr Formica's 100 volunteers improved, even though some had suffered from debilitating fatigue for two years or more.

Another reason why a high-raw, low-grain diet counters fatigue and lifts the spirits is that it affects blood sugar levels. It stops the terrible ups and downs which are associated with Syndrome X and responsible for that mid- to late-afternoon tiredness that has you reaching for strong cups of coffee and sweet snacks. The same low blood sugar levels can be responsible for feelings of depression and anxiety too. American physician John Douglass MD and others who recommend a high-raw diet for diabetics do so in part because raw fibre helps to stabilise blood sugar levels and insulin. It does the same for someone suffering from persistently low blood sugar levels, and abolishes the mood swings and other symptoms that characterise hypoglycaemia.

Out with Allergies and Addictions

Another cause of mood swings can be food allergies. It is not uncommon, for example, for wheat and milk products to cause catarrh, digestive problems and feelings of chronic lethargy and tiredness. A lot has been written in the popular and scientific press about food allergies and special diets to deal with them, regimes in which the 'offending' food is left out. What few people are aware of (although Bircher-Benner discovered the fact more than 50 years ago) is that a tendency towards food allergies is significantly reduced by a high-raw diet which eliminates wheat and milk. Other allergies such as skin rashes, hay fever and rheumatic conditions can also be reduced by a vegetables-only regime.

FREEDOM FROM ALLERGIES

Allergists such as H. Rinkel and T. Randolph have written extensively about the addictive aspects of food allergies: the allergic person actually develops a craving for the very thing he is allergic to. The craving masks the allergy, provided the body's resistance is high enough but, when resistance weakens, all the symptoms of the allergy develop. Douglass finds that a high-raw diet is also an effective weapon against allergies and the addictive patterns that accompany them. Even common addictions such as cigarettes and alcohol seem to lose their force after a few weeks on a raw diet. At first Douglass was most unwilling to believe that raw foods lessen addictive cravings, but his patients insisted that after a few weeks of high-raw eating they simply did not want as many cigarettes or drinks as before. Willpower did not come into it. Douglass concluded that in some mysterious way, raw foods must sensitise the body both to what is good for it and what is bad for it. Experimenting with specific raw foods and their effects, he found that some, such as sunflower seeds, were particularly effective in suppressing cravings associated with addiction.

Help for Smokers

Sunflower seeds are an excellent source of vital nutrients. They contain most of the B-vitamins, vitamin E and also many essential fatty acids, and weight for weight twice as much iron and 25 times as much thiamine (a B-vitamin) as steak. Douglass found they were particularly good for people trying to wean themselves off cigarettes, so much so that he recommends that his would-be non-smoker patients carry a handful of raw shelled sunflower seeds around with them and every time they feel the desire to smoke, to pop a few into their mouth and munch until the desire subsides. In a few weeks, he says, the desire to smoke seems to fade. How does he explain this David and Goliath effect, the humble sunflower seed versus the ogre nicotine?

STOP SMOKING EASILY

It seems that sunflower seeds contain ingredients which mimic some of the effects of nicotine. To an extent, therefore, they give smokers some of the gratification they seek from nicotine. Nicotine exerts a mildly soothing, sedative effect on the nervous system; so do sunflower seeds because they contain various sedative oils, and also plenty of B-vitamins, always good for the nerves. Nicotine triggers the release of glycogen from the liver, producing a temporary increase in brain activity; sunflower seeds produce a similar lift. Nicotine raises the level of adrenal hormones in the body; sunflower seeds also stimulate the adrenal glands. Sunflower seeds are non-allergenic, and

> effectively break through the smoker's pattern of addiction without themselves becoming the target of a new allergy.

Times of Stress

High-raw, low-grain living also makes you much more resistant to stress. Resilience is not so easily destroyed by having to drive in rush-hour traffic or stay up all night to finish a piece of work. You seem able to gear up or gear down to whatever is demanded. This, at least in part, has to do with the way eating 50–75 per cent of your foods raw alkalinises the body.

Balanced body chemistry is not merely a recipe for keeping calm and collected, but a fundamental necessity for health. Over-acidity lies at the root of many illnesses, particularly arthritis and rheumatism. Every food you eat tends to be either acid-forming or alkaline-forming. If your diet contains a lot of coffee, sugar and convenience foods but only a few fresh vegetables and fruits, you are consuming foods which are mainly acid-producing and you will tend to feel stressed very easily. You get this nervy feeling because your body has used up its alkali reserves in an effort to balance the acid-forming foods you have eaten.

Stress Free

Unfortunately the compounds that the body produces in response to stress are also acidic. A combination of acid-forming foods and periods of stress sends the body's acid levels up and up. So it is important, for overall health and as an antidote to stress, to eat plenty of alkaline-forming foods. A desirable ratio of alkaline- to acid-forming foods would be 80 per cent alkaline to 20 per cent acid, four to one in favour of the alkaline. Sugars, grains, junk food and excess meat are all acid-forming. Raw, non-starchy vegetables and fruits are alkaline-forming. When you know you are going to be exposed to situations you find stressful, eat an even greater percentage of alkaline-forming foods.

Conquer Jet Lag

To my mind one of the most unpleasant and unavoidable forms of stress is jet lag, when the body's inner biochemical rhythms get out of sync after crossing several time zones. This does not happen when you fly north or south, of course, only if you fly west or east. The symptoms of jet lag include confusion, exhaustion during the day and sleeplessness at night, and that awful 'spaced out' feeling of not quite knowing where you are. When I increased the level of raw vegetables in my diet, I noticed that I felt all these unpleasant things to a much lesser degree. Then I began to experiment with various ways of eating before, during and after long-haul flights to see if I could improve things further. Finally I hit on a method which works wonders. Others who have tried it report similar relief from time zone troubles.

FLY EASY

This is what I do. The day before a flight I eat lightly, and raw foods only, with the emphasis on salads and fruits, which are alkaline-forming, rather than nuts and seeds, fish and meat, which are more acid-forming. On the day of the flight I eat only a little. I drink lots of water or take some fresh fruit or vegetable juice. This does two things: it helps your digestive system prepare itself for the change in mealtimes at the end of your journey, and keeps you from having to eat the pretty horrendous meals most airlines serve. The day after the flight I eat raw food only with a little fish or microfiltered whey. The following day I go back to my normal way of eating, which is about 75 per cent raw. I end up able to sleep at night, well-oriented in time and space, and able to work productively – in short, feeling like a human being rather than a wrung-out dishcloth.

Key to Self-fulfilment

Twenty-five years ago the idea that what you eat could be a major player in enabling you to fulfil your life would have made me laugh. I would have dismissed the notion as nothing more than a fantastic invention of some strange Californian cult. But when I began experimenting with raw foods and found they affected me so profoundly, I started to wonder. I ploughed through ancient treatises on the relationship between diet and the mind, from the Vedic teachings that form the basis of India's traditional Ayurvedic medicine, to Szekely's translations of Essene teachings. I was not altogether surprised to find that the kind of diet most of these writings recommend for increasing mental and spiritual awareness is one very close to what I had been eating.

If I had not read so many meticulously charted clinical reports on high-raw eating, I might have been tempted to dismiss the positive effects of raw foods as yet another demonstration of the placebo effect – 'a little of what you fancy does you good'. But vast experimental evidence – mountains of it – suggest otherwise.

Fulfilling the Blueprint

Raw-food pioneer Dr Max Bircher-Benner (*see Energy Raw and Free*) believed that live foods could not only help cure illness but that they also form an important part of a self-realising and self-healing system which helped his patients in every conceivable way to fulfil their individual potentials. Bircher-Benner initiated a school of medical thinking, treatment and outlook which envisaged, and still envisages, the patient as an indivisible whole, as a psycho–physical personality, in order to promote the realisation, as far as possible, of the potentialities and original 'blueprint' given them at their creation. A high-raw diet, he insisted, helped people fulfil their potential in every area of their lives.

Raw Food Versus Ageing

A high-raw diet bolsters the immune system. It prevents immune re-actions in the gut which create food cravings as well as digestive problems. It also helps colonise the intestines with 'good guy' flora which produce important B-complex vitamins and help protect against cancer of the bowel. The protection it gives against degeneration and acute disease conditions in clinical terms alone is another strong indication that it strengthens the body's immune responses. A high-raw, low-grain diet helps keep you looking and feeling young. It can even reverse some of the age-related changes that have already taken place in your body in medically measurable ways.

Cancer studies, such as those carried out at the University of Texas, have shown that wheat grass inhibits mutations in DNA. Research at the Linus Pauling Institute discovered that a high-raw diet lowered radiation-induced cancer in mice, supporting the thesis that raw foods sharpen up an organism's ability to distinguish 'self' from 'other' and destroy the 'other'. Raw foods are full of myriad anti-ageing factors quite apart from all the antioxidants they contain. There is a special enzyme in the body called superoxide dismutase (SOD) which discourages the formation of 'rogue' molecules called superoxides and free radicals which do serious oxidative damage to every part of the body. Raw foods are full of it.

THE ANTI-AGEING ENZYME

SOD occurs in every single cell in your body. So far, four different forms of it have been identified, three of which play protective roles. It plays an important part in preventing cancer and protecting us from radiation damage. Intravenous injections of SOD have been used to treat arthritis, muscular dystrophy, cancer and radiation poisoning. Researchers are highly enthusiastic about its ability to protect cell DNA and other body systems, especially the immune system, from the damage associated with ageing. The theory is that SOD in fresh raw foods boosts the body's own production of SOD.

Raw foods are very rich in SOD. Together with other enzymes present in raw foods, it gets to work on substrates formed as soon as food is chewed, to form other active compounds important for health.

The Proof of the Pudding

The changes that take place when you eat a high-raw diet speak for themselves. Skin loses its slackness and puffiness and seems to cling to the bones better. The true shape of your face emerges where once it may have been obscured by excess water retention and poor circulation. Lines soften. Eyes take on a clarity and brightness one usually associates with children and super-fit athletes.

The rejuvenation that can be achieved on a high-raw diet is not just skin deep. It happens at the physiological and biochemical level as well. On a high-raw, low-grain diet, most of the tests used to assess age-related change – serum cholesterol, serum lipids, blood pressure – change for the better. In the diet-oriented clinics of Europe and the United States, a high-raw diet has been used for generations to heal degenerative diseases associated with ageing. Impotence and other sexual dysfunctions, which tend to increase with age, often right themselves. Flagging sexual interest rekindles. Raw diets can even reduce the severity of senile dementia.

Long-lived Cultures

Virtually all long-lived cultures – the Hunzakuts, the Georgians, the East Indian Todas and the Yucatan Indians – live on a low-calorie diet

LOW-CALORIE HEAVEN

Diets based on fresh raw vegetables, fruits, seeds, nuts and good-quality proteins are by definition low in calories. When you eat most of your food raw you do not need so many calories. Nor do you want to eat as much as you would on a 'normal' diet. Partly this is because a high-raw diet contains such a lot of fibre, and partly because it does not over-stimulate the digestive system, create food allergies and make you want to eat more and more.

rich in fresh, uncooked foods. So did the 'primitive diet' cultures that Dr Weston Price, famous American researcher, visited in the 1920s and 1930s (*see Raw Beginnings*) and in whom he found low incidences of degenerative illness.

A high-raw, low-grain diet makes it possible for me to work harder and more effectively, to maintain a more equable attitude to other people and to experience a heightened sense of enjoyment from day-to-day life. Bircher-Benner's statement about how such a diet was an important tool for self-realisation and self-healing which 'helped the patient in every conceivable way' – not just by banishing the symptoms of disease – no longer sounds as far-fetched as it once did. So we keep an open mind. Raw foods may indeed help human beings to fulfil their potential, not only for high-level health and good looks but in many other ways too. I figure only time will tell.

POWERHOUSE SLIM

Weight control is easy on a high-raw, low-grain diet, so easy in fact that anyone who has a habit of going on and off weight-loss diets and achieving only temporary 'success' will rejoice to know that you can lose weight steadily without even counting calories.

Weight loss the Powerhouse way banishes the cravings for food – especially carbohydrates and sugars – which make us fat. It also improves nutritional status, fostering a steady loss of unwanted fat. Best of all it keeps energy high, makes your flesh firmer and skin smooth. It lifts your spirits as nothing else can. Ordinary weight-loss diets are notoriously poor nutritionally. Going on and off them creates sub-clinical deficiencies that lead to illness, fatigue and 'hidden hunger'. This in turn triggers bingeing and disturbs insulin balance, leading to bad eating habits and more weight gain.

NURTURING APPROACH

The raw approach to weight loss works with nature rather than against it. It does not mean starvation – it means superb nutrition and slow, steady weight loss. You do not have to count calories, buy special foods, weigh out bird-sized portions on kitchen scales or feel deprived when you do not eat and guilty when you do. Some raw foods are particularly good for losing weight. Sprouted seeds and grains form the ideal basis for delicious main meals. Fresh juices provide an excellent way to stock up quickly with minerals. Living foods vibrate with special energy, which affects you both physically and mentally. They give you strength, clarity of mind, confidence and a sense of well-being that make you want to do what is best for your body.

Calm in the Storm
A familiar problem to dieters is irritability. Flare-ups of temper and

rapid changes in mood are often due to an over-acidic system. The more acidic your system, the more irritable you feel. Uncooked foods, particularly fresh fruit and vegetables, have a counteractive alkalinising effect. This means that you feel calmer, more resilient and less tired while you are losing weight. As a result of overeating, eating too many nutritionally 'empty' foods or depleted foods, or eating too few potent ones, the digestive system becomes overloaded. This leads to deficiencies in important enzymes needed to break down foods fully and provide nutrients for cell use. No matter how much you eat you feel yourself plagued by a constant hunger. Ongoing stimulation to the digestive organs results in excess acidity of the stomach and long-standing inflammation of the intestines, which further increases the cravings for more food. To digest foods we rely on enzymes – plenty of them – of just the right kind. Eating the wrong food, or eating too much, depletes your body and stresses the whole enzymic system. This can lead to food allergies and result in subclinical vitamin and mineral deficiencies, which in turn reinforce the vicious circle of hidden hunger. A high-raw, low-grain diet is fabulous for weight loss for another reason, too. It protects from the world's most threatening epidemic – Syndrome X – and corrects insulin disturbance so you lose weight naturally.

POWERFUL PROTEIN

Once you have plenty of raw fruits and vegetables, no food is more important than protein when it comes to enhancing overall health and balancing weight. Every molecule of muscle in your body is made from the proteins you eat. Muscle is the engine which turns food calories into energy and burns fat. Enhance the quality of your muscle and you enhance the vitality of your whole body. You also enhance sex hormones, improve your skin and gain strength and power. Protein foods help ground you. So much so that they can play an important part in your living out your dreams, and even help to make your sense of spirituality a day-to-day part of ordinary life, rather than something rarefied. When you improve both the quality and quantity of the proteins you eat you can completely transform, regenerate and rejuvenate not only the way your body functions, but also the way you look.

Fat Fighter

Powerhouse eating fights fat naturally in many different ways:

STRONG BONES NEED PROTEIN

Too much protein makes bones weak – right? Wrong. New research examining the relation between bone mineral density (BMD) and protein intake in post-menopausal women shows that women who eat the most protein have a significantly higher BMD than those who consume less. Anyone at risk of osteoporosis needs plenty of good-quality protein to look after bone health.

BALANCE THE GENETIC SCALES

The Powerhouse way of eating for human health has emerged out of our biological inheritance and genetic makeup. When you provide the body with a diet and lifestyle to which it has been genetically adapted, you are giving it what it needs to restore balance where it is needed as well as healthy form and harmony. What this means is that we need to make major shifts in both the ratio of proteins to carbohydrates and fats that we are taking as well as the types of food we consume. That is what Powerhouse eating does.

THE ADDICTION TRAIL

In the so-called civilised world, human beings are fatter than ever. What's worse, we grow fatter still with each year that passes. An over-weight body with its bloated flesh, flabby muscles and knotty deposits beneath the skin is also a body with an inherited tendency to store fat. A wonderful thing about losing fat the high-raw, low-grain way is that you do not end up looking drawn and flabby. Skin and muscles become firm and the whole body undergoes a process of rejuvenation.

The more industrialised and commercial our societies have become, the more processed carbohydrates we have eaten and the more our blood sugar and insulin levels soar. These foods are also highly addictive. Eat them and you want to eat more. Called carbohydrate craving, it's a constant or intermittent hunger that people on a high-carb diet know only too well. You eat one biscuit and suddenly you find yourself scoffing the whole packet. Such behaviour is not the consequence of a lack of willpower, but the result of imbalances in the body caused by a high-carb diet.

Glycaemic Help

If you are eating a diet high in grains, a major ally in combating

Syndrome X is the Glycaemic Index. The GI, the result of many years of research, is a rating system for carbohydrates that enables you to choose the ones offering a gradual conversion into glucose. By eating these carbs, you help your body release insulin more slowly and keep your levels of insulin lower. And the benefits are not confined to the loss of body fat. Once you improve insulin control using GI, you help reduce serum cholesterol, prevent and even reverse hypertension, improve your overall health and increase your energy. Good glycaemic control even slows the formation of cross-linking collagen in the skin, which causes wrinkles.

The Glycaemic Index is an extremely useful tool, so use it by all means (you will find it in two of my books, *Age Power* and *The X Factor Diet*). However, your body handles raw food quite differently from cooked grain products; when you are eating 50–75 per cent of your foods raw, the GI of these foods is not something you need worry about.

LOW-GRAIN LEAN

Generally speaking, the more carbohydrate-dense foods you eat – that is legumes, whole grains and starchy vegetables – the more insulin you will produce. The more insulin you produce, the more weight you will tend to gain – particularly if you have a genetic tendency to store energy as fat in your body. By contrast, low-carbohydrate-dense vegetables like broccoli, spinach and Chinese leaves have four to 10 times less carbohydrate than grain-based foods, legumes and starchy vegetables. This means you can eat a lot of low-carbohydrate-dense foods without having to wrestle with insulin-related health problems.

Do it Now
What I find especially exciting is that, armed with an understanding of how insulin works, you can begin steadily changing your life for the better. Right here, right now. Powerhouse eating has already changed my own life and the lives of many others for the better. Since puberty, despite eating a healthy diet, I had always been heavier than I felt was right for my body. After the menopause it got worse. Now, I feel better

and look leaner than I did 20 years ago. It has been like tapping into a fount of boundless energy. Now I have a sense that my brain and body will support, with grace instead of strain, all the creative projects I want to take on now and in the future.

The culprits that trigger Syndrome X are grain-based and sugar-based, particularly the refined kind. Although the human body runs on glucose as its principal fuel, it was never designed to deal with a diet high in convenience foods. Most of the calories we eat come from high-density carbohydrates that pour sugar into the bloodstream when we eat them. Even the so-called 'good' carbohydrates such as whole-grain breads and brown rice can cause insulin resistance if eaten to excess. This mix can be more dangerous if you also have nutritional deficiencies, generally eat too much, ingest too many highly refined and processed foods, drink too much alcohol, smoke and/or have a sedentary lifestyle.

THE RANDLE EFFECT – FATS VS. CARBS

In the standard Western diet, a lot of fats and carbohydrates are eaten together. This is bad news. Fats effectively reduce the cells' ability to use blood sugar released by the carbohydrates. So while the fats are being burnt as fuel, there's excess glucose swirling around the bloodstream. More insulin is released to deal with the glucose which ultimately causes the glucose to be stored as fat. This is the Randle effect. It throws any overweight, insulin-resistant person into a terrible cycle in which hunger and carbohydrate cravings lead to overeating, followed by an inevitable increase in blood sugar and insulin levels, leading to body fat deposits and more cravings. When your body is unable to use the foods you are eating for energy, it only knows how to store it as fat in your belly, hips and thighs. The irony is that for a long time we have been blaming dietary fat for all this when the phenomenon is actually caused by a high carbohydrate intake in the presence of fats.

Eaten on their own or together with protein but without an abundance of carbohydrates, natural fats do not cause the laying down of fat in the body. This is perhaps the most difficult thing for those of us who have been highly schooled in the low-fat, high-carb approach to weight loss to grasp, yet it is absolutely essential to understand.

Banish Cellulite

With a high-raw, low-grain diet, cellulite becomes a thing of the past. Sound too good to be true? That's what I thought until I watched it happen before my very eyes. Cellulite is a sign that internal pollution is present in your body. This not only reduces your energy, it mars physical beauty as well. Whether or not you care passionately about having smooth sleek thighs, if you see cellulite developing, listen to what your body is telling you: something needs attention.

SCREWED-UP ECOLOGY

Looked at under a microscope, cellulite tissue reveals that a number of abnormal changes have taken place in the living tissue of your thighs. They include:

- ❑ Distended lymphatic vessels in the upper skin
- ❑ Loss of elastin in the fibres
- ❑ Slowed circulation of blood and lymph
- ❑ A sclerotic hardening of connective tissue
- ❑ Trapped fluids and wastes
- ❑ A stasis in the tissue like a polluted swamp
- ❑ A network of distorted collagen bundles which can pinch nerve fibres and eventually cause pain
- ❑ Poor exchange of life energy
- ❑ A deadened quality – all sure signs of poor body ecology

Pollution Disorders

Just as the planet has an ecology on which its health depends, so does your body. Its every cell, every vessel, every tissue, interacts in highly complex ways, either directly or obliquely, with every other part. All of your organs, glands and systems speak to each other chemically via the metabolic processes which break down nutrients to make them available for cell use, produce energy for movement, and eliminate wastes. They also communicate via subtly energetic pathways. Some of these were charted long ago through acupuncture and are still used in the application of pressure at specific areas in Oriental medicine, as well as in techniques like shiatsu and reflexology.

This ability of the living body to take in and break down nutrients, to channel them into life-sustaining metabolic processes and to eliminate wastes is all part of maintaining its ecology through what is now known as *the living matrix* (*more about this in Chapter Two*). The problem is that pollution in our air, water and food continues to increase, placing real burdens on the immune system. So does the average or even 'good' diet when it is low in fresh raw vegetables and high in cereals, convenience foods, sugar and other high-glycaemic foods. Such foods deplete your body of nutrients, diminish your energy and build fat stores – particularly in women thanks to their high oestrogen levels.

Bad to Worse

The availability of a good balance of essential nutrients in our over-processed foods continues to decline. One of the many obvious consequences of this decline is the production of cellulite in women's flesh. When the body's ecology is good, then your whole body works well and you have plenty of energy. You don't develop cellulite. And, what is most frequently forgotten, you also experience a high level of awareness and autonomy – you find it easier to be your own person and to make your own decisions from a position of mental clarity and physical power.

When you support and rebalance your body with high-raw, low-grain eating, and eliminate the drugs, convenience foods and debris from your system, you not only banish cellulite, you also empower yourself and make it easier to maximise all of your potentials.

MICRO-MAGIC

Capillaries are minute blood vessels which form the vast network of microcirculation throughout your body. It is their responsibility to deliver oxygen-rich blood for use in the cells. So important are these fine vessels that nature has supplied you with incredible lengths of them. If you were to attach all the capillaries in your body end to end they would measure some 60,000 miles in length – more than twice around the world. The state of your capillaries also determines to a great extent the functional age and condition of your body as a whole, for these transport systems are the arbitrators of cell nutrition, respiration and elimination. It is through these capillaries that nutrients and oxygen are carried to the cells all over the body – organs, skin, brain and glands – and wastes eliminated. Without good micro-circulation, metabolism cannot take place efficiently.

Fair Exchange

Over the years, the capillaries of people living on the average Western diet of highly processed foods become twisted, distended and highly porous. When this happens, substances can seep through the capillary walls and deposit themselves where they shouldn't be, and where they can interfere with proper oxygen exchange and impede nutrient delivery and waste elimination. This can gradually starve cells, tissues and organs of all they need to function properly and can also lower cellular metabolic activity. The same degenerative process underlies the build-up of cellulite in women. Such changes in microcirculation can not only lower overall vitality – since none of your body's parts are receiving sufficient oxygen and nutrients for healthy metabolic functions – but also predispose us to degenerative illness and to rapid ageing. A high-raw way of eating helps restore normal microcirculation.

GOOD TENSIONS

The interchange of chemicals and energy between the micro-circulation and the cells takes place through two thin membranes and a fine space between cells. It happens only because the cells and capillaries have what is known as 'selective capacity'. This means they are able to absorb the substances they need and to reject what is harmful or unnecessary for metabolic processes. This selective capacity is the result of antagonistic chemical and micro-electrical tensions in the cells and tissues of all living systems. The stronger the tensions, the more intense these antagonisms, and the healthier and more vital your cells and your body as a whole will be, and the more efficiently it will function.

Professor Hans Eppinger and another German scientist, Karl Eimer, discovered that a high-raw diet steadily increases the cells' selective capacity by heightening electrical potentials between tissue cells and capillary blood. This, too, improves the ability of your capillaries to regulate the transport of nutrients. It also helps detoxify the system, removing any 'sticky marsh' of waste products present – another factor encouraging the build-up of cellulite. Powerhouse eating restores your body's natural ability to detoxify, improve the selective capacity of cells, rebuild the body's enzymic systems, and aid metabolic rejuvenation.

SMOOTH OUT

But raw foods do something else of even more direct benefit to cellulite: they strengthen the capillaries. Italian biochemist S.B. Curry, at the University of Milan, examined thigh tissue from four dozen women of all ages and compared it with thigh tissue from women with cellulite. He found that in women with cellulite, blood plasma had escaped from weakened capillaries into the spaces between the cells and encouraged the formation of cellulite.

The vastly complex living system which is your body has a magnificent ability to regulate itself. It takes into account the food you eat, the air you breathe, the stresses you are under, the physical demands made upon you, your age and all the other factors that come into play in your life. It does this provided of course it is not *over*burdened by excess fatigue, stress or pollution, and provided its metabolic processes have at their disposal a full complement of the essential nutrients on which they run. Powerhouse eating provides them. Your body does the work of eliminating cellulite, step by step, from within.

Eat 50 to 75 per cent of your foods raw. Choose the rest from wholesome microfiltered whey, fish, game, organic meat, and naturally produced soya products such as miso and tofu. You will notice a dramatic improvement in how you look, feel and function within the first couple of weeks. It is likely to be a few weeks before the burden of toxicity which you have been carrying has fully cleared, and it will probably be a few months before even deeper benefits begin to show themselves. So be patient. Your body has a magnificent ability to heal itself. Take action now to help it work its wonders. You won't look back.

WILD WOMAN

Powerhouse eating can transform a woman's life. A high-raw, low-grain diet is the way the world's most exclusive and expensive health farms stay in business. Two weeks on it can make you look and feel 10 years younger – flesh is firmer, lines are softer, and skin, eyes and hair glow with health. For many it resolves PMS and menopausal difficulties as well as making mood swings a thing of the past.

Other typically female problems such as stubborn cellulite, excessive menstrual flow and chronic fatigue often seem to melt away, leaving you with the sense that you do not need pills, potions or plastic surgery to look and feel great.

WIDESPREAD DEFICIENCIES

An astonishing number of women suffer from nutritional deficiencies, as many large-scale studies carried out in Europe and America show. One three-year research project found that calcium and iron deficiency are widespread in women; one in two women lacked calcium, and nine out of 10 were deficient in iron. This is likely to be a conservative estimate since the levels of these and other nutrients used to define health in the study were nowhere near those a competent nutritionist would recommend to anyone wanting to look and feel their best.

Women eating the typical Western diet often incur zinc deficiency as well, particularly if they are on the Pill. Vitamin deficiencies are also common. These can only be partially corrected by taking vitamin pills. Vitamins and minerals are synergistic – each complements the actions of others. *All* the essential nutrients are necessary for high-level health. The average diet does not offer enough of these or the right balance of vitamins and minerals to build long-lasting energy, vitality and good looks. Fresh raw foods can, especially when you include sprouted seeds and grains which you can grow in your own kitchen window, seaweeds, green supplements and freshly prepared vegetable juices.

Beauty Nutrients

Certain vitamins and minerals – available in far greater quantities on a high-raw, low-grain diet than when living on 'normal' fare – are essential to maintaining strong shiny hair and nails and protecting your skin from early ageing. Vitamin C and the flavonoids, for instance – those brightly coloured substances with quite exceptional properties for health and beauty – also guard the integrity of collagen in the body. Collagen is the fibrous protein which gives your skin its firmness and contour. Both are present in good quantities in raw fruits and vegetables. Most of these, like other water-soluble nutrients, can be completely destroyed by heat. The mineral zinc, plentiful in pumpkin seeds, sunflower seeds and some sprouted seeds, is needed to maintain healthy collagen too, as well as to make new collagen. Women who have insufficient zinc get stretch marks on their breasts and stomachs when they are pregnant. These often show up more when you lose weight. Vitamin A is made in abundance in the body when you are supplied with the carotenoids from fresh green vegetables and carrots, and helps regulate oil balance in your skin.

ANTI-AGERS

Vitamin A is an important anti-ager in other ways too. Like vitamins E, C and some of the B-complex vitamins, it is a natural antioxidant. This means it is important in protecting the skin – indeed your whole body – from age-related changes.

Antioxidants have ways of combating oxidative reactions caused by radiation, chemicals and free radicals which cause damage to cells' genetic material, proteins and lipids. It is just this kind of damage that makes skin grow old rapidly. Uncooked foods are also full of enzymes such as superoxide dismutase (SOD) and catalase which help prevent the free-radical damage that causes cell damage and skin ageing. When you eat these foods your body makes use of them.

Seeds of Beauty

Sprouted seeds and grains, which you can easily grow on your kitchen windowsill or in your airing cupboard (*see Free, Wild and Cautious*) are the richest known source of naturally occurring vitamins. They are also the most prolific of all foods: just 125 grams of mung seeds will produce a kilo of bean sprouts. Sprouts come in all shapes and colours, from the tiny curlicue forms of mustard to the round yellow spheres of chick-peas. Easy seeds, grains and pulses for sprouting include: mung beans, adzuki (aduki) beans, wheat, barley, fenugreek, lentils, mustard, oats, pumpkin, sesame, soya beans and sunflower. When a seed sprouts, enzymes which have been dormant in it spring into action, breaking down stored starch and turning it into simple, natural sugars and split-ting long-chain proteins into amino acids. This is why you can eat sprouted grains when the unsprouted variety is not so good. Sprouted grains are living foods complete with enzymes which are very easily digested, whereas cooked grains not only have no enzymes but also deplete your own body's enzymes – it has to use its own enzymes to digest them. Unlike their sprouted counterparts, unsprouted grains are high in starch, which the human body has difficulty processing. As a result, eating a lot of cooked grain foods produces in most people a semi-toxic state where your body retains water, making skin puffy and reducing energy levels. Sprouted grains bring life to your system. Large amounts of cooked grains deplete your system. Sprouted seeds have many times the nutritional goodness of the seeds from which they have grown. Gram for gram, they provide more nutrients than any other natural food. And they are great for beautiful skin.

Plant Hormones are Great

To reap the rewards of high-raw, low-grain eating, choose foods high in phyto-hormones – compounds in plants whose molecular structure is akin to the body's own hormones. Unlike dangerous xenoestrogens – 'foreign' oestrogens found in petrochemically derived herbicides, pesticides and plastics – plant hormones are 'weak' in their actions. They 'fit' with a woman's metabolism. Your body recognises them, and knows how to use them. When weak oestrogens from plants bind with oestrogen receptor sites in your body, they protect you from the nega-tive effects of environmental xenoestrogens and oestrogens in drugs. They help the body to readjust its own hormonal balance naturally. This is why a diet high in soya bean products such as tofu plays an important part in protecting Japanese women from hormone-related diseases. Vitamins, minerals and phyto-hormones in fresh foods should be eaten as close as possible to the state in which they come out of the ground, or carefully and naturally fermented such as some Japanese soy products or German Sauerkraut. This enables them to supply enough phyto-hormones to mitigate most of the symptoms that plague women in industrialised countries, from fibrocystic breast disease, PMS and hot flushes to osteoporosis.

GREEN MEANS STRENGTH

Some of the best hormone-rich foods to add to your diet, both as protection against health problems and for the sake of overall vitality, are the green foods: spirulina, chlorella, the seaweeds and green barley (*see Nature's Supplements*). Eating green foods and taking green supplements every day can slowly, over a period of months, help to replenish what may have been lost for many years. This is something that is very difficult to achieve in any other way, for in order for minerals to be well assimilated they need to be highly bio-available – your body needs to be able to make use of them easily. Most vitamin and mineral supplements are not bio-available. Seaweeds, chlorella, spirulina and green barley are also wonderfully cleansing foods, helping to detoxify the body of excess oestrogens as well as other pollutants, and they are excellent energy enhancers.

You can buy powdered green foods such as spirulina, green barley and chlorella and mix a tablespoon of them into a glass of juice. Sprinkle seaweeds liberally on your salads. The natural tendency of the human body is to strengthen and heal itself, and it relishes the nutritional elements that can help it to do so. Green foods have much to offer.

SHORTER TIME OF MONTH

Women on a high-raw, low-grain diet report that menstrual problems such as bloating, premenstrual tension and fatigue improve greatly after two or three months. For some of them, the improvement is so dramatic that they are not aware of their periods until they arrive. This is something I discovered myself, and at first I thought I was unique. Then I spoke to numerous other women who said they had had a similar experience. Heavy periods become lighter – a period that ordinarily lasts six or seven days can be reduced to as few as one or two.

American gynaecologist C. Alan Clemetson first become interested in the possibility of regulating menstrual flow with substances that occur in foods when a young Italian patient told him she could easily cure her excessive menstrual bleeding by sucking lemons. It was the standard remedy for the problem in her home village, she said. Surprised and disbelieving, Clemetson could not quite quench his curiosity.

Bioflavonoid Link

Many years later, Clemetson had an opportunity to study the relationship between the bioflavonoid levels in the blood and menorrhagia – very heavy periods. His research established three things: first, the capillaries in a woman's body weaken briefly just after ovulation each month and again, more markedly, for a few days before menstruation. Second, women who have heavy periods have considerably weaker capillaries than women whose flow is normal. Third, lots of citrus flavonoids and vitamin C over a period of three or four months significantly reduced the excessive bleeding in the majority of women he tested. After his study was completed he suggested to his patients they eat three oranges a day, with plenty of pith, because it is the pith which contains the bioflavonoids. Many of them found this was enough to maintain their lighter periods.

Several flavonoids are oestrogenic. They mimic some of the effects of the female sex hormone oestrogen, including oestrogen's ability to strengthen the fragile capillary walls. When oestrogen levels are highest, as they are at ovulation – around 10 days after bleeding ceases – and again seven days later, oestrogen appears to replace the bioflavonoids in the capillary walls of the uterus. When oestrogen levels drop most markedly, as they do in the three days after ovulation and again just before and during menstruation, the bioflavonoids re-enter the capillary walls, giving them some of the protection withdrawn by dropping oestrogen levels. It is because the bioflavonoids partly compensate for the fall in oestrogen that they help to reduce the menstrual flow. If oestrogen levels never varied but were always high or always low, menstruation would not occur. It is only a sustained fall in oestrogen that brings on the breakdown of the uterine wall and bleeding.

C IS FOR COLLAGEN

Vitamin C powerfully complements the action of the bioflavonoids, but just in case you are tempted to rush to your nearest health-food store for supplements instead of increasing your intake of fresh raw foods, there is something you should know. Several studies show that pure ascorbic acid (vitamin C) is not as effective in treating capillary fragility and permeability as are fruit and vegetables containing the vitamin. This is important for beautiful skin too. Zinc, vitamin C and the flavonoids are all central to your body's ability to make new collagen. The bioflavonoids in food greatly strengthen many of the health-protecting qualities of vitamin C. Their presence also improves the storage of vitamin C in the system.

Oestrogens in Raw Foods

Clemetson also studied 36 other commonly eaten foods in the nut, fruit and vegetable category to see if any of them had oestrogen-like effects. Were any of them capable of inducing the kind of changes that occur when the hormone itself is given? He discovered that almonds, cashews, oats and apples were. Other researchers have observed similar hormonal effects from raw foods.

GOOD GUY OESTROGENS

Oestrogen drugs in HRT are potentially dangerous, as are the xenoestrogens in the air we breathe and in the pesticides in our foods. But in the same way that medicine now recognises that there is a good-guy cholesterol and a bad-guy cholesterol in relation to protecting the body from heart disease, so are there 'good' oestrogens and 'bad' oestrogens. According to Herman Aldercreutz, nutritional chemist at the University of Helsinki, and others, a number of weaker natural oestrogen-like ingredients in fresh plant foods actually help protect us against cancer of the breast and reproductive system, by binding with oestrogen receptor sites so that dangerously strong oestrogenic compounds are not so readily taken up.

Cancer Protectors

Many of the best protective foods contain oestrogen-like compounds called isoflavones. They are found in many of the soya-based foods eaten daily in the Orient such as tofu, tempeh and miso, as well as in legumes such as lentils. This, plus the fact that Japanese women also eat a great variety of land and sea plants that continually help to detoxify the body, may explain why Asians still have very low rates of breast cancer and few menopause-related problems compared to Europeans and North Americans. However, when Japanese women move to the United States and take up a Western diet, they rapidly develop the same diseases we have.

A number of other edible plants, including pomegranates and French beans, contain phyto-oestrogens of a different kind that also boast protective properties.

PLANT HORMONE SUPPORT

So many fresh foods are rich in hormones which help support human health when we eat them. Include them often in your meals. The fresher they are the better: yams, peas, papayas, bananas, cucumbers, raw nuts, bee pollen, sprouted seeds and grains and the herbs liquorice root, red clover, sage, sarsaparilla and sassafras. Raw fruits and vegetables, green vegetable juices, figs and garlic, dates, avocados, grapes, apples, seaweed, wheat germ and chlorella can all be helpful in countering menopausal and menstrual problems. Grapes, cherries, citrus fruits and red clover are excellent sources of bioflavonoids, which also have weak oestrogenic activity and help counter hot flushes and mood swings and prevent heavy and irregular menstrual flow. Plant foods high in phyto-hormones are good insurance against cancer too since they help prevent oestrogen-dominance in the body.

Natural Fibre and Calcium

The fibre found in raw plants is protective against oestrogen dominance and cancer via another mechanism. Breast cancer is highly related to oestrogen levels. Women eating the Powerhouse way, which is high in raw fibre, excrete a much higher level of oestrogen than other women and have much lower levels of the hormone in the blood. In Britain and the United States, the use of milk products has also been correlated with breast cancer. Sea plants and green vegetables, spirulina and chlorella are far better sources of calcium than cheese and milk.

TWO

RAW TRUTH

Living foods vibrate with a special quality of energy. This energy, when regularly taken into your body, changes you physically as well as mentally, bringing strength, clarity of mind, confidence and a sense of well-being which makes you want to do what is best for your body. It also heightens your senses so that the smells, tastes and textures of foods become a source of growing delight. Before long a large piece of pizza and a rich chocolate dessert lose their appeal.

COOKING MAY DAMAGE YOUR HEALTH

Everyone knows that cooked foods have the ability to sustain life. What is increasingly questioned is whether cooked foods enhance health. Unless the genetic inheritance of a person is exceptionally adaptable, a diet high in cooked foods tends to lead to slow but progressive degeneration of cells and tissues, ultimately leading to premature ageing and the development of degenerative diseases.

Many essential nutrients are detrimentally altered or destroyed by cooking. Numerous studies show that food processing and cooking – particularly at high temperatures – bring about changes in the nature of proteins, fats, sugars and fibre which render the foods containing them not just 'less health-promoting', but maybe even harmful. Distinguished German nutritionist, H. Glatzel, puts it this way: 'No other medium besides warmth, in its various applications, accomplishes such significant alterations in the structure and substances of raw foods.'

Tales of War
If you had been a prisoner of war in Japan during World War II, you would have been fed on a diet of cooked brown rice, vegetables and a little fruit. It was a regime containing a mere 729–826 calories a day per 154lb/70kg of body weight. Compare this with the minimum recommended requirements:

	Daily prisoner of war diet	Daily minimum recommended intake
Protein	22–30g	60–70g
Carbohydrates	164–207g	200–400g
Fat	7.5–8.5g	10–11g
Calories per 154lb/70kg body weight	729–826	2150

In 1950 it occurred to Dr Masanore Kuratsune, head of the Medical Department of the University of Kyushu in Japan, that the Japanese prisoner of war diet might be an excellent way to validate previous studies comparing the effects of raw and cooked foods. The guinea pigs he chose were himself and his wife. Both followed a raw version of the diet (including raw rice) for three different periods: 120 days in winter, 32 days in summer and 81 days in spring. During this time Mrs Kuratsune was breastfeeding a baby. Both she and her husband continued to do their usual work. Both continued in good health. In fact, Mrs Kuratsune found that nursing was less of a strain than before the experiment. Then they both switched to eating the same diet in cooked form and . . . all the symptoms of the hunger disease that so devastated the inmates of Japanese prisoner of war camps – oedema, vitamin deficiencies and collapse – rapidly happened. They were forced to abandon the experiment. The grossly inadequate diet that had maintained their health to start with, even the health of a nursing mother, did drastic damage when it was eaten cooked.

DANGER: COOKED FOOD

'The World Health Organisation began a three-day emergency meeting in Geneva last week to evaluate the recent discovery that certain popular starchy foods, from potato chips to bread, contain a chemical that can cause cancer. Never before has the agency assembled so many experts, so quickly, to evaluate food safety. "This is not just another food scare. This could give cancer, in foods, and in significant amounts," Jorgen Schlundt, head of The World Health Organisation's Food Safety Program, told ABC News.' ABC News.com on 25 June 2002

Vitamin Wipe Out

Vitamins – a word which did not enter the dictionary until 1934 – are organic substances which the body must have in very small quantities to carry out its thousands of building-up and breaking-down operations. The body can manufacture some vitamins itself. Vitamin D is one – provided of course you get enough exposure to sunlight. Others must be taken in with food.

Vitamin C and the vitamins in the B-group are water-soluble. This makes them especially vulnerable to cooking. As well as being very sensitive to heat, they leach out of food when it is soaked, blanched or boiled. Putting a cabbage into cold water and bringing it to the boil destroys 75 per cent of its vitamin C content. Cook fresh peas for five minutes and you wipe out 20–40 per cent of the thiamine present (one of the B-vitamins) and 30–40 per cent of vitamin C. Other B-vitamins in vegetables especially at risk are folate, riboflavin and inositol. Often, the remnants of these fragile nutrients get thrown away with the cooking juices. Untreated milk contains 10 per cent more B-vitamins (B_1, B_6 and folate) and 15 per cent more vitamin C than the heat-treated pasteurised product people drink. Sadly, the unhealthy condition of cows has necessitated governments throughout the world making it illegal to sell unpasteurised milk.

Vitamins A, D, E and K are fat soluble. They are less at risk, and can remain relatively stable up to about 212°F (the boiling point of water). Nonetheless, up to 50 per cent of vitamin E in food can be destroyed by frying or baking. Even the A-vitamins and the carotenoids can be destroyed at high temperatures.

PROCESS AND DESTROY

Essential nutrients are also lost in food processing, canning and preserving. The American expert in trace elements and minerals, Henry A. Schroeder, discovered that commercially frozen vegetables are seriously lacking – by as much as 47 per cent – in some of the important B-vitamins such as pantothenic acid and B_6 found in their fresh counterparts. Canning inflicted even greater vitamin losses – up to 77 per cent. Grains lose between half and almost all of their vitamin B_6 and between a third and three-quarters of their pantothenic acid when they are processed and refined.

Aminos Deformed

A protein is a chain of amino acids. Your body assembles and uses about 50,000 different proteins each day. All are made from just 22 amino acids. Strung together in special sequences, amino acids make up all the proteins there are in the universe. Only eight to 10 of them appear to be absolutely essential for human nutrition since, given enough amino acids, your body is able to make the rest. Our body needs all of these essential aminos all the time.

When protein foods like meat, fish, eggs and tofu are heated, some of their amino acids become so 'denatured' (changed in their molecular structure) that digestive enzymes in the gut can't process them. A few amino acids such as glutamine can be destroyed completely. Damaging proteins by cooking can make us want to eat more because we don't feel 'nourished' by what we have just eaten. About 10 per cent of the proteins in whey – the liquid fraction of milk – are denatured during pasteurisation. Seventy per cent becomes distorted during UHT processing. Cooked proteins can also chemically bind with vital minerals rendering them unavailable for use by the body.

GET OUT OF THE KITCHEN

Four kinds of damage to amino acids occur as a result of heating and processing protein foods:

❑ Under high heat some proteins become resistant to digestion so that the bio-availability of the amino acids they contain is reduced.
❑ Lysine (one of the essential amino acids) can be lost when you heat proteins, especially in the presence of reducing sugars – as in the pasteurisation of milk.
❑ When protein is exposed to treatment with alkali, as it is in many food-manufacturing processes, lysine and cysteine (a natural antioxidant and another essential amino acid) residues cannot easily be eliminated from your body and toxic amino products can be formed.
❑ When oxidising chemicals like sodium dioxide are used in food processing, methionine from the protein can be lost. Methionine is another of the natural antioxidant amino acids, important as a protection against cross-linkage and oxidation damage to the cells and in methylation-fuelled detoxification.

Food toxicologist Leonard Bjeldanes and his colleagues at the University of California in Berkeley found that cooked eggs and beef contained substances which can cause genetic mutations. The longer and hotter the cooking, the greater the activity of these substances. Frying and grilling were worst, roasting less so. We need to cook our foods carefully.

Protect Your Enzymes

Raw foods are rich in natural enzymes. These are destroyed when a food is cooked. Orthodox nutrition still pays little attention to these enzymes in the belief that they are wiped out by the digestive processes and therefore have no beneficial effects. But researchers such as Kaspar Tropp in Würzburg and Nobel laureate Artturi Ilmari Virtanen in Finland have shown this is simply not true. Virtanen – the teacher of Finnish chemist Johan Bjorksten, one of the most famous researchers in the world – discovered that although many of the enzymes in raw fruits and vegetables are broken down in the mouth as a result of chewing, their substrates react chemically with substances in saliva to produce new chemical compounds beneficial to the health of animals and man. The one thing we know for sure is that the beneficial enzymes in raw food are severely altered or destroyed by cooking.

Beware Hot Fat

When fats are heated to high temperatures, the molecular structure of their constituent fatty acids changes dramatically so they can become non-assimilable, poisonous, even carcinogenic. The heat processes used in the manufacture of margarine, cooking oil and countless convenience foods convert valuable 'cis' fatty acids, which the body needs and can make use of, into 'trans' fatty acids, which the body can't. It is now possible to eat nothing but fat and end up with a fatty acid deficiency. It is also why fatty acid deficiencies have become widespread in populations fed on high-fat convenience foods.

LOSS OF INFORMATION

Other important substances such as essential oils in plants, the chlorophyll, the flavonoids, carotenoids and important phytonutrients can be changed or destroyed by heat. Such substances are part of the chemical and energetic information biologically necessary to support our best genetic expression and to slow degeneration.

Although unsaturated fats such as those found in flax, hemp, corn, sunflower, safflower, soya and wheatgerm oil are necessary in small amounts for health and life, they become potentially poisonous when subjected to heat. Dr Rakel Kurkela at the University of Helsinki found that oils that had been exposed to heat contained numerous poisonous compounds. Some of these are powerful oxidisers which bring about damaging structural changes to cell membranes, cell nuclei and proteins. Others, such as malonaldehyde, are directly cancer-inducing. If you must fry food, olive oil and coconut oil are the safest oils to use. Olive oil is a monounsaturate, making it less susceptible to degeneration. Coconut oil is a saturated fat which makes it highly stable. However, they should never be heated to smoking point.

WAY TO GO

Cook foods on a low heat and never overcook them. Wok frying and teppenyaki grilling are good ways to cook meat and vegetables. Almost all of the dangerous bacteria we associate with raw meat lives on the outside of the meat. Choose your meats carefully – buy organic whenever possible. I like to sear my meat by cooking it very quickly on both sides on a teppenyaki grill. This way I have killed off the bacteria and can benefit from the almost uncooked 'inside' of the meat.

Beware Digestive Leucocytosis

Research done by Paul Kouchakoff at the Institute of Clinical Chemistry in Lausanne throws an intriguing sidelight on our relationship with cooked foods. Kouchakoff discovered that the body recognises cooked and processed foods as 'harmful invaders' and does its best to wipe them out. Simply put, white blood cells (leucocytes) rush to the scene of the invasion – the gut – as soon as cooked food enters the mouth. This phenomenon is called *digestive leucocytosis*. Until Kouchakoff's work it was thought to be a perfectly 'normal' reaction to the ingestion of all food. Kouchakoff demonstrated that when food is eaten raw, digestive leucocytosis does *not* occur. Neither do the number of white cells in the bloodstream increase. Processed and cooked food, by contrast, trigger white cell mobilisation. He also found that leucocytosis does not occur if you eat something raw before you eat something cooked.

The implications of leucocytosis are these: every time white blood cells flock to the intestines to deal with cooked food the rest of the body is left undefended. Continual red alerts – three or more times a day, year in, year out – put considerable strain on the immune system. Raw foods leave the white blood cells free for other tasks and save the body the effort of a defensive action, thereby strengthening its resistance to disease. This is why it is good advice to begin every meal with something raw.

RAW BEGINNINGS

Many pioneers of high-raw eating discovered its health-promoting qualities as a result of personal health problems – illness which only high-raw or temporary all-raw diets could cure. These pathfinders often attracted the opprobrium of their professional colleagues, yet when they used their skills patients responded with infinite gratitude. Many of them, who expected to be ill for the rest of their lives, found themselves cured.

Born in 1867, the Swiss physician Dr Max Bircher-Benner is one of the most famous great European pioneers of nutritional science. He came upon the potential of uncooked foods when, as an overworked young doctor, he was seized with an attack of jaundice. It sent him to bed for several days and made it impossible for him to eat anything. His wife, peeling apples for dinner one day, slipped a small piece of raw fruit between his lips. He found it pleasant and, unlike all the other food that had been offered to him, digestible. Several days and many well-chewed apples later, he had completely recovered.

PYTHAGOREAN WHISPERS

Bircher-Benner was called on to treat a patient who was unable to digest anything. She was starving slowly and very weak. He mentioned the case to a colleague who had an interest in ancient history. Did he know, his colleague told him, that in 500 BC Pythagoras wrote of curing a similar condition by giving nothing but mashed raw fruit, a little honey and goat's milk? Bircher-Benner was sceptical, despite his own experience with raw apples. Such a 'cure' broke all the rules. Bircher-Benner had been taught – as most health professionals still are today – that raw foods are difficult to cope with if you have an ailing digestive system. But since everything else had failed he decided to try Pythagoras' remedy. His patient ate the raw foods he gave her. Tests carried out the next day indicated she had digested them well. He was surprised that a digestive system which could not handle cooked food thrived on the same foods eaten in a raw state.

Spurred on by what he had seen, Bircher-Benner began to investigate the special properties of 'living foods' as he called them, in the treatment of other illnesses. Regardless of the type or seriousness of the disease, his living-food treatments were an enormous success. The clinic which he founded in Zürich in 1897 (and now sadly closed) remained one of the most highly respected centres for nature-healing in the world for almost a century.

Defeating the 'Incurable'

Bircher-Benner foresaw all too clearly the epidemic proportions degenerative diseases have now reached in the industrialised West. Not long before his death in 1939, he wrote: '. . . we were oppressed by an overwhelming burden of incurable disease which hangs over our lives like a dark cloud. It is a burden which will not disappear until men become aware of the basic laws of life. As it is we doctors have to concentrate so much of our attention upon the task of keeping the incurable alive with the aid of artificial "crutches" that the divinely ordered rule of our profession – the healing of the sick and the prevention of disease – is forced more into the background. Neither the profession nor the public seems to see the tragedy of the situation.'

SELF-REALISING HOLISM

Bircher-Benner was a proponent of holistic medicine long before the phrase was coined. He insisted that a patient be treated as an indivisible whole – a psycho–physical personality – with the end in mind not only of curing illness but also of promoting the realisation of a person's full potential. He saw each human being as unique, as having been born with a 'blueprint' that had to be realised. And he found that a diet high in uncooked foods along with regular exercise played a central role in this self-realising, self-healing process.

The Hell of Migraine

The ailment that German physician Max Gerson suffered from was migraine. Dr Gerson, a near contemporary of Bircher-Benner, also went in search of food remedies when all other possibilities had been exhausted. Severe migraine ran in Gerson's family. At times his own headaches and the nausea that accompanied them would sentence him to lying in darkened rooms, unable to do a thing for days on end. Medical experts whom he consulted insisted that there was no cure for migraine. Probably his headaches would disappear by the time he was 40 or 50, they told him.

Gerson was too young and far too passionate about his work to wait that long. So he started to experiment with his diet. First he tried milk, reasoning that since it is perfect for babies, it might be easy to digest and healing for him. But on a milk diet he only grew sicker than ever. Then he turned to fruit. If his monkey ancestors had lived healthily on fruit and nuts and green vegetables, he figured, maybe he could do the same. He began with apples, then cautiously extended his regime to include other fruits. At first he had a couple of excruciating migraines, as his body began to detoxify. Then they disappeared altogether. His headaches stayed away, except when he added new items which disagreed with him. He ate masses of fresh raw fruit and vegetables for the rest of his life. Freed from migraine so long as he continued to eat high-raw, Gerson rose to be, in the opinion of his one-time patient Albert Schweitzer, 'one of the most eminent geniuses in medical history'.

Gerson's 'Migraine Diet'

When Gerson hesitantly suggested his apple diet to a young man who came to him suffering from migraine and whom nothing had helped, the doctor did not expect dramatic results. Nevertheless the young man reported that on the diet his headaches also vanished. He reported something else as well: another ailment from which he suffered, a kind of tuberculosis of the skin, called lupus, had also disappeared. Before the advent of antibiotics, lupus was completely incurable.

UNIVERSAL HEALING POWER

Nobody in the history of medicine had ever reported a lupus lesion healing. Yet on Gerson's 'migraine diet' other lupus sufferers, sent to Gerson by the same patient, also got well. Max Gerson treated them all without charge, hardly daring to consider that the diet he had come upon was a serious therapy. Then in 1928 Albert Schweitzer's wife came to Gerson suffering from severe lung tuberculosis. She too made a complete recovery on his migraine diet. It was then that Gerson truly began to believe that his diet was much more than a mere cure for migraine. It was a way of eating that restored an ailing body's ability to heal itself. That explained why it was so effective across a whole range of ailments.

Gerson went on to use uncooked fresh foods and juices pressed from raw vegetables and fruit to treat everything from mental disorders to coronary heart disease. In time, he became most famous for his treatment of cancer. His book *A Cancer Therapy: Results of Fifty Cases*, first published in 1958, is still the *vade mecum* of all physicians using natural and metabolic treatments for cancer.

Gerson believed that the starting point for all illness, cancer included, is an imbalance of sodium and potassium – usually too much sodium and too little potassium. Correct that, he insisted, by eating potassium-rich raw foods, which invigorate and cleanse the body as well as improve respiration at the cellular level, and you mobilise the white blood cells to fight and destroy cancer cells. Gerson's raw food regimes have enabled many 'terminal' cancer patients to fight and destroy their cancers.

Physician, Heal Thyself

Many other physicians and healers have cured themselves of serious illness by eating a diet high in uncooked foods. As a last resort Danish physician Kristine Nolfi turned to raw foods in an effort to beat her own breast cancer. She won. Then she taught her patients about this natural form of healing. Her success was so great (as was the fury her treatments unleashed among her orthodox peers) that she gave up using drugs altogether and started the Humlegaarden sanatorium in Denmark which she directed until her death in 1957, after which her work was continued by Dr F. Skott Andersen.

On the American front, expert on raw juice and raw food therapy, Dr Norman W. Walker, discovered the healing potentials of a high-raw diet when it helped him rid himself of the excruciating pains of neuritis. He went on to write numerous books on how to use foods and juices to create high level health, and lived to be 117 years old. Naturopath Ann Wigmore, founder of the Hippocrates Health Institute in Boston, travelled the world lecturing and writing about how raw foods transformed her life when she was in her 50s and seriously ill.

CLEARING BODY POLLUTION

German scientist Arnold Ehret suffered from heart disease, kidney trouble and Bright's disease until he discovered that fasting and fresh fruit could cure him of all those things, at a fraction of the cost of all the treatments he had tried previously. Convinced about the health-destroying effects of the wrong kinds of food, in particular of the 'internal pollution' they cause in the colon, he developed the famous Mucusless Diet which he taught to wide acclaim in Europe and America.

Free, Wild and Wonderful

Another pioneering advocate of a high-raw diet was the American dentist, Weston A. Price. From 1920 to 1940, Price travelled the world studying primitive societies – looking at the development of teeth and bones, the incidence of dental caries, and the general physical and mental health of isolated cultures. He examined the dietary patterns of many different peoples – from the Loetschental Valley people high up in the Swiss Alps to the rugged Gaels on Harris in the Outer Hebrides. The results of his work came in the form of a now classic book, *Nutrition and Physical Degeneration*, published in 1945. It carefully documents his findings, complete with photographs and statistics. Price's main conclusion was bleak indeed: processed foods pose appalling dangers to human health. He argues that human health is related to the wholeness and freshness of the foods we consume, and that a high level of health is almost impossible to achieve unless a diet is rich in uncooked foods. In recent years, palaeopathologists working to establish the kind of diet human beings are well adapted to strongly affirm Weston Price's findings.

Price discovered that despite great differences in the specific foods they ate, peoples who were largely free of mental and physical diseases, had good skeletal structure and few, if any, dental caries, had many things about their diet in common. It was what he called a 'primitive diet', a diet of simple, fresh foods, many eaten raw, which were gathered and used immediately. These peoples ate minimal grains, no sugar or manufactured foods and spread natural fertilisers on any crops they grew. They knew nothing of fungicides or insecticides.

BAD NEWS

Our 'modern diet' consists of a wide variety of foods, many of which are tinned, frozen and preserved. Even our fresh foods are adulterated: lettuce is plunged into chemicals like N-6 Benzyl-adenine to keep it fresh, apples have been sprayed with as many as 18 different chemicals. The staples of the modern diet are different too. They are not the fresh fruit and vegetables, seeds and a few grains that Price's isolated cultures ate. They are foods made with massive quantities of refined flour and sugar, and dairy products made from pasteurised milk. Each of us takes in several pounds of chemical additives each year, the effects of which are now even questioned by those professionals who still advocate the standard 'well-balanced' British and American fare of meat-and-two-veg.

When Price visited the remote Loetschental Valley in Switzerland in 1932, its 2,000 inhabitants had only one route to the outside world, a winding single-track railway. Examining their records, which went back some 2,000 years, Price found there had never been a case of tuberculosis among them. They had no policeman or jail; no doctor or dentist – there had never been any need for them. Price realised that diet is more than physiological in its effects; it strongly influences behaviour and environment too. His fieldwork complete, Price went back to America advocating a return to simple fresh foods grown in organically fertilised soils.

FRESH, ORGANIC, HIGH-RAW

Like Gerson and Bircher-Benner and so many other advocates of dietary change, Price found that his colleagues ostracised him. His approach was too radically simple and too ecological to be swallowed by a scientific community committed to high-technology procedures and intent on reducing disease to a matter of single causes and single effects. Yet, like the findings of McCarrison over the past 40 years, Price's intuitions have been increasingly confirmed by epidemiological research all over the world.

Pottenger's Amazing Cats

Further confirmation of the healing and health-enhancing effects of a high-raw or all-raw diet came from the work of American physician Francis M. Pottenger more than 50 years ago. His clinical discoveries about fresh foods and their effects on health paralleled Price's studies. Pottenger noticed that when he fed cats on scraps of raw meat, the animals were much healthier and more resilient than cats fed on cooked meat. So remarkable did this seem to him that he decided to conduct controlled studies to explore the phenomenon. Protocol in his experiments was carefully controlled, met the most rigorous scientific standards of the day, lasted for 10 years, and spanned several generations of animals.

What's New Pussycat?

Pottenger fed part of his colony of 900 cats on pasteurised milk, cooked meat and cod liver oil. He found that animals fed on these cooked foods developed a high incidence of allergies, sickness and skeletal deformities. As one generation begat another, the cats produced smaller litters of weaker, low-birth-weight animals. Pottenger fed the other group of cats in the same way, but the meat was raw and the milk was unpasteurised. The raw-food group of animals remained healthy, had good skeletal structure and were normal in their behaviour. Their offspring also remained healthy through several generations. The offspring of the cooked-food group, like the people Price studied on the standard modern Western diet, increasingly showed pronounced abnormalities in physiology and behaviour. Pottenger discovered that cooked foods can interfere with the normal behaviour of an animal and that the life-damaging effects of eating cooked foods are passed on from generation to generation. Finally he concluded that the inherited damage induced by eating cooked foods requires four generations of animals nourished on raw foods to correct.

Raw Energy Does It

Pottenger began his study of the effect of nutrition on human health and to look at the effect that dietary change has on both health and disease. He was particularly interested in the damage brought about by eating a diet of chemically fertilised, processed foods, and proteins denatured by heat. He was not only a fine laboratory technician, he was also a first-rate physician.

From his clinic in Los Angeles, Francis Pottenger's reputation for astounding cures of resistant illness grew rapidly and brought him worldwide recognition. He insisted on treating his patients on a diet of raw foods which included raw vegetable juices and even a raw liver 'cocktail' which was much admired for its curative properties. Before antibiotics existed, Pottenger became famous for being able to heal all manner of chronic and acute diseases without drugs – from tuberculosis and syphilis to arthritis, heart disease and many forms of cancer. My own grandmother's life was saved by Pottenger. She swore by the power of his amazing raw liver and vegetable juice cocktail for 25 years afterwards. As a small child I visited her in his clinic. Little did I know that my experience of this would foreshadow spending most of my life exploring the whys and wherefores of the raw healing phenomenon.

ANCIENT TEXTS

In the early 20th century, a young French philologist named Edmond Bordeaux Szekely came upon the writings of the Essenes, a monastic sect that flourished on the shores of the Dead Sea at the time of Jesus, while researching in the archives of the Vatican. These ancient texts appear to enshrine wisdom more ancient still, and give specific instructions about health and healing, stressing the use of fasting and raw foods to achieve potent mental, physical and spiritual health. Szekely's translation of the Essene manuscripts (originally into French) was published in English in 1937. It attracted wide attention. The French writer Romain Rolland, winner of the Nobel prize for literature in 1915, was so fascinated by the prescriptions of the Essenes that, with Szekely, he became co-founder of the International Biogenic Society, dedicated to researching, applying and propagating the teaching of the Essenes. Until his death in 1979, Szekely gave yearly or bi-yearly lectures all over the world to teach the 'biogenic' way of life.

Healing Traditions

The European tradition of using uncooked foods to heal and to promote high-level health continues to thrive. In Sweden, Professor Henning Karstrom and many eminent colleagues continue to research and to teach about eating uncooked foods. In Finland, the volume and complexity of the research done by scientists such as A.I. Virtanen and Pentti K. Hietala into the specific biochemical properties and physiological effects of raw food is quite staggering. The Finns have had a special interest in raw foods for farm animals as well as for humans. In Britain, Australia, New Zealand and South Africa there are many physicians and naturopaths who quietly continue to help their patients heal themselves on high-raw diets. Even in America, where high-tech, pill-oriented medicine is strongest, the use of uncooked foods is growing – one of America's most prestigious medical corporations, Kaiser-Permanente, boasts a Health Improvement Service which uses high-raw diets to treat conditions such as obesity, high blood pressure and diabetes. All over the world, live foods and juices are part of the 'gentle' treatment of cancer.

Nevertheless the principles of healing underlying the use of raw foods are still foreign to the training doctors receive. Unfortunately, in most medical schools no more than a couple of hours' training is given in nutrition. British and American doctors are at a disadvantage when it comes to reading the scientific literature, for much of it is not in English, a reflection of the more serious attention paid to the subject elsewhere. But the present health crises in the Western world and a growing demand for a 'whole person' approach to health and illness continue to change all this. High-raw, low-grain eating is a way of living whose time has come.

LIVING MATRIX HEALING

The philosophy behind all natural methods of healing, including high-raw or all-raw diets, is that sickness – whether 'caused' by viruses, germs or genetic changes – is the result of disturbances in the body's natural energetic, biochemical and physiological balance. Once these disturbances can be corrected then the body's own healing abilities – which are virtually infinite – will often clear the 'cause'.

When Professor Hans Eppinger, chief doctor of the First Medical Clinic of the University of Vienna, and his colleagues investigated how uncooked foods can successfully treat resistant illnesses such as heart disease, hypertension, kidney and blood diseases, alcoholism and arthritis, they found that a high-raw or all-raw diet improves functioning on a cellular level in an important way. It raises micro-electric potentials throughout the body. Electrical potentials in tissues are considered a direct measure of the 'aliveness' of cells. Where an increase in these potentials occurs, metabolic functions are heightened, congestion and swelling in tissues decrease, cell respiration or oxygenation increases, the body's overall resistance to illness becomes heightened and a speeding up of the healing processes occurs.

THE LIVING MATRIX

'The living matrix is a continuous and dynamic "supramolecular" webwork extending into every nook and cranny of the body: a nuclear matrix, within a cellular matrix, within a connective tissue matrix. In essence, when you touch a human body, you are touching a continuously interconnected system, composed of virtually all of the molecules in the body linked together in an intricate webwork.'

Dr James L. Oschman

Life's Tapestry

In the early 1990s, scientists D.S. Coffey and K.J. Pienta developed revolutionary new ways of understanding and measuring how all living systems function in health and disease via the 'tissue matrix system' – *the living matrix*. They discovered that this living matrix is a multi-dimensional, molecular continuum – a dynamic communications network which even has semi-conductor properties. It is a structural, biochemical, energetic, oscillatory informational network which integrates all of the body's parts and activities. The physiological and regulatory processes on which the health of the body depends take place within your living matrix. Support its functioning with proper nourishment and it will reward you not only with a healthy body, but radiant vitality too. The word matrix means 'womb'. Your living matrix is the womb out of which health and healing continues to be born.

New England scientist Dr James Oschman, author of the paradigm-breaking book *Energy Medicine . . . The Scientific Basis*, is another of the pioneers whose work is important to natural healing. An articulate and exacting researcher, Oschman has evolved scientific explanations and ways of measuring the beneficial effects on the body of such diverse practices as yoga, the Chinese qigong, the laying on of hands, and Reiki healing. Like a diet high in raw foods, they too influence the living matrix. When your matrix functions with a high degree of energetic order, your body is vital and resistant to degeneration and heals easily.

LIGHT SOURCE

Meanwhile, Professor Fritz Popp in Germany and Professor Hugo Niggli in Switzerland, together with scientists from Russia, Japan and Australia, have long studied how subtle light energy – *biophotons* – behave in living tissue and charted their importance to health. The fact that a high-raw, low-grain diet enhances health is in no small part due to the quality of biophoton energy it imparts to the body. Measuring the nature of this ultra-weak but super-important biophoton energy with the help of high-tech equipment, they are able to identify healthy as opposed to diseased tissue in plants and animals. Biophoton measurements have scientifically verified the vast superiority of fresh, organically cultivated foods and the health-giving energy they carry as compared to conventionally grown foods. This complexity of energetic order is imparted to a person eating them.

The findings of these scientists, together with the work of the other raw-food pioneers, challenge the traditional view of how we nourish our body. We know that it is possible to supply the body with a plethora of what it needs to make its *own* transformation happen from within by activating its own natural regeneration power and that of the living matrix itself. There is no greater power for healing than the body's own. High-raw, low-grain eating helps it happen.

Look After Your Matrix
Your own gene expression is governed by the quality of the fluid your cells are bathed in within the living matrix. This depends on the way you eat, handle stress and use your body, as well as on the load of chemical toxicity your body carries. Exposed to high levels of pollutants from water and chemicals in food and household products, and living on the standard modern diet, the body gets into trouble. Follow a diet which supplies a high level of order to the cells and tissues and you strengthen the whole organism.

VITAL TENSIONS

Health, indeed life itself, depends on the constant interchange of chemicals and energy between the bloodstream – which via the capillaries supplies the tissues of the body with oxygen and nutrients and carries away cellular wastes – and cells. This interchange takes place between two thin membranes and a fine interstitial space. It occurs in a living organism only because the cells and capillaries have what is known as *selective capacity*. This means they are able to attract the substances they need and reject what is harmful or unnecessary. Selective capacity is the result of antagonistic chemical and micro-electrical tensions between cells in a living system. When you die, of course, it is lost completely. The stronger the tensions – the more intense these antagonisms – the healthier and more vital your body will be.

Ill health is characterised by a decrease in chemical and micro-electrical tensions and a loss in selective capacity. This in turn leads to a lowering of cell metabolism and a slowing down in cell reproduction, a weakening of the capillary walls and the gradual development of a sticky 'marsh' which builds up in the intestinal spaces from excess waste products. This marsh, or tissue sludge, encourages degeneration, favours the development of bacteria in the tissues and supports the kind of genetic damage associated with ageing. It also further lowers cell metabolism.

In this way the vicious circle of chronic illness develops. The actual appearance of symptoms may take some time. In the meantime the person feels chronically fatigued and lacklustre. He or she is living in the twilight zone of 'half-health', unaware that something is wrong because as yet there are no clear disease symptoms.

DEFEAT DISEASE

At the University of Vienna, scientists discovered that raw food steadily increases selective capacity by heightening electrical potentials between tissue cells and capillary blood. This improves the ability of capillaries to regulate the transportation of nutrients, and gradually detoxifies the living matrix, removing the sticky marsh that further lowers vitality. A raw diet breaks through that vicious circle of disease, replacing it with a 'circle of health'.

Clear Arthritis

Take arthritis. Many people believe that the stiffness and pain of arthritic joints are an inevitable part of growing old. Experts in the use of uncooked foods insist that it is not. They view arthritis as a toxic condition which builds up as the result of poor dietary habits. A cleansing regime based on fresh, uncooked foods gives the body a chance to dispel the misery-causing toxins responsible for painful joints, to improve cellular exchange and to increase cellular vitality so that the condition can heal. Dr Lars-Erik Essen of Sweden's Vita Nova clinic, famed for his successful treatment of arthritis, prescribed short fasts of three to five days followed by a high-raw cleansing diet. Dr Carl Otto Aly, a disciple of Are Waerland, founder of the Swedish Health Movement, uses a low-protein, high-raw diet temporarily for healing. In Britain, general practitioners like Dr Gordon Latto and Dr Phillip Kilsby, who taught me how to heal myself of endogenous depression in my early 20s, became famous for having cured many resistant cases of crippling arthritis with high-raw diets. They claimed, as do their European colleagues, that raw regimes stimulate the body to heal itself.

RAW FOOD CURE

Diabetes is another widespread ailment which improves through high-raw, low-grain eating. It is an illness in which the pancreas does not produce enough of the hormone insulin. Insulin works rather like a key, making cell membranes permeable to energy-giving glucose. Without enough of it, glucose accumulates in the blood and eventually overflows into the urine. As well as having to manage their illness for many years, diabetics are faced with a higher risk of heart disease and cancer. A high-raw diet, requiring no 'special' diabetic foods, can often not only reduce the amount of insulin a person needs but, in some cases, eliminate the need for it altogether.

The Schweitzer Experience

Dr Albert Schweitzer was a severe diabetic. By the time he sought the help of the raw-food pioneer Max Gerson, he was seriously ill and taking huge doses of insulin. Gerson put Schweitzer on a regime of raw fresh vegetables with lots of vegetable and fruit juices. Ten days later, Gerson judged it safe to reduce his patient's insulin by half. A month later, Schweitzer needed no insulin at all. His diabetes never returned and he remained healthy and active until his death in 1965 at the age of 92.

More recent evidence that diabetes yields to high-raw treatments comes from Dr John Douglass, head of the Health Improvement Service at the Kaiser-Permanente Medical Center in Los Angeles. Some of his patients have been able to stop using insulin altogether. Others have reduced its use to a minimum. One of his star cases, a brittle juvenile diabetic, was weaned off insulin and eventually off oral anti-diabetic drugs as well by a 90–100 per cent raw diet. Douglass still insists that some diabetics need to restrict the amount of fresh fruit they eat, because fruit contains a lot of sugar and is too high on the glycaemic index. One of his patients who failed to respond to his high-raw diet was found to be eating 18 bananas a day!

The Fibre Factor

The efficacy of raw diets in diabetes is thought to be related to fibre. Almost by definition, a diet of raw fruits and vegetables is a high-fibre diet. As far as the diabetic is concerned, the most desirable property of fibre is that it slows down absorption of glucose into the blood-stream. David Jenkins at Oxford, and others, have shown that after a high-fibre meal, blood sugar does not rise as much as it does after a low-fibre meal. If the level of insulin in the blood is low, or if the patient is trying to make do with less injected insulin, slowly absorbed glucose does not swamp its limited capacity to make cell membranes permeable.

Douglass has also speculated that because fibre passes through the gut in 18 to 24 hours when it is consumed in large quantities (for the average Western cooked diet throughput time is 80 to 100 hours) there is less chance of the body being damaged by waste products in the colon. The longer wastes stay in the colon the more likely they are to decompose, producing gases which diffuse into the bloodstream and interfere with the way the sugars are metabolised.

Redox Matters

There is another general attribute of raw foods as valuable in treating ill health as in improving good. It may play an important part in treating diabetes. This is the very active nature of many of the energetic and biochemical substances which live foods impart to the person eating them. By definition, molecules which are highly active are also unstable. They have a high tendency to lose electrons to and acquire electrons from other molecules. A chemist would say that they have 'high redox potentials'. Vitamin C has this tendency *par excellence*. So do many other molecules – vitamins, proteins, enzymes, fats, minerals and unknown factors – in raw food. In effect, they ginger lazier molecules into action, encouraging greater energy exchange. When the same food is cooked, the chemical activity of many of its ingredients is drastically diminished.

GREAT POTENTIAL

Douglass believes that the redox potential of uncooked foods – their ability to awaken relatively inert molecules – is another important factor in their potential for healing. Like vitamin C, they encourage optimal electrical exchange, imparting liveliness to the body's cells and systems and enhancing health by doing so. He points out that 'Optimal electron transport speed can't occur in denatured protein since its molecular matrix has been altered.'

Researcher, Dr Chiu-Nan Lai, who has carried out many studies to determine the protective properties of chlorophyll in uncooked foods, describes it this way: 'Raw food has a higher redox potential than cooked food. Cooking destroys the oxygen-containing enzymes as well as plant tissues rendering the food more anaerobic. Putrefying bacteria which require a low redox potential environment to grow will thrive on dead tissues but not on living tissues. Raw food then is more clean.'

Cancer Fighters
The higher redox potentials of raw foods and the way they enhance the functioning and order of the living matrix are major reasons why they form the foundation of all the 'gentle' approaches to cancer treatment and prevention. A report from the United States Academy of Sciences on the relationship between diet and cancer is based on a survey of some 10,000 research papers. It recommends greater emphasis on fresh fruit and vegetables in the diet. Vitamins A, C and E, which occur in good quantity in fresh leafy green vegetables and fruit, are known to discourage cancer. A great deal of recent research has shown that the retinoids (forms of vitamin A) inhibit chemically induced malignant growths of the breast, bladder and skin in humans. Vitamin C, the survey cautiously comments, may 'lower the risk of cancer, particularly gastric (stomach) and oesophageal (throat) cancers'.

RAW FOOD PLUS C

In more than three years of research at the Linus Pauling Institute in California, a raw-food diet – fresh apples, pears, tomatoes, carrots, wheat grass, sunflower seeds and bananas – was found to have cancer-preventing properties at least equal to those of a normal diet plus massive amounts of extra vitamin C. Even more spectacular resistance to cancer was achieved when the all-raw diet was supplemented with huge doses of vitamin C. Vegetable fibre has also been shown to be protective against certain kinds of cancer. And specific vegetables – Brussels sprouts, cabbage, cauliflower and broccoli – contain compounds which have been shown to lessen the effects of environmental cancer-causing agents.

It is the belief of those who treat cancer by biological methods rather than by drugs and radiation that malignancy is not something which descends out of the blue on a helpless victim. It is the final stage of slow poisoning of the living matrix, especially of the liver, by metabolic wastes and environmental pollutants. Often this slow poisoning is the result of an unbalanced diet, a diet excessively weighted towards convenience foods and junk fats and other refined and processed foods. An excess of protein and a deficit of vital nutrients can cause all sorts of mayhem within the living matrix. Tired cells are bad at picking up oxygen and nutrients and eliminating wastes, pushing the whole sodium–potassium, acid–alkaline balance of the body in a direction which breeds malignant changes.

Get Balanced

This sodium–potassium balance and food oxygenation of cells are as important in the prevention and treatment of cancer as they are in raising heath to its highest potentials. Sodium and potassium work together to maintain an osmotic pressure between intracellular fluids (those within cells) and extracellular fluids (those outside the cells). Potassium compounds predominate mainly in the cells of muscles, soft tissues, organs and blood vessels. Sodium is found more in the blood plasma and interstitial fluids between cells. The better each predominates in its own sphere, the greater the balancing tensions between them and the more vital an organism will be.

CHOOSE ORGANIC

Sodium and potassium are nutritional antagonists. When there is an excess of one, the balance is disturbed and health suffers. Imbalances between sodium and potassium almost always err on the side of too much sodium and too little potassium. Many people in Britain and the United States appear to suffer some degree of potassium deficiency because of the foods they eat and the way they are cooked and processed. Organically grown foods consumed raw are high in potassium and low in sodium. In artificially fertilised foods, the sodium content is higher and the potassium content lower. When food is cooked, sodium is added to it in the form of salt. Processed foods are flavoured with massive amounts of salt. Excess salt, together with antibiotics and other drugs, causes sodium to be drawn into the cells and potassium to move out of them as active sodium-extruding mechanisms are impaired or break down.

Cells Suffer

As the vital difference between the inner and outer environment of a cell decreases, every single process in it begins to suffer. Unable to absorb or excrete efficiently, it ceases to carry out vital manufacturing operations, toxic wastes build up inside it and all sorts of rubbish accumulates outside. The symptoms of this clogging up and slowing down at cellular level are fatigue, lowered immunity and finally disease. Raw foods, with their high potassium content, appear to be able to throw this insidious process into reverse.

Expert in the dietary treatment of cancer, Dr Max Gerson insisted that the beginnings of all chronic illness lie in this loss of potassium from the cells as a result of a gradually developing sodium–potassium imbalance in the body. This imbalance, he claimed, results in serious disturbances in the body chemistry. For not only is potassium an important nerve conductor, it also acts as a catalyst for many body enzymes and is essential for proper muscle contraction, including contraction of the muscles of the heart and the muscles involved in digestion. Potassium is also vital for the conversion of glucose into glycogen in the liver. A healthy liver will contain twice as much potassium as sodium. Too little potassium causes cardiac abnormalities and can also result in high blood pressure. Low levels of potassium are associated with chronic fatigue. Potassium has an affinity for oxygen; enough of it encourages good cell respiration or oxygenation. This is another important factor in the prevention and treatment of cancer and another reason raw foods bring so much power for health to the body.

A KEY TO GOOD HEALTH

The way a diet of raw foods increases cell oxygenation is just as important in the healing of a sick body as it is in protecting against illnesses, including cancer. In the development of most chronic illness, regardless of the specific disease, lowered cell respiration is evident. Another expert in cancer, Nobel laureate Otto Warburg, Director of the Max Planck Institute for Cell Physiology in Berlin, discovered that while normal cells use oxygen-based reactions as their source of energy, cancer cells are different. They appear to derive their energy from fermentation via a glucose-based chemistry instead. Other researchers, such as Heinrich Jung and P.G. Seeger, confirmed Warburg's work and showed that cancer, like many other degenerative diseases, arises from a disturbance in cellular respiration which results not only in a lowering of energy but also in a serious disturbance in metabolism on the organism as a whole. When normal cell respiration is restored by raw diet, the vitality of the whole organism and its immunity to disease is increased.

Quite a short time on a high-raw, low-grain diet does several things. It eliminates accumulated wastes and toxins. It restores optimal sodium–potassium and acid–alkaline balance. It supplies and/or restores the level of nutrients essential for optimal cell function. It increases the efficiency with which cells take up oxygen, necessary for the release of energy with which to carry out their multifarious activities. With all these desirable and interactive functions to their credit, it is hardly surprising that raw foods have proved effective against many forms of cancer.

ANTI-CANCER DIETS

A typical anti-cancer regime consists of organically grown food – food that has not been treated with fungicides, insecticides and artificial fertilisers (some of which have carcinogenic residues) or with additives, colorants or preservatives. Approximately 80–90 per cent of food is eaten raw and protein intake is temporarily reduced. Too much protein while a body is undergoing the deep detoxification necessary for healing can not only lead to excessive nitrogenous wastes, but can also put strain on the pancreas, the organ responsible for manufacturing protein-digesting and cancer-fighting enzymes. Many scientists consider the loss of pancreatic function to be a major cause of cancer. A strong, well-functioning pancreas is particularly good health insurance. Many nutritionally-oriented therapists also insist that in cancer patients it is important to 'save' most of the enzymes the pancreas produces for combating malignancy rather than digesting protein.

Anti-cancer diets are also free of junk fats. No more than 10–20 per cent of daily caloric consumption comes from fat, all of it consumed unheated and derived directly from freshly hulled seeds, nuts and certain fruits and vegetables. Margarine and processed vegetable oils are regarded with the greatest suspicion. Raw egg yolks from free-range eggs are allowed, but the only milk products used are those made from fresh raw milk – kvark, a raw, unheated, home-made cottage cheese, and home-made, unheated yoghurt, for example. Goat's milk is thought to contain more anti-cancer and anti-arthritic factors than cow's milk.

Fermented Foods

Fermented foods – fermented grains and juices, sauerkraut, nut and seed 'cheeses' – also play a part in most cancer-treatment regimes. The lactic acid in them encourages the development of helpful gut bacteria (*Acidophilus*) which destroy their more harmful relatives (the *Escherichia coli* bacteria which meat encourages are potentially harmful) and improve digestion and assimilation. Because they are 'pre-digested', fermented foods require less effort from an already ailing digestive system. German cancer researcher, Dr Johannes Kuhl, one of the first to explore the beneficial effects of lactic acid in cancer treatment, insists that as much as 50–75 per cent of the daily diet can, with benefit, be taken from naturally fermented raw foods.

ALKALINISING THE BLOOD

Sprouted seeds and grains also figure in most cancer regimes. They cleanse the body of toxic wastes, are exceptionally high in essential vitamins, minerals and enzymes, provide easily assimilated proteins and tend to alkalinise the blood.

The alkalinity of raw foods is a particularly powerful ally in cancer treatment too. Amongst other things, it helps the pancreas to produce its cancer-fighting enzymes. According to the distinguished cancer specialist Hans Neiper, the biggest challenge to the cancer healer is to find ways of breaking down the protective mucous envelope with which cancer cells surround themselves. Pancreatic enzymes have the power to destroy this mucous barrier, rendering cancer cells vulnerable to attack and liquidation by the body's immune system. Certain substances in raw fruit and vegetables such as the phytonutrients and the enzymes chymotrypsin, trypsin, and the bromelains also appear to carry this power.

Live Juices

Live raw fruit and vegetable juices are an essential part of anti-cancer diets. Raw juices do most of the excellent things that solid raw foods do but in a way that places the minimum strain on the digestive system. The concentrated vitamins, minerals, trace elements, enzymes, sugars and proteins they contain are absorbed into the bloodstream almost as soon as they reach the stomach and small intestine. American immunotherapist and cancer expert Dr Virginia Livingston urges her patients to drink fresh raw juices as often as possible and recommends two pints of carrot juice a day. Other juices she favours are apple, cabbage, cucumber, spinach, tomato and beetroot. Of course huge quantities of fresh fruit and vegetables are needed to produce juice by crushing or centrifuging. The Gerson cancer diet, for example, which prescribes ten 8oz/225ml glasses a day of fresh carrot, apple and green vegetable juices, uses some 1,800lb/820kg carrots a year, 125lb/57kg green peppers, 145 cabbages and upwards of 1,300 oranges.

Non-nutritional treatments, such as heat therapy, cold therapy and laser therapy, depend on the use of external agents to kill malignant growths. They do little to help the body train its own defensive guns on the offending tissue or build up enough resistance to prevent malignancy recurring. High-raw, low-grain eating can.

ENERGY RAW AND FREE

Nutrition is not only about biochemistry. The state and quality of living energy – biophotons, sunlight-quanta, electromagnetic information – which a food carries plays an enormous role in determining the health of your capillaries and cells, your organs and tissues – your life as a whole. Now this is hot stuff, so far ahead of conventional nutritional thinking that it makes heads spin. Yet it is a truth that has been known for centuries to experts in natural healing. And raw foods are at the heart of it.

Most of the study of what a high-raw diet can do to detoxify, restore and rejuvenate the body comes out of Austria, Germany, Switzerland and Scandinavia. This may be why we know so little about it in English-speaking countries like Britain and the United States. In Europe there is a long tradition of healing and age retardation using organic foods – a high percentage of them uncooked. For more than half a century, European scientists have carried out elaborate clinical and laboratory studies to determine how, on a cellular level, fresh foods are able to work wonders for the health of human beings.

Not by Chemistry Alone
The revitalising properties of a high-raw diet cannot be wholly explained in terms of vitamins, minerals and phytonutrients. Max Bircher-Benner, who became famous worldwide for his raw-food 'cures', insisted that the vitality that raw foods imparts to your body depends on their 'aliveness', something which defies chemical analysis. It cannot be tracked down by computing the calorific value of so many molecules of fat or carbohydrate, or by isolating and cataloguing all the different nutrients in a piece of food, or by measuring the level of those nutrients in the blood.

QUANTUM POWER

Bircher-Benner claimed that fresh, live plants – fruits and vegetables, seeds and herbs – contain a special form of energy directly derived from the sun during photosynthesis. When we eat plants this special energy passes into us. He sought support for his theory from physics, in particular from the second law of thermodynamics, which forms the foundation of classical physics.

Free Energy – Open Systems

In physics, the first and second laws of thermodynamics focus on the nature of energy in the universe, in an attempt to explain events in the universe by studying the kind of energy changes which accompany them. The *second law of thermodynamics* is particularly important in relation to physical health. It is called the law of *entropy*. It states simply that, left to their own devices, things in the universe become disordered: iron rusts, buildings crumble, dead flowers decay, and we humans degenerate and eventually die. This is described in scientific language by saying that everything tends towards *maximum* entropy. 'Entropy' means a state of disorder – chaos if you prefer – in which all useful energy has been decreased.

DEFY THE LAW

What is so remarkable about a living human being – and what has been a great puzzle to some of the world's finest scientific minds – is this: despite the second law of thermodynamics, we, like other living organisms, are able to remain highly ordered. In fact, so long as we remain alive, our bodies are maintained in a condition of fantastic improbability, despite the endless destructive processes continually going on in and around us. More than that, there is every indication that a healthy body, regardless of age, is continually involved in creating yet more order. This we do both individually, thanks to the repair functions of our cells and enzymic systems, as well as from an evolutionary point of view since, with time, living species differentiate into ever more complex and highly structured organisms. This is only possible because the living body is an *open system* – able to access *free energy* from the air it breathes, the food it eats, the physical, emotional and spiritual experiences it gathers.

Negentropic Wonders

Unlike the rocks and nails in the inorganic world, living organisms like your body are capable of both becoming and remaining superbly ordered. They have a capacity for re-creating balance and restoring health when things get out of whack. This is how we maintain our bodies at a high degree of health. This 'ordering ability' makes no sense within the paradigms of classical Newtonian physics: there should be little difference in the chemical and physical processes taking place in a living body and those of a corpse – since both follow the same scientific laws. Yet, there is every difference in the world. In life, internal processes are able to maintain the system in quite exceptional harmony (in scientific terms a high degree of negative entropy or *negentropy*), despite the fact that events leading to maximum entropy in the universe as a whole should destroy it.

PENETRATING THE MYSTERY

In the words of Nobel laureate Albert Szent-Györgyi, who spent most of his life trying to penetrate the mystery of life energy: 'Life is a paradox . . . the most basic rule of inanimate nature is that it tends toward equilibrium which is at the maximum of entropy and the minimum of free energy. The main characteristic of life is that it tends to decrease its entropy. It also tends to increase its free energy. Maximum entropy means complete randomness, disorder. Life is made possible by order, structure, a pattern which is the opposite of entropy. This pattern is our chief possession, it was developed over billions of years. The main aim of our existence is its conservation and transmission. Life is a revolt against the statistical rules of physics. Death

> means that the revolt subsided and statistical laws resumed their sway.'

From an energetic point of view, ageing is the process which transports a body from its youthful, healthy, highly ordered, homoeostatic state towards maximum entropy – illness, degeneration and death. To protect your body from this destructive process, you need to give it all the help you can to support your natural capacity for order on an energetic level.

Sunlight Quanta

Bircher-Benner pointed out that when we eat fresh raw plants themselves we appear to receive the very highest order of energy possible direct from our food. A very high order of the sun's energy – he called it sunlight quanta – is converted by plants through photosynthesis and then stored in them, and the quality of this energy is degraded by all kinds of physical and chemical processes such as wilting, cooking or processing. The power of this form of free energy in the environment is a major player, enabling us to resist illness, degeneration and disintegration. In effect, it disproves the famous second law, turning classical chemically based assumptions about nutrition on their head.

DRINK ORDER

Some 40 years later, Austrian physicist and Nobel laureate Erwin Schrödinger confirmed Bircher-Benner's hypothesis with his own theory. Schrödinger tried to state it in terms that were acceptable to physicists: 'What is that precious something contained in our food which keeps us from death? That is easily answered. Every process, event, happening – call it what you will – in a word, everything that is going on in Nature means an increase of the entropy in the part of the world where it is going on. Thus a living organism continually increases its entropy – or as you may say, produces positive entropy – and thus tends to approach the dangerous state of maximum entropy, which is death. It can only keep aloof from it, i.e. alive, by continually drawing from its environment negative entropy . . . What an organism feeds upon is negative entropy . . . which is in itself a measure of order. *Thus the device by which an organism maintains itself stationary at a fairly high level of orderliness (= a fairly low level of entropy) really consists of it continually sucking orderliness from its environment.*

Bircher-Benner believed, as did Schrödinger, that to stay healthy the body has to continually 'drink order'. To live at the peaks, we need to take in the fresh living matter raw foods provide. They have the highest-quality nutritive energy – energy which has never been debased by oxidation, spoiling processes or heating.

Although many scientists are aware of Schrödinger's concept that living organisms feed on negative entropy and the idea is discussed in virtually every textbook on biophysics and biochemistry, it continues to be largely ignored by orthodox nutritional teaching. Until recently, few researchers had investigated exactly how much negative entropy or what degree of orderliness exists in raw foods. One notable exception is Professor I.I. Brekhman of the Far East Scientific Centre Academy of Sciences of the USSR in Vladisvostock, who won the coveted Lenin prize for science in recognition of his work.

Information Brings Order

Brekhman coined the phrase 'structural information'. By this he means something very close to Schrödinger's 'order'. He claims that not only are the nutrients which can be measured chemically – vitamins, minerals, proteins, etc. – important for health, so is the complexity of the way they, and other as yet unidentified factors, are combined in a particular food and the quality of energy that food carries.

YOU ARE AN OPEN SYSTEM

Energetically, your body is an open system. It continually exchanges energy with its environment – through the foods we eat, digest, assimilate and excrete, as well as the company we keep, ongoing radiation and electromagnetic fields we are exposed to, the way we exercise – even the thoughts we think. As such we are constantly processing mechanical, biochemical and energetic *information* which comes to us and flows from us. We need a constant supply of the right kind of information from the outside world to keep our bodies functioning optimally, and we need to be able to dissipate any disorder and chaos – entropy – that has built up within our bodies and our lives.

Unanswered Questions

Life processes which cannot be explained within a particular scientific discipline have a long history either of being ignored or misinterpreted. It is often easier to bury your head in the sand. Yet these unanswered questions are central to an understanding of the ageing process. For when control processes go awry, disorder invades the organism and degeneration ensues. They are also biology's most intriguing problems, and therefore make many biochemists very uncomfortable indeed, simply because they are unanswerable in biochemical terms. Where can we find the answers? Or at the very least, where should we be looking?

Free Exchange

Brekhman has studied energy exchange in relation to his main interests: food and natural medicines such as ginseng and Siberian ginseng. These are plants with a long history of use, which scientific research has shown have non-specific abilities to strengthen an organism's vitality. Brekhman and his team confirmed that the heating and processing of foods can decrease the quality of structural information they bring to an organism and thus their health-supporting and age-retarding properties. Fresh foods carry a much higher degree of the structural information your body can beneficially use than do cooked or processed foods.

They also found that foods high in 'structural information' enable animals – us included – to carry out physical tasks for significantly longer periods than processed foods low in structural information. This is true even when the foods compared are equal in calories and are, by orthodox biochemical standards, supposed to be supplying an organism with the same amount of energy. The structural information a particular food or herb carries is measured in what Brekhman calls 'significant units of action'. To retard the process of ageing and degeneration then, both the quantity and quality of this information must be as close to the ideal needs of our organism as possible – in other words, as close to what we as human beings have been genetically programmed to thrive on. In Schrödinger's terms, it needs to supply a high degree of *orderliness*. Brekhman has been particularly interested in natural pharmacological substances, like healing herbs, which supply a high degree of structural information to an organism and therefore support a high level of health and energy.

Unravelling the Mysteries
Cutting-edge biophysics confirms that Schrödinger and the rest are right. And if an organism has to 'drink order' to stay alive, and if the reason why raw foods are such powerful forces for health is that the structural information they carry is particularly high and appropriate to the purposes of the living body, then we need to ask two questions: first, what is the nature of that order? Second, in what form is it conveyed through the foods we eat?

These questions make orthodox biochemists and nutritionists uncomfortable, for their answers can never be found in a chemical analysis of these foods. You come closer when you enter the realms of microbiology and speak of electron transfer and the 'aliveness of cells'. You can focus on some extraordinary properties which uncooked foods have but still you are only describing the shadows on the wall. Few scientists are comfortable with the sense that it is not the nature of reality they are delineating but merely its phantasmagoric ever-changing forms, frozen in a moment in time. They mistake the shadow for the thing itself. They assume that since we know a carrot or a slice of calf's liver contains such and such nutrients and so many calories, and since we can produce those nutrients chemically in a laboratory, then by adding a little simple carbohydrate to supply the calories, we can make a food that is just as good as the one we are copying.

CONSCIOUSNESS ENERGY

From the point of view of quantum physics, as human beings we are not only immersed in an energy field, our body, our mind, our whole being are energy fields. These fields are constantly contracting and expanding as our thoughts, diet and lifestyle change. The aim of any form of natural treatment, from dietary change or detoxification to hydrotherapy, exercise and meditation, is to enhance positive bioenergies in an organism and to create greater order in your body, biochemically, psychologically and spiritually.

Dyed in the Wool

Despite revolutionary developments in high-level physics, most biochemists are still committed to the traditional atomistic notion that the universe is built out of elementary particles and that all of life can ultimately be understood by taking it apart and putting it back together. Before scientists of any discipline can begin to answer either of our questions, they must first examine the underlying assumptions on which their methodologies are based and ask if these assumptions are still appropriate for what they are trying to discover.

New Energy Paradigms

As far back as the 1960s the Polish priest and biophysicist Wlodzimierz Sedlac wrote prolifically, describing biological structure in energetic ways. His work set in motion an energy revolution which, I believe, is helping to topple the chemical and mechanical paradigms that too rigidly still define human health. Cells he described as *diode resonators.* Mitochondria work as *intracellular interferometers,* and *inductance emission coils.* Cell membranes can be considered *biophoton resonators.* In Germany, the brilliant physicist Fritz Popp showed that, when stimulated by a laser emission from the mitochondria, DNA emits far UV light. In fact our cells give off powerful light energy. When they are dividing or dying they also emit UV light radiation. It is the *coherence* between UV light and electromagnetic organisation which appears to give each cell its ability to vibrate at specific frequencies.

LIVING MATRIX

Cells behave much like radiotransmitters, enabling them to communicate within the superconducting semi-solid plasma of the body's liquid crystal matrix – the *mesenchyme* – now more

> commonly known as the living matrix. Doctors and scientists working with natural treatments have claimed for over 150 years that the living matrix is the seedbed of health and youth. Look after the state of the living matrix – your body's biological terrain – and the rest of the body will look after itself.

Mathematics, biophysics and wave mechanics describe biological systems as kinetic, electrical, magnetic, gravitational and mass energies. All these terms fit into the cohesive field theory of universal energy at the leading-edge of modern physics. They help us to understand some of what enhances the ability of negentropy to preserve health and also what can undermine it from an energetic point of view.

Out with Splintered Thinking

The approach to health taken by physicians who emphasise a diet high in uncooked foods in many ways parallels that of scientists working in high-level physics. Both replace the Newtonian reductionist view of reality with a quantum perspective of a dynamic universe. The Newtonian view is based on the classical dualism which underlies the methodologies of biochemistry and nutrition. This became an important premise on which modern medicine is based when it was formalised in Descartes' philosophy.

Descartes divided reality into two separate and independent realms, that of mind and matter – *res cogitans* and *res extensa*. This Cartesian dualism made it possible for scientists to treat matter objectively, as something completely separate from themselves to be taken apart, analysed and categorised. Such a paradigm of reality has been enormously *useful*. It has made possible the isolation and control of micro-organisms behind much widespread disease in the late 19th and early 20th centuries, from tuberculosis to typhoid fever and smallpox.

In the realm of biochemistry and nutrition, this dualistic thinking has enabled scientists to establish the nutritional causes of simple deficiency diseases such as beriberi and scurvy and to isolate the 'missing' substances without which disease symptoms appear. And following such an assumption about the nature of reality, biochemists have been able to isolate, quantify and categorise the 50 or more nutrients so far known to be necessary for life.

But every dominant paradigm has its limitations. In the realm of biology and physiology, such thinking has led to the notion that the human body is little more than a machine made up of a lot of different parts which can be analysed into a collection of cause-and-effect relationships. From this world view comes the notion of disease as an outside entity – a cruel act of fate caused by some external threat like a microbe – something which we are neither responsible for, nor able to help ourselves with.

WANTED: A SCIENTIFIC REVOLUTION

In *The Structure of Scientific Revolution*, Thomas Kuhn insists that every dominant paradigm eventually expands to the limits of its methodologies and becomes no longer useful. That is just what is happening right now in the field of biochemistry, nutrition and medicine.

Newtonian physics and Cartesian dualism, useful though they have been in the research which led to the control of epidemic diseases and illnesses caused by gross malnutrition, are inadequate to deal with the kind of chronic illnesses which have been called the 'diseases of Western civilisation' – coronary heart disease, cancer, diabetes, arthritis, gastric ulcers, emphysema, etc. They are also practically useless if science is to discover ways of helping men and women to live at a state of high-level health – not just free of overt symptoms of disease but feeling positively good and having a high resistance to the process of ageing. The achievement of such goals involves myriad interrelated considerations in our lives: our relationship to stress, our psychological orientation, social and environmental factors and, most important of all, our nutrition. These influences are all too diffuse and complex to fit into any world view based on Cartesian dualism. When we continue to try and make them fit, as too many still do in their search for answers, we not only falter amidst masses of interesting but unconnected facts, but our efforts lead nowhere.

HOLISM MATTERS

To answer the questions posed, medicine and nutrition are being forced to expand their atomistic notions. They have to move beyond the limits of the Newtonian–Cartesian world view and discover new paradigms. Scientists need to acknowledge that the 'bits' which they continue to treat as separate entities are not descriptions of reality as it is but, as physicist David Bohm says, 'ever-changing forms of insight', which can only 'point to or indicate a reality that is implicit and not describable or specifiable in its totality'. Finally, they have to develop awareness – however subtle or oblique – of that implicit reality, and the way everything within the living body, as within the universe itself, is interrelated.

The late David Bohm was one of the world's most highly respected quantum physicists. A protégé of Einstein, he has written the classic textbook on quantum theory used in English-speaking universities. In another of his books, *Wholeness and the Implicate Order*, he comments: 'People are led to believe that . . . fragmentation is "the way everything really is" and therefore do not look for alternatives. But it is not in fragmentation . . . that the understanding of life is to be found . . . life is the flow of that implicit order that animates the dead forms of the objective world, and as such, life is both whole and never identical to any of the forms of existence. Therefore there is no use looking for it among the bits and pieces of those forms.' Modern biologists, he says, have little awareness or appreciation of the revolutionary character of modern physics. Most continue to believe that 'the whole of life and mind can ultimately be understood in more or less mechanical terms through some kind of extension of the work that has been done on the structure and function of DNA . . . In modern physics,' he continues '. . . parts are seen to be in immediate connection . . . their dynamical relationships depend in an irreducible way on the state of the whole system (and indeed on that of broader systems in which they are contained, extending ultimately and in principle to the entire universe). Thus one is led to a new notion of unbroken wholeness which denies the classical idea (that the world can be analysed into separate inde-pendent existing parts).'

UNBROKEN WHOLENESS

In their desire to penetrate the mysteries of raw energy, biochemists and nutritionists are beginning to acknowledge that the healing powers implicit in foods are greater than the sum of their parts as measured in terms of nutrients and calories. They will also have to recognise that foods interact with the human organism as part of an *unbroken wholeness* before they can even begin to tackle seriously the issues involved.

There are scientists who now work within this new dominant paradigm. They range from a growing number of forward-thinking physicists and biochemists to healers and soil chemists concerned about how to grow stronger and more successful crops. They acknowledge interrelatedness that under the influence of Cartesian dualism and Newtonian physics we have long ignored. And in their laboratory experiments, some of them still formative, valuable new techniques and approaches for studying the raw-energy phenomenon might be found.

Whichever way you look at it, the power of a diet high in raw vegetables and fruits points far beyond the parameters of nutritional chemistry. Now we enter the realms of sheer energy.

ENERGY BREAKS THE RULES

Energy. This is where Quantum Nutrition breaks all the rules. Biological science has at last begun to penetrate the mysteries of life energies. Until now, energy has remained the province of mystics, sages and leading-edge physicists. When it comes to creating optimal levels of vitality and protection from ageing, on a high-raw, low-grain diet, energy is where it's at.

Most scientists now accept that animal tissue has electrical – and therefore electromagnetic – properties. The notion that plants, as living organisms, also possess electrical properties is less well accepted. But happily the idea that these energies can interact with those present in a body that consumes them is no longer regarded as sheer lunacy.

Ask Any Rat

Eminent scientist Albert Szent-Györgyi, who won a Nobel prize for his work on oxidation and for isolating vitamin C, asked himself a question more than 50 years ago. He has spent almost every working moment of his life since in an attempt to answer it. He is often quoted as having posed this question at a dinner party: 'What is the difference between a living rat and a dead one?' According to the laws of classical chemistry and physics, there should be no fundamental difference. Szent-Györgyi's own reply was simple: 'Some kind of electricity.'

Energy Equations

More and more is known about the electromagnetic properties of plants. Electromagnetism is one of the media through which we 'drink order'. It was the Russian-born engineer Georges Lakhovsky who first suggested, some 70 years ago, that the cells of plants and animals are microscopic oscillating circuits, which emit as well as absorb electromagnetic energy. At about the same time an American scientist, E.J. Lund at Texas State University, invented a method of measuring minute electrical potentials in plants. He went on to demonstrate that plants generate tiny electrical currents and emit electromagnetic waves. These electrical phenomena not only vary with the health of the plant concerned. They also appear – at least in part – to direct and organise plant growth. Bud formation, for instance, is heralded by changes in electromagnetic radiation long before there is any detectable rise in the level of auxins – the hormones which mediate plant growth.

LIFE AS A PHENOMENON

American scientist and surgeon George Crile, who founded the Cleveland Clinic, published a fascinating book called *The Phenomenon of Life*. In it he suggested that it might be possible to diagnose illness long before the symptoms of it appear by monitoring the electromagnetic characteristics of the person concerned. This idea was based on the fact that physical changes in cells are preceded, and maybe even controlled, by electromagnetic changes.

L-Fields Direct

In the 1950s, two Yale University professors, philosopher F.S.C. Northrop and doctor Harold Saxton Burr, suggested that electromagnetic fields which surround living organisms might be the source of organisational controls governing growth and species characteristics. To demonstrate this theory Burr began measuring what he called the 'life fields' or L-fields around seeds. He discovered that altering a single gene in a parent plant would bring about significant changes in the fields of its seeds. He also found that by measuring the intensity of L-fields around seeds he could predict how healthy or unhealthy plants grown from them would be. If the seeds are subjected to chemicals or heat their fields get weak.

The subtle energies which a fresh living food emits are certainly one important medium through which a living organism 'drinks order'. We draw on structural information of a high quality for human health when we eat fresh raw foods. But we incorporate information which in electromagnetic terms becomes distorted, decreased and less appropriate to the needs of the human organism when these foods are cooked. Subtle energies given off by a cooked leaf or vegetable are markedly different from those of its raw counterpart.

Radiant Beauty

One possible method of making such measurements is by Kirlian photography, a technique which was originally discovered in Russia by an electrician and amateur photographer Semyon Kirlian and his wife Valentina. They found that they could reproduce on photographic paper, without the need for camera or lens, a remarkable luminescence that seemed to emanate from all living things but which was ordinarily invisible to human senses. One of its American practitioners, H.S. Daki, describes how the Kirlian technique works: 'It is a technique for making photographic prints or visual observations of electrically conductive objects with no light course other than that produced by a luminous corona discharge at the surface of an object which is in a high-voltage, high-frequency electrical field.'

There are many problems associated with Kirlian photography. The most important is that the parameters for using it as a scientific method of measurement need to be meticulously controlled, otherwise you can end up with artefacts that yield little in the way of scientific information. When used correctly, however, Kirlian photographs yield both beautiful and useful information. A drop of spring water radiates splendidly while a drop of ordinary tap water shows little luminescence. Scientists are still unsure about just what kind of luminescence they are picking up in their photographic plates, but the potentials of Kirlian photography are many. Dr Thelma Moss at UCLA in California carried out excellent and well-controlled studies on foods and herbs, healers and healing, using the technique. It continues to be investigated by official Russian institutes using newly developed techniques, many of which are applicable to nutrition or to the diagnosis and treatment of illness.

SPIKES OF LIGHT

When the Kirlian method is carefully controlled and used to photograph plants and foods – comparing cooked foods with their raw counterparts or the leaf from a healthy plant with a leaf from an ailing or damaged one – researchers get consistent results. They find that the luminescent discharge, or corona, recorded on film from the raw or healthy plant is significantly stronger, more radiant and wider than that from a cooked or damaged plant.

When I examined Kirlian photographs taken by British researcher Harry Oldfield, I was stunned by the differences. His photographs compared the corona produced by a raw carrot or cauliflower with what was produced after these vegetables had been cooked. The former radiated brilliant spikes of light, harmoniously surrounding their shapes. The latter showed only the dimmest evidence of a corona discharge.

Crystals Speak Volumes

Chromatography is another tool for measuring the energy radiated by living organisms. However, it is more often employed in chemistry, biology, medicine and industry as a means of analysing complex compounds and substances such as the amino acids in protein, and for detecting impurities.

RAW CHROMO TESTS

European chemist Ehrenfried Pfeiffer used chromatography to measure energy differences between fresh and cooked foods and between natural and synthetic vitamins. Early in his career Pfeiffer was asked by the German educationist and mystic Rudolph Steiner to search for a chemical reagent that would reveal what Steiner called 'the formative etheric forces in living matter'. After experimenting with different substances, Pfeiffer discovered that when he added extracts of living plants to a solution of copper chloride and let it evaporate slowly, it produced a pattern of crystallisation typical of the species of plant used and also revealed the life-strength of the plant. Strong crystallisation patterns indicated health; weak ones, ill health.

Later, when he had settled in the United States, Pfeiffer refined and simplified his crystallisation method, eventually using treated circles of filter paper with a developer and a wick positioned in the centre to absorb the liquid being tested. From the crystal patterns which formed as the filter paper dried he was able to detect differences between two apparently identical seeds, one damaged by heat or chemicals, the other not. He could also describe accurately the condition and shape of the plant from which the seeds had come.

RAW LIFE

If chromatograms are another measure of the special energy of life force – call it what you will – in foods, it would be impossible not to conclude that fresh foods have many times the 'aliveness' of their heated and processed counterparts. Even the addition of minute quantities of common food preservatives have disrupted crystallisation patterns. It is little wonder that they can have the same effect in the body.

Pfeiffer always considered vitamins to be 'biological' rather than 'chemical' agents. He successfully demonstrated big differences between natural vitamins and their synthetic analogues. His vitamin chromatograms are interesting, sometimes remarkably beautiful, to look at. Commercially made vitamin C and the same vitamin in fruit look completely different. Synthetic vitamin A and the vitamin A found in cod liver oil also produce different crystallisation patterns. Man-made vitamins lack the vivid colours, strong clear patterns, radial lines and fluted edges of their natural counterparts. Similar differences appear when one compares fresh foods with cooked or processed foods. Other scientists have obtained similar results working with Pfeiffer's methods.

Dowsers' Skills

While Pfeiffer was working with chromatography and various scientists in Russia and the West were looking at the differences in foods via Kirlian photography, a French engineer named André Simoneton had been using a dowsing technique. He had learned this from André Bovis, who was well known for the experiments carried out on pyramids. Bovis found that he and others (Simoneton included) could tell with the use of a pendulum how fresh a food was from the power of the subtle radiation picked up by dowsers. To measure these radiations he designed what he called a *biometer* – a simple device graduated arbitrarily in centimetres to indicate 'microns' and 'angstroms' – which offered a range of measurements between zero and 10,000 angstroms. Using Bovis's version of this traditional dowsing technique, Simoneton and others found they would get consistent measurements of the freshness and vitality of the food. Simoneton discovered that fresh raw fruits and vegetables had a reading of between 8,000 and 10,000 angstroms on his meter and would make the pendulum spin at high speed. Other foods such as cooked vegetables or pasteurised milk radiated so little energy that they did not make the pendulum spin at all.

Just what kind of wavelengths Simoneton was picking up remains unknown. But because of his background in engineering, he realised that the fact something was there that could be measured consistently on a scale meant that it could be of value to human health. Simoneton went on to measure a great variety of foods over many years and recorded his findings. He claimed the technique could measure both a food's vitality and its freshness. A food such as milk which measures 6,500 angstroms when fresh loses as much as 40 per cent of its radiation after 12 hours. At the end of 24 hours, a mere 10 per cent of its radiation remains. Simoneton discovered that pasteurising milk destroyed all its radiation as did tinning fruit. Cooking most vegetables rendered them 'lifeless'.

HOW DO YOU RADIATE?

Simoneton reasoned that if foods give off various levels of whatever emanation he was measuring, so must other living systems. He began to measure wavelengths from human beings. He found that a healthy person gives off radiations of about 6,500 angstroms while the measurement of cancer patients is much lower. He also discovered that people ill with degenerative diseases such as cancer will demonstrate a wavelength below 4,000 a long time before they show symptoms of the disease.

In a fascinating book *Radiation des Aliments*, Simoneton records his work. There he developed the hypothesis that the radiance in the foods you eat either contributes to your body's own radiance and overall vitality – in which case they are above 6,400 angstroms – or diminish it. To stay optimally healthy, he calculated we need to eat mostly fresh raw fruits and vegetables, nuts and fresh fish because these foods best contribute to, rather than detract from, the body's own life energy.

More than the Sum of its Parts
Simoneton's work could easily be dismissed. After all, it is based on dowsing for which there is, as yet, no scientific explanation. But what is significant about it, as well as about the work of scientists in Kirlian

photography and Pfeiffer's chromatograms, is the underlying assumptions – the dominant paradigm – on which they have based their work. Unlike the *atomists* who believe that truth is only to be found by pulling something to pieces and viewing it as nothing more than a collection of 'bits', these researchers have postulated the existence of an energetic principle underlying both life and health and a subtle but pervasive interconnection between mind, body and environment. Not only is the living body holographic in the way it functions, so is the living universe of which it is a part.

THE WHOLE IS GREATER

Pfeiffer insisted that, as Goethe taught, 'The whole is more than the sum of its parts.' In a booklet which he wrote just before his death he says: 'One can . . . take a seed, analyse it for protein, carbohydrates, fats, minerals, moisture and vitamins, but all of this will not tell its genetic background or biological value . . . a natural organism or entity contains factors which cannot be recognised or demonstrated if one takes the original organism apart and determines its component parts by way of analysis.'

Enter Biophotons

Early in the 20th century, quantum physics established that wave particles in living systems behave as biophoton light energies. These light energies regulate and control enzyme activities, cell reproduction and the creation of vitality in living systems. Experiments, such as those reported in the March 1995 issue of *Scientific American* by Brumer and Shapiro, have helped establish the importance of particle/wave reactions in organisms. Like light bulbs, all atoms and molecules give out radiant bioenergies, both good and bad, when it comes to their effect on the human body. Science is beginning to understand how the interference wave forms from negative sources – generated either by internally manufactured toxins or by external exposure to environmental pollutants – can disrupt the body's harmonious biophoton energies and undermine homoeostasis on which our health depends.

What are Biophotons?

Biophotons are fine emissions of light which all living systems – from the cells of your skin to the cells of living plants – send out as well as receive. They cannot be seen by the naked eye. They *can* be measured by special equipment developed by researchers in various countries. Biophoton light is ultra-weak yet ultra-important. It is stored in the cells of your body – within the DNA molecules of the nuclei and else-where in your living matrix. Scientists at the International Institute of Biophysics in Germany, in Japan and Russia have determined that biophoton emission is a ubiquitous phenomenon characteristic of living systems. This dynamic web of light released and absorbed via the living matrix of the body may even turn out to be the primary means by which the biochemical processes of life are regulated. The intensity and order of biophoton emission and the ability of living cells to store light carry important information about the functional state of a living organism. The more light cells can store, the better. Diseased cells, such as cancer cells, do not have the ability to store light. They can even be damaged by it.

Biophotons Revealed

German biophysicist, Professor Fritz Popp, and Professor Hugo Niggli in Switzerland, together with scientists from Russia, Japan and Australia, have long studied how subtle light energy – biophotons – behave in living tissue, and have charted their importance to health. Measuring the nature of this ultra-weak but super-important biophoton energy with the help of high-tech equipment, they can now identify healthy as opposed to diseased tissue. Biophoton measurements of live foods have verified the vast superiority of fresh, organically cultivated foods and the health-giving energy they carry when compared to conventionally grown foods. The complexity of energetic order and all the information it carries is imparted to a person eating them.

In experiments stretching over almost two generations, Professor Fritz Popp and his colleagues demonstrated that measuring biophotons can provide sensitive information about conditions within a cell in a living body and the functioning of its defence mechanisms. Philip Coleridge Smith, a surgeon at the University Medical College in London, recently told *New Scientist* magazine he believes, in time, that it will be possible to identify inflammation in leg tissues to warn of an ulcer.

Electron Energy Transfer

Expert in the use of essential fatty acids in health and the treatment of cancer, Dr Johanna Budwig in Germany believes that live foods act as high-powered electron donors and as solar resonance fields, attracting, storing and conducting the sun's energy throughout the body. Certainly the greater our store of light energy and the higher its order, the greater the power of our overall energy field, and the healthier we are – consequently the more vitality we experience. Live foods, including cold-pressed flax oil which Budwig uses a lot in her treatments, are high on the list of effective electron donors. They bring quantum life energy into our body when we eat them.

LIGHT – THE ULTIMATE NUTRIENT

'Light,' says Popp '. . . can initiate or arrest cascade-like reactions in the cells, and genetic cellular damage can be virtually repaired within hours by faint beams of light.' The more vital your body, the more ordered is the activity of your biophotons and the longer your cells are able to store light. The food you eat carries light energy and information to the body.

Research into biophoton emission is now used in industry and in medicine – especially in the wellness movement where it is raising the whole approach to colour therapy to a new level of effectiveness. Until biophotons, electron transfer, electromagnetism and other subtle energy emanations are taken into account, explanations about why raw foods have such extraordinary capacities to promise high-level health will, at best, remain frustratingly inadequate. Once they are, research into the whys and wherefores of healing with uncooked foods could lead to the expansion of other areas of consciousness not even directly related to nutrition or health.

In the meantime, used wisely, a diet rich in simple foods like fresh fruits and vegetables, organic, home-grown sprouted seeds, natural unheated dairy products, nuts and seeds – available to everyone – can alleviate a great deal of human suffering. It may even make possible the use of much dormant human creative energy submerged under a sea of mesohealth. You don't need to understand the theories behind high-raw, low-grain eating to reap its benefits.

THREE

FORCE FOR CHANGE

It has only been in the last two or three decades that researchers have begun to explore and identify in detail the bioactive compounds in foods that have antioxidant, anti-cancer and anti-ageing properties. They are able to enhance immune function, strengthen various organs, even lower excessive blood pressure and cholesterol. The list of functions that the nutraceuticals in foods can impart is a very long one indeed.

PLANT POWERS

Expanding nutritional awareness has brought with it a brand-new vocabulary – words like 'nutraceutical' and 'phytochemical'. What we are talking about are compounds in foods which have specific health-protective and health-enhancing effects on the body, substances or compounds that we do not produce for ourselves. But they *are* available to us when we eat plants – especially in a fresh, raw state.

Uncooked foods contain numerous substances, in addition to vitamins and minerals, whose beneficial effects on living organisms are just beginning to be acknowledged – volatile essential oils, natural antibiotics, plant hormones, pigments like the bioflavonoids, chlorophyll and the anthocyans, even special kinds of fibre with anti-ageing and anti-cancer properties.

Plant Powers

In most vegetable foods there are active substances which exert a positive effect on human health. But the biochemistry of plants is extremely complex, and for the most part the effects of plant substances on the human body are only beginning to be charted. Some of these substances – most of which are destroyed or drastically altered by heat – appear to be particularly important for health. Various types of fibre and pigment which occur in good quantity in a diet rich in raw fresh vegetables and fruits have well-proven, but little-understood, properties for encouraging high-level health. Some, such as chlorophyll, the anthocyans and pectin, even help protect the body against damage from airborne pollutants and radiation. They may also be useful in preventing cancer and in retarding ageing. And for every known health-enhancing property of a plant-based substance there are likely to be dozens still unknown.

WHOLE AND RAW

Nutritionists are increasingly aware that vitamins and minerals, essential fatty acids, proteins, carbohydrates and sugars are only a very small part of eating for high-level health. The latest research indicates that there is no way we can take vitamin and mineral supplements yet continue to eat highly processed foods and still stay healthy. Why? Because the ability of food to enhance health is finally being recognised. Not only does enough vitamin C prevent scurvy, and enough calcium and magnesium help build strong bones; foods also contain important phytochemicals. The only way to reap their benefits is to eat whole foods. Second – also as a result of this recent research – the focus of eating for health is no longer in eating less of this or that; it is about eating more. More what? More fresh raw foods, raw vegetables, fresh fruits, nuts and seeds together with fish, organic poultry and organic meat.

Protection from Illness

Russian scientists such as Professor I.I. Brekhman and I.V. Dardymov of the USSR Academy of Scientists in Vladivostock have devoted decades to the study of herbs and plant foods which have the ability to increase the human body's 'non-specific resistance' to disease and ageing. They have shown that certain plant-based substances which occur in the foods we eat and in the plants we use for healing not only passively affect the body in specific ways – increasing the flow of digestive juices or calming mucous membranes in the intestines, for example – but also in more general ways by strengthening the organism as a whole.

RAW PLANTS DO IT BEST

Unlike pills which you can buy at the corner pharmacy to stimulate one body system and harm another, these substances come to us in raw foods and herbal remedies in a context chemically balanced by nature. As such they offer a synergistic potency for high-level health. The presence of these naturally synergistic factors in uncooked foods may help explain why, as Swedish expert in raw-food therapy Dr Henning Karstrom says,

'Even though you get all 50 known nutrients in your diet – i.e. vitamins, minerals, essential amino acids, fatty acids etc. – your health will still suffer unless you also include large quantities of uncooked and unprocessed foods.'

Let's take a look at just a few of these raw food plant factors and what is known about them.

Aroma of Health

A plant's fragrance may be due to as many as 50 different aromatic compounds which can be extracted as an essential oil or essence. Mint, the skin of citrus fruits, and many other strongly smelling herbs and fruits, are particularly rich in essential oils. The benefits of many of these essential oils, which our palaeolithic ancestors got good quantities of in their diet, are amazingly varied. Some relieve irritation because of their mild antibiotic properties. Others relieve muscular spasm and pain – until quite recently, clove oil rubbed on the gums was the standard remedy for toothache. Taken by mouth, others relieve coughs and sore throats, stimulate the action of the liver and gall bladder, mildly stimulate peristalsis (rhythmic contraction of the gut), and reduce fermentation and decomposition in the gut, protecting the colon from cancer-promoting chemicals. Some can also be inhaled as decongestants or used to induce changes in mood and alertness, as in aromatherapy. But perhaps the most important of their effects is that they stimulate the salivary glands and intestines to secrete digestive enzymes.

BITTERS FOR GOOD DIGESTION

Bitter factors, contained in fresh plant juices, are also principally digestive in function. They boost the secretion of digestive enzymes, exert a calming effect on the smooth muscle of the gut, and encourage better assimilation of nutrients. Plants particularly rich in bitters are mugwort, wormwood (formerly an ingredient of absinthe), angelica, sweet flag and St Benedict's herb, but they also occur in respectable amounts in many commonly eaten plants. Many aperitifs, digestifs and liqueurs contain bitters.

Hormone Boosts

Plants, like animals, depend on hormones to provide a chemical messenger service. In fact, in plants, hormones take the place of a nervous system. The gibberellins are a class of plant hormones which appear to have beneficial effects on the human immune system. Another plant hormone, abscisic acid, which is plentiful in avocados, lemons, cabbage and potatoes, obligingly helps the body to use gibberellins. Meanwhile, the gentle oestrogen-like hormones in many plants (in good quantity in sprouted soya beans) help to protect the body from dangerous petrochemically derived hormone mimics in our food and air which cause havoc in reproductive processes.

So similar is the structure of some plant hormones to human hormones that it is reasonable to believe, as many researchers do, that they probably boost their actions. Secretins, another group of hormone-like substances in plants, are thought to stimulate the pancreas and the production of hormones associated with a youthful skin.

Enzymes Carry Life

In many ways, the most important of all the health-giving plant factors are the enzymes. These are completely destroyed by cooking. Enzymes are essential triggers for the metabolic machinery of every living thing from daffodil to buffalo. Some are extraordinarily powerful. The pepsin produced in your stomach, for instance, can break down the white of egg into its protein sub-units called peptides in just a few minutes. It would take hours to do the same thing in a laboratory through chemical manipulation, and then only if the egg white was first boiled in strong acid or alkaline solution.

HEALTH PROTECTORS

There are tens of thousands of enzymes working away in the human body – some 50,000 in the liver alone – breaking down the foods we eat and helping assimilate it, building new tissue and repairing it, and manufacturing more enzymes so that the work essential to life can continue. The human body grows old quickly when enough metabolic errors accumulate to injure the synthesis of its enzymes.

Most experts in the use of high-raw diets for healing insist that the enzymes in raw foods are central to the healing process because they help support the body's own enzyme systems. Each food we eat raw, whether it be a banana or broccoli, contains just the enzymes and co-factors (vitamins or minerals linked to enzymes) needed to help our body break down and assimilate that particular food. When we destroy these enzymes by cooking or processing, the body has to make more of its own enzymes to properly digest and assimilate what we eat. Unless you have inherited a particularly virile enzyme-replication system, without the enzymes from raw foods your body's own enzyme-producing abilities tend to wane as the years pass. Ensuring that your body has an outside supply of enzymes can help you live longer, look more youthful and stay healthier.

ENZYME HELP

Freeze-dried plant enzymes are commonly used as nutritional supplements. When eaten with protein foods they assist with digestion and assimilation. Bromelain, from pineapple, is one of these. So is papain, from pawpaw. Chemically, papain startlingly resembles pepsin, the protein-digesting enzyme produced by the stomach. It is capable of digesting 35 to 100 times its own weight in protein. Raw pawpaw has also been used to heal wounds; the papain in it digests the dead tissue which retards the healing process.

Orthodox doctors used to dismiss such arguments, claiming that exogenous food enzymes – those which come to us through the foods we eat – are not necessary food ingredients. Some say that enzymes (which are mainly proteins) are no more important than any other proteins – only useful as a source of amino acids from which the body can build new proteins. They insist that the notion of enzymes affecting health in any way is nothing more than a fantasy of ill-informed food faddists. European research indicates that they are wrong.

Professor Artturii Ilmari Virtanen, Helsinki biochemist and Nobel prize winner, showed that enzymes in uncooked foods get released in the mouth when vegetables are chewed. When these foods are crushed the enzymes come in contact with their respective 'substrates' and they form entirely new physiologically active substances which, because of their high biological activity, are vastly important for health.

Great Allies

Other studies have shown that even the assumption that all enzymes in raw foods are denatured by digestion in the stomach is false. Extensive tests by Kaspar Tropp in Würzburg, and by Chalaupka and others, have shown that the human body has a way of protecting enzymes as foods pass through the digestive tract so that between 60 and 80 per cent of them reach the colon intact. There they bring about a beneficial shift in the intestinal flora – the bacteria that live in the colon – by attracting and binding whatever oxygen is present. This removes the aerobic condition responsible for fermentation, putrefaction and intestinal toxaemia, all of which are associated with the development of degenerative diseases including cancer. By eliminating free oxygen in the colon, food enzymes help create conditions in which the 'good guy' lactic acid-forming bacteria can grow.

Beware Dysbiosis

A healthy colony of intestinal flora – the right kind of bacteria and the right quantity – produces vitamin K in the intestines as well as almost all of the B-complex vitamins. When the 'good guy' bacteria are destroyed as a result of taking antibiotics or if they are replaced by colonies of harmful bacteria then you get a condition known as dysbacteria or dysbiosis, an 'insidious menace' to health. Dysbacteria suppresses the immune system, creates digestive disturbances and causes chemicals to form from bile acids, which are poisonous to the body and can lead to disease.

THE GOOD GUYS

The right kind of intestinal flora is important to protect from cancer and premature ageing. Diet strongly influences the enzyme activities and the types of micro-organisms which proliferate in the intestines. When dysbacteria is present and health-damaging putrefactive bacteria are allowed to grow, they can produce histamine which causes allergies. They also give off large quantities of ammonia and other chemicals which irritate the lining of the intestines and pass into the bloodstream causing toxicity of the body and predisposing it to serious illness. The enzymes in uncooked food protect against all this.

Plant Fibre – Life Saver

Essential oils, hormones, bitters and enzymes are not the only wonder-working plant factors. Two other categories of plant substances are of vital importance: 'plantix' and plant colorants which form the core of nutraceuticals or plant factors known to parallel vitamins in their importance to human health. Flavonoids, carotenoids and anthocyans are all plant colorants. So is chlorophyll. If you have never heard of plantix, you have a perfectly good excuse. The word was coined by researchers at the Syntex Laboratories in California in order to dispel the common idea that bran is the only kind of plant fibre available. You may be pleased to know that you need never stare another spoonful of the flaky stuff in the face again.

Fibre is what is left when all the nutrients in food have been taken out of it. But to think of it as inert, as nutritionists did for a long time, would be far from the truth. Fibre, particularly raw fibre, actively affects the gut. Plantix or plant fibre is much more than bran, which is mostly cellulose. It is also lignin (the woody fibre that keeps trees upright), pectins, gums, mucilages and hemicellulose, a relative of cellulose. These are substances which are just now being seriously studied.

KEY TO FIBRE

Here is a list of different plant fibres, each of which is important for health in its own unique way:

Cellulose: You find cellulose mostly in the outer layers of fruits and vegetables as well as in some nuts and grains. It has been shown to prevent constipation, haemorrhoids and varicose veins.

Gums and mucilages: These kinds of fibre, which you find in sprouted seeds, grains, beans and many seaweeds, lower blood cholesterol as well as help regulate glucose levels. They are particularly useful in clearing heavy metals, such as lead, from the body and removing other toxins.

Haemocellulose: Found in vegetables, grains and fruits, a high level of haemocellulose in the diet has been shown to lower the risk of colon cancer by clearing many carcinogens from the intestines. It is also believed to help in weight loss.

Lignin: Found in fruits and vegetables as well as in brazil nuts, lignin helps prevent the formation of gallstones, lowers LDL cholesterol and reduces the risk of colon cancer. It can even help decrease the need for insulin in adult-onset diabetes.

Pectin: This soluble fibre slows down the absorption of nutrients from meals. This means that it helps decrease appetite and is therefore useful for anyone wanting to shed excess fat. It also reduces the risk of heart disease, eliminates many toxins from the body – including dangerous heavy metals – and helps lower LDL cholesterol. You'll find pectin in citrus fruits and other fruits and vegetables as well as in dried peas.

Get Enough

Plenty of plant fibre in your diet brings you at least five major benefits:

1. More vigorous peristalsis (sequencing of food through the gut). This decreases transit time through every part of the gut, especially through the colon, and so reduces opportunities for harmful substances to damage the mucous membranes lining it.
2. More bulk in all parts of the gut. This aids peristalsis and therefore transit time. It also makes you feel fuller longer, an important consideration if you are trying to cut down on snacks between meals. Bulk also ensures a stately and steady rate of nutrient absorption. By the same token, harmful substances, diluted by the amount of fibre around them, get into the walls of the gut less easily.
3. A low population of bacteria of the undesirable variety. These cause putrefaction of various substances in the faeces, produce cancer-causing substances from bile acids, and give off large quantities of ammonia and other chemicals which irritate the bowel lining.

4. A flourishing population of beneficial or good guy micro-organisms in the gut, including those which synthesise the important B and K vitamins.
5. A reduction in the amount of fat absorbed during digestion, very useful if you want to lose weight or stay the weight you are.

A diet high in uncooked plant foods provides you with many kinds of fibre, each with its own protective powers for high-level health. Such findings are of particular importance in the context of modern urban life in which we are increasingly exposed to the destructive effects of the chemical pollutants and toxic substances we take in through our foods and in the air we breathe. Like radiation, these poisons encourage the kinds of damage to the body's proteins, cell membranes and specific genetic materials which are associated with ageing. They also appear greatly to contribute to body toxicity, which in turn leads to the development of many common ailments from migraine to cancer. The plantix in raw foods helps protect against their damaging effects.

COLOUR HAS CLOUT

Scientists estimate that each of the 60 trillion cells in the human body suffers 10,000 damaging free-radical 'hits' each day. And this is on the rise as a result of increasing chemicals in our environment. It has long been known that raw vegetables and fruits have powerful antioxidant capacities to protect against such damage, but the health-enhancing properties of raw vegetable foods go way beyond this.

Already scientists have discovered hundreds of bright-coloured health-enhancing phytochemicals that inhibit blood clotting, lower cholesterol, detoxify the body of wastes and poisons, reduce inflammation and allergies – even slow the growth rate of cancer cells. These amazing nutraceuticals, most of which were completely unknown 10 years ago, work synergistically: the wider the variety of fruits and vegetables you eat, the greater will be the protective health-enhancing benefits for you.

Bright and Beautiful

Although carotenoids are by no means the only health-enhancing phytochemicals nestling within brightly coloured vegetables, they are probably the most highly researched. These plant pigments, found in the protein complexes of plants, are responsible for many of the bright colours of various fruits and vegetables. You find carotenoids in green plant tissues as well, but in this case they tend to be covered by a thin layer of chlorophyll. Their presence only becomes evident after the green pigment has degraded, as it does when you cook the plant, or when it begins to die in autumn.

COLOUR UP

Many health-enhancing plant factors are found in common foods, from berries, citrus fruits and grapes to broccoli, cabbage, spinach, carrots, soya beans, onions, garlic and tomatoes. They occur in spices and herbs – from red pepper to basil, oregano, parsley and mint. You will find lots of phytochemicals hidden within the red, yellow, orange, green and blue colours of the vegetables our ancestors ate. But in the average Western diet of manufactured convenience foods, they are as scarce as hen's teeth. It is these rainbow-coloured plant factors which give the autumn leaves and flowers their colour as well as imparting the wonderful fragrances to fruits and vegetables. Phytonutrients usually come packaged together in groups within the same plant, to impact the body at deep physiological and biochemical levels. And they are always best gleaned not from supplements, but rather eaten from whole, mostly raw, foods.

Epidemiological studies show that the more we eat of fresh fruit and vegetables rich in carotenoids, the more our risk of cancer is diminished. Part of this is due to carotenoids' powerful antioxidant activity. They help protect the body from free-radical damage, which is associated with the development of degenerative conditions from arthritis to coronary heart disease as well as premature ageing. Carotenoids, like some of the vitamins, such as A, C and E, are able to quench free radicals and deactivate them, thereby inhibiting excessive free-radical reactions in our body, and protecting us from damage.

POPEYE WAS RIGHT – EAT SPINACH

Scientists estimate that there are more than 600 naturally occurring carotenoids in our foods. They are certainly the most widespread pigments found in nature. The most well known include lutein, lycopene, alpha-carotene, zeaxanthin and beta-carotene. Eat more spinach and leafy greens – such as silver beet, kale or collards – and you tap into a rich supply of zeaxanthin and lutein to protect the eyes and probably the brain, too, from degeneration. In one study of 356 older people reported in the *Journal of the American Medical Association*, research found that eating good quantities of these leafy green vegetables – the equivalent of a large spinach salad each day – reduced the risk of macular degeneration by 43 per cent. This is an age-related retinal disease that has you holding the menu at arm's length in order to read it.

The most highly studied carotenoid is beta-carotene. In fact, so enthusiastic were the scientists who first discovered the effects of beta-carotene about its ability to protect our health, that nutritional supplement companies were quick to jump on the bandwagon and produce supplements with high levels of beta-carotene – touting them as a cure for just about everything. The problem is that these commercially minded chemists lost track of one of the most important principles of natural health and healing: synergy.

Beta-carotene, like the other flavonoids and phytochemicals, vitamins and minerals, exists in a very fine balance with other health-enhancing compounds found in nature. The moment you separate one chemical out and take it on its own without acknowledging this fact, you not only undermine some of its ability to enhance health, you may also create a situation of imbalance. This is why a few years after nutritionists oversold beta-carotene, there were a number of health warnings about taking too much of it. In one study, for instance, beta-carotene supplementation on its own was shown to interfere with vitamin D absorption. Another indicated that taking excessive amounts of beta-carotene can reduce the body's ability to absorb another very important carotenoid – lycopene. What matters most in nature, as in human health, is balance. All of the carotenoids, together with the vitamins, minerals and other plant factors for health, work best just the way nature provides them – in splendid and highly complex balance, which we can neither fully understand nor replicate. The message is clear: build your daily meals around the colourful vegetable kingdom by eating salads, drinking juices and preparing them in ways that preserve as much of their innate life-enhancing abilities as possible.

A Little Light Magic

Among the most therapeutically exciting of all the precious compounds in plants are their pigments: chlorophyll, the anthocyans and the bioflavonoids. Living plants perform the incredible feat of converting light energy into chemical energy – photosynthesis. This would not happen unless they contained chlorophyll, the pigment which gives foliage its green colour.

> # LIFE BLOOD
>
> In 1930, Nobel prize winner Dr Hans Fischer pointed out that chlorophyll closely resembles haemoglobin, the pigment that gives human blood its colour and oxygen-carrying capacity; the difference between the two pigments is that chlorophyll has a core of magnesium and haemoglobin a core of iron. So close is this relationship that when crude chlorophyll is fed to anaemic rabbits it restores normal red blood cell counts within 15 days and is apparently completely non-toxic.

Chlorophyll that has been chemically refined to remove 'impurities' has no corrective effect on anaemia. On the contrary, it probably poisons the bone marrow, the site of red cell production. Spinach, cabbage and nettle juice, all rich in chlorophyll, have been used with excellent results to treat anaemia in humans. Cabbage juice is especially good at healing stomach ulcers. At the age of 50 my mother suddenly developed stomach ulcers which nothing would heal. She began to drink raw juices several times a day and used a lot of cabbages in making them. In three weeks the ulcers were gone. They never returned.

Chlorophyll Protects

Chlorophyll has an impressive record in the treatment of heart disease, arteriosclerosis (hardened arteries), sinusitis, osteomyelitis (inflammation of the bone marrow), pyorrhoea (infected and bleeding gums) and depression. It may also help block the genetic changes which cancer-causing substances produce in cell nuclei, judging by research with bacteria at the University of Texas Systems Cancer Center and elsewhere. Taken internally by mouth or rectally by enema, chlorophyll curtails the activities of harmful protein-destroying bacteria and of enzymes which cause proteins to putrefy in the gut. It also makes human saliva more alkaline, an advantage if you are eating carbohydrates. For these and many other reasons, chlorophyll and other raw juices containing substantial amounts of chlorophyll are often prescribed in the treatment of allergies and malabsorption problems.

Another group of pigments, the anthocyans, have figured mainly in the treatment of cancer and leukaemia. Raw beetroot contains a particular anthocyan in large quantities – cancer patients drink the juice of just over 1kg of beetroot daily, a little before each meal. The name most often associated with the use of beetroot juice to both cure and prevent radiation-induced cancers is that of Dr Sigmund Schmidt, a tireless antinuclear campaigner in the international courts.

The Amazing Troubleshooters

The flavonoids are pigments which occur in particularly high concentration in the pith of grapefruits, oranges and tangerines, and in lesser amounts in all raw plant foods. However, they are highly active and unstable and easily destroyed by heat and exposure to air. This is why orange juice contains very little of them. To get the benefits of the bioflavonoids – and there are many – leave a little pith on citrus fruits when you peel them.

GLAMOROUS DISCOVERY

The existence of this particularly glamorous group of colorants, the flavonoids, was discovered in 1936 by Nobel laureate Albert Szent-Györgyi, the Hungarian biochemist who first isolated vitamin C. A complex of exotically named substances makes up the group: hesperiden, rutin, vitamin P, flavones, flavonals, the so-called methoxylated bioflavonoids nobiletin and tangeretin, eriodictyol, and so on. Since the 1930s a great deal of research has been done in the Soviet Union, United States and Europe which has demonstrated the potent health-enhancing and health-restoring effects of the flavonoids.

In plants themselves the flavonoids play a disease-preventing role. The extraordinary thing is that they display the same talent in humans. Nobiletin and another closely related bioflavonoid appear to have even wider anti-inflammatory powers than cortisone. Others, either on their own or in combination, actively combat infectious bacteria, viruses and fungi. Rutin, a bioflavonoid found in buckwheat, is known to lift depression. Even in relatively small doses (50mg), it significantly alters brain waves; its effect is a curious combination of sedative and stimulant, rather like that of certain substances in ginseng. Rutin is one of several bioflavonoids that also prevent superficial bruising and broken blood vessels in the skin. Nobiletin and tangeretin boost the activity of a certain group of enzymes (mixed function oxidases) which specialise in ridding the body of drugs, heavy metals and the unburnt hydro-carbons in car exhausts. Indirectly, therefore, these two bioflavonoids are cancer-preventing – only one of the reasons why so many forms of cancer yield to raw diets.

END SLUDGED BLOOD

Experiments have demonstrated that the methoxylated bioflavonoids – especially plentiful in oranges and tangerines – significantly reduce the clumping together of red blood cells. This is not a normal tendency, but it means that blood flows less easily, clots more readily, transports less oxygen and may occasionally block tiny blood vessels, causing death of areas of tissue in vital organs. In one trial in which patients with 'sludged blood' ate three or four oranges or five tangerines a day for three weeks, blood viscosity decreased by an average of six per cent.

The wide-ranging effects of the bioflavonoids have not been anywhere near fully investigated. One of the most interesting things about them is they seem to be most active and most useful when an organism is under the worst stress. This has led researchers to speculate that one of their main actions must be to correct the wide fluctuations in body functions which occur during illness and emergencies. In fact, the bioflavonoids as a whole have such a broad range of defence actions in the body that many of the protective qualities of raw foods can probably be attributed to them.

Green Magic
Green foods regenerate and rejuvenate your body. As such, they are powerful anti-agers. The old adage 'eat your greens if you want to stay young and healthy' has become a scientific fact. And the fun of it all is that, so far, advanced nutritional scientists know that green works wonders, although as yet we only partly understand why.

Green foods are superfoods. Not only do they help clean up your body and continue to detoxify, they also help to protect it from future damage by offering a high level of synergistic nutrients, immune enhancers and specific phytochemicals – both identified and as yet unidentified – each of which works its own energy magic.

GREEN SUPREME

Dark-green vegetables such as broccoli, Brussels sprouts, collards, kale, kohlrabi and mustard greens have hit the headlines, thanks to an overwhelming abundance of medical and scientific evidence that they help prevent cancer. What prevents cancer also prevents ageing.

Prestigious medical journals such as the *Federal Proceedings Report* and the *Journal of the National Cancer Institute* report that sulphorophane and other plant factors in the brassicas inhibit the growth of cancer tumours, detoxify the body of poisonous and environmental chemicals, prevent colon cancer and increase the body's own supply of natural anti-ageing compounds. They also help lower LDL cholesterol, improve elimination and fight yeast infections such as *Candida albicans*. Adding a couple of florets of broccoli – better still the new broccoli sprouts – or a few leaves of kale to a salad, a soup or a glass of vegetable juice, turns a food that is good into something that is superb. But start slowly and gradually build up on your greens, especially if you have a sweet tooth or are addicted to sugar. In the beginning, the taste can seem pretty strong. Build up gradually and you will find that your wild craving for sugars and carbohydrates has actually been transformed into a new craving for greens.

SUPERGREENS

So powerful is the life support offered by green superfoods that the Japanese – who lead the world in nature-based health products – pay premium prices for them. Freshwater algae such as spirulina and chlorella, as well as freeze-dried young green plants like wheat grass and barley, are carefully prepared at low temperatures to produce powdered foods which can be stirred into a glass of water or vegetable juice. Prepared in this way they preserve most of the living properties of raw foods. The Japanese themselves call them wonder foods, for they are packed with minerals, amino acids (in a form that your system soaks up the moment you swallow them), and most important of all, enzymes, the very stuff of life itself.

While the physical by-products of stress – like most pollutants in our food and water – tend to be acid, green foods alkalinise your system. This restores balance and creates a feeling of being calm and in control during highly demanding times.

Delicate Wonder
Chlorophyll is one of the most important elements in green food when it comes to what it can do for human health. To get the benefits from it you need to eat the foods raw, for chlorophyll is delicate and easily damaged by heat. This is one of the reasons why all the good green superfoods are processed at low heat.

BROCCOLI – SUPER SPROUTS

By now, everyone knows how good broccoli is for you but the seeds of broccoli are infinitely better. In fact, recent scientific research carried out in the United States indicates that they contain 60 times the level of sulphorophane – the most widely acclaimed phytonutrient in the war against cancer and ageing – than the broccoli itself.

Sea Greens
Sea vegetables, too, are a wonderful source of anti-ageing power. If you have never used sea vegetables for cooking, start now. They are not only delicious, bringing a wonderful spicy flavour to soups and salads, they are also the richest source of organic mineral salts in nature, especially iodine. Iodine is the mineral needed by your thyroid gland. As your thyroid gland is largely responsible for the body's metabolic rate – which tends to decrease with age – iodine is very important for energy. Sea greens have other properties too (*more about this in Foods That Heal*), which make them a welcome addition to any meal.

TRACE ELEMENTS

Seaweeds are also full of trace elements that are essential to the body, but in minute quantities. When boron, chromium, cobalt, calcium, iodine, manganese, magnesium, molybdenum, phosphorus, potassium, silicon, silver and sulphur (to mention only a few elements) are not present in the body, metabolism can experience big problems. Unlike the chalk which is added to bread to 'enrich' it with calcium, and most of the mineral supplements you can buy in pill form in stores, the minerals in sea plants, like the minerals in all of the important green plants, are organic. This means that your body can easily make use of them to build energy.

Get to know seaweeds and make use of them. Not only will they support a more youthful metabolism, but you will also find that your nails and hair and the rest of your body will be strengthened by a rich supply of minerals and trace elements that support the energy-producing enzymes in the body. Seaweeds are readily available these days in health-food stores and food shops. Make good use of them and they will care for you well. Try:

Arame	Kombu
Dulse	Laver Bread
Hiziki	Nori
Kelp	Wakami
Mixed sea salad	

Even Tea Helps

Last, but by no means least, of the powerful anti-virus, anti-cancer, anti-ageing green superfoods is green tea – the most popular of Asian drinks. For centuries green tea has been celebrated for its health benefits. It is literally riddled with antioxidants including polyphenols – bio-flavonoids that act as super antioxidants to neutralise free radicals, lower cholesterol and blood pressure, block cancer proliferation, inhibit the growth of bacteria and viruses, improve digestion and help prevent ulcers and strokes.

All of the more than 300 varieties of tea grown come from the leaves of the same plant – *Camellia sinensis*. The three types of tea – black, oolong and green – vary only in the way that this plant is processed. The flavonoids green tea contains – mainly catechins with a ridiculously long name, epiglallocatechin-3-gallate (EGCG) – are degraded soon after harvesting in most teas. However, in the case of green teas, the degradation process is prevented by steaming or pan-frying the leaves, inactivating the enzyme that brings this degeneration about. Most researchers believe that it is this EGCG catechin that is primarily responsible for green tea's anti-ageing, disease-preventing abilities.

DRINK A CUP

Drinking green tea regularly may protect against cancer and ageing by preventing damage to DNA. Many studies indicate that drinking green tea regularly can help lower cholesterol and reduce the risk of heart disease and stroke. In several studies, green tea has been shown to prevent the clumping of blood which contributes to arteriosclerosis and raises the risk of a heart attack. To reap the benefits of green tea, you need to drink it strong. This is a process most people have to ease themselves into, for full-strength green tea has quite a bitter taste and a strong kick. Start weak and once you have become accustomed to the taste, increase the strength of the tea you are drinking. There are no known side-effects to drinking green tea except, in very large quantities, when the small amount of caffeine it contains (usually 20 to 30 mg per cup compared to 150mg in a cup of coffee) may create an experience of nervousness or insomnia.

When looking for green tea it is best to go for the finest traditional green teas or for gunpowder green tea, which you used to be able to find only in Asian speciality markets but which you can now get in most supermarkets. An average cup of green tea contains 40 to 90mg of EGCG. If you dislike the taste of this green powerhouse, you might like to go for supplements of green tea extract. In this case, read labels and limit your dose to somewhere between 350 and 500mg of polyphenols a day. This is about what you would get in four to five cups of brewed green tea.

The widespread drinking of green tea is now believed to be one of the reasons why the rates of cancer in the Orient are so low compared with those in the West. Try changing from your usual cup of tea or coffee to drinking green tea. Your body will thank you for it.

FOODS THAT HEAL

For decades the study of the relationship between food and health revolved around amassing information about how many vitamins and minerals, how much protein and carbohydrate and what kind of essential fatty acids humans require to stay healthy. Popular nutrition focused on urging us to take high-potency, man-made nutritional supplements. Predictions were that by the year 2000 we would all be taking pills instead of bothering to make meals. We are still told mostly about what we shouldn't eat: lower your saturated fat intake, eat less meat, and so on. Forget it.

Now is the time to eat *more*. More what? More wholesome natural plant foods together with plenty of good-quality fats and proteins. The focus of nutrition has shifted from an obsession with food groups and vitamin pills towards an understanding that our foods are functional in their own right. Individual foods often carry healing power and health-giving properties – coconuts, mangoes, mushrooms, garlic, fish. So much is this the case that many are now called *functional foods*. Their actions are well backed up by medical research. Get to know the health benefits of common foods. Then make use of them and thrive.

Health Payoffs

Garlic, for instance, is rich in organo sulphur compounds. These phytochemicals lower cholesterol levels, reduce blood clotting and lower blood pressure. Soya beans contain protease inhibitors as well as phytic acid, which helps lower cholesterol levels and protects against cancer. Broccoli is rich in indoles and *sulphorophane* which helps prevent breast cancer.

FOODS THAT HEAL

So powerful are the health-enhancing properties of some phytochemicals found in natural foods that even the United States Food and Drug Administration – the FDA, a highly conservative

---

and rather industry-supporting government body – has come out in favour of their consumption. The FDA now insists that edible fruits and vegetables 'exhibit a potential for modulating human metabolism in a manner favourable for cancer prevention'. As anyone worth their salt in nutritional biochemistry will tell you, whatever helps prevent cancer is also going to help prevent other degenerative diseases – even premature ageing.

Out with 'Health Foods'

The age of 'health foods' is coming to an end. It is no longer appropriate for us to do as we did in the 1970s and 80s – hold our nose and pile in our morning yoghurt with bran, in the belief that although it tastes disgusting, it's doing some good. Self-denial is being shoved aside thanks to beautifully grown – preferably organic – foods, prepared in ways that are not only delicious to eat but are also rich in the nutraceuticals which enhance health. It is time to lay to rest forever the notion that for something to be good for you it has to taste revolting. Healthy meals are not only radiant with colour and form, but delicious and fun to prepare as well. Instantly edible and perfectly portable, even simple fruit packs a big punch with its store of phytochemical compounds.

BANANA TRUTHS

If you were looking for an almost-perfect fast food, you could not do better than bananas. Bananas have so many things to offer for health that it would be hard to list them all. They relieve both constipation and diarrhoea, reduce the risk of stroke and heart disease, lift spirits, heighten energy and lower blood pressure.

Banana Boost

Bananas are also one of the richest sources of potassium, which few of us get enough of these days since convenience foods are virtually devoid of it. Potassium helps regulate blood pressure and enhances your body's ability to deal with stress. It also helps to get rid of water-logging, especially in women at the time of a period. And it balances the excessive amounts of sodium many people get from eating highly salted foods. Ripe bananas – especially organic ones – act as natural antacids. In fact, they strengthen the lining of the stomach. Some research shows they may even help kill harmful bacteria in the gut. And they are a great source of pectin – a soluble fibre that helps eliminate harmful chemicals from the body. Always use bananas ripe – never green. If your bananas ripen all at once, peel them and pop them into the freezer.

THE SURPRISING COCONUT

Coconut oil is rich in a special kind of fat known as medium chain triglyceride (MCT). It is often used to feed racehorses and has been shown to reverse arteriosclerosis, improve glucose metabolism, lower body fat and even lower serum and liver cholesterol, while raising HDL, the good cholesterol. Coconut oil is nature's richest source of MCT – over 50 per cent of its fat is made up of MCTs. MCTs also encourage fat burning and can play an important role in weight loss.

Cranberries Protect

Cranberries are another of those wonderful red/orange/yellow fruits rich in flavonoid antioxidants and high in flavour. Native Americans have used them for centuries as a food and as a medicine. They have anti-fungal properties and are anti-viral too, except in the case of *Candida albicans*, which they don't seem to touch. Cranberries, fresh or dried, also help prevent as well as treat many urinary infections such as cystitis. They knock out the *Escherichia coli* bacteria that glue themselves to the walls of the intestine and the bladder. An as yet unidentified phytochemical in cranberries appears to prevent them from sticking. Cranberries also boast a natural antibiotic – *hippuric acid.* Eating them carries it into the bladder and kidneys.

Mangoes Lift Depression

Mangoes have long been called food for the gods. It was Paramahansa Yogananda who wrote in his *Autobiography of a Yogi*, 'It is impossible for the Hindu to conceive of heaven without mangoes.' He may have known nothing of the biochemistry of this sensuous fruit, but he certainly got right its uplifting qualities. Mangoes are rich in anacardic acid – phytochemicals that bear a strong resemblance to the drugs used to treat depression. This makes them a great way to start the day – especially if you can get them tree-ripened and organic.

Asparagus Soothes Digestion

Asparagus has long been used in Ayurvedic medicine as a remedy against indigestion. Not long ago, researchers compared the therapeutic effect of asparagus with a commonly used drug in the prevention of nausea and hiatus hernia, heartburn and gastric acid reflux. They discovered that asparagus was just as effective as the common drug remedy, yet had no side-effects.

Asparagus also has great diuretic properties. It stimulates the digestion and has been used to alleviate rheumatism and arthritis. A member of the lily family, asparagus was used by the ancient Greeks to treat kidney and liver troubles. It is one of the best natural remedies for PMS-related bloating and a top source of folic acid, the antioxidant glutothione, and vitamin C. All three are associated with a reduced risk of cancer, age-related degenerative diseases and heart disease.

FENNEL FOR PMS

As well as containing potassium, fennel (bulb fennel) also contains phyto-oestrogens. These are the natural plant hormones that help protect us from the onslaught of dangerous oestrogens in the environment and from the negative effects of oestrogen-based drugs, which are given far too often to women. As a result, fennel is a useful vegetable in helping not only to regulate menstruation but also to clear PMS. It even stimulates the flow of breast milk in nursing mothers. When you buy fennel, look for the fattest stems – they have more flavour and contain more phytohormones.

Mushrooms are Magic

When it comes to the more exotic varieties of mushroom – those widely used in the Orient that are now becoming popular in the West – you could hardly do better than to make them a daily part of your meals; raw or grilled, added to home-made sausages or sauces, or even gently braised in a little butter. These include oyster mushrooms, enoki mushrooms and tree ears, as well as the immune-boosting medicinal mushrooms, shiitaki, maitake and reishi. These 'big three' have been used in Japan for over 4,000 years to nourish and cleanse the body, and bring a high level of energy. You may find it difficult to get hold of maitake and reishi mushrooms, but the rest are readily available either in Oriental shops, health-food shops or good supermarkets.

IMMUNE POWER

Among the many potent immune-building compounds which Asian mushrooms contain is one called *lentinan*, which strengthens the body against infection and degeneration. Studies have shown that lentinan is more effective than prescription drugs in fighting flu. It has even been shown to slow down the destructive effect of the AIDS virus and the growth of cancer.

Eating Oriental mushrooms is also good for your heart. Shiitakes contain more than one compound which helps reduce cholesterol levels. In one study when a group of women were given a mere 75 grams of shiitakes a day, their cholesterol levels dropped by an average of 12 per cent. As far as the reishi mushroom is concerned, this powerful fungus is able to do all of the above, and more. Scientists have discovered that it is rich in an anti-cancer compound called *canthaxanthin* – a particular carotenoid – as well as other substances including lanostan, which helps protect against allergies, thanks to its ability to inhibit the release of histamines in the body.

Onions Boost Immunity

Onions help prevent thrombosis and lower raised blood pressure. They also inhibit the growth of cancer cells – probably thanks to their high flavonoid content, including quercetin as well as coumarin and ellagic acid. Use them whenever you can. They not only improve the flavour of the food you prepare, but eating them is also a sure-fire way of protecting yourself against acute illness as well as bringing long-term strength and support to the immune system.

Peppers Protect

Peppers go back at least 7,000 years in their many forms: bell peppers, pimentos, cherry peppers, paprika, piquin, Anaheim, jalapeño, chilli, cayenne and aji, to name a few. They became part of European fare when Colombus returned from their native New World and introduced them to the court. By the mid-16th century they were being widely cultivated in Spain and Portugal. All peppers are rich in vitamins C and E and the carotenoids, helping protect against degeneration and the damaging effects of toxic chemicals in the environment. The hotter peppers are rich in the alkaloid capsaicin, which appears to decrease pain, enhance digestion and even detoxify the body, protecting it from flus and colds. Eat peppers raw as crudités, bake them and add them to stews and soups. Their magnificent colour and health-enhancing capacities are truly a wonder to behold.

Tomato a Day

Two recent research projects – one carried out at Harvard University and the other at the Cancer Research Center in Hawaii – showed that men and women who eat large quantities of tomatoes are less than half as likely to die of cancer than those who don't. In people who had cancer already, eating good quantities of tomatoes doubled participants' survival time. No one knows yet exactly why this is, except that tomatoes are very rich in lycopene, one of the powerful, plant-based antioxidants, which improves mental as well as physical functioning and at the same time reduces the risk of degenerative diseases. Lycopene is one of the few phytochemicals that is actually absorbed more readily by the body when tomatoes are eaten cooked instead of raw. Tomatoes also contain good quantities of glutathione, another potent antioxidant, which helps enhance immune functioning, slows down premature ageing and even helps prevent macular degeneration.

Seeds for Life

Nuts, like almonds and seeds, are high in fat. But surprisingly the fat they contain helps decrease cholesterol levels and plays an important part in preventing cardiovascular disease. The two essential fatty acids prevalent in most nuts and seeds are linoleic acid and alpha linolenic acid. Linoleic acid is pretty easy to find in fresh foods; alpha linolenic acid is not so easy, since it is destroyed quickly in food processing. Fresh walnuts, linseeds and rapeseeds are full of it.

EAT FAT

The essential fatty acids found in seeds and nuts – from almonds and sesames to sunflower seeds, pumpkin seeds, macadamias, pecans and walnuts – are important for the regulation of reproductive functions in the body. Get too little of them and your hair, nails and skin will suffer as well. If you have a tendency to allergies or menstrual disorders, insufficient fatty acids will make you highly prone to attacks.

There are other virtues to nuts and seeds too. Walnuts help lower blood cholesterol levels and reduce blood lipids, as do almonds. Macadamias, which are rich in a monounsaturated fatty acid, are linked to a reduction in high blood pressure and strokes in people who eat them in quantities. Brazils are rich in selenium too, so much so that a single brazil nut offers enough of this vital antioxidant to meet the recommended daily allowance. This important mineral has been shown to enhance immunity and protect the body from free-radical damage. Nuts and seeds are also rich in isoflavones and in lignans. Recent studies show that pumpkin seeds may help reduce enlarged prostate glands because they are rich in specific amino acids that help clear symptoms of prostate trouble.

PUMPKIN EATERS

Pumpkin seeds are richer in zinc than any other plant – important for good immunity, for growth, for wound healing and to make sure your senses of taste and smell work as they should. They are also a good source of iron, phosphorus, potassium and magnesium and boast a huge amount of fibre – 10 grams in each 25 grams of seeds – as well as some vitamin A. Sunflower seeds are a rich natural source of vitamin E and linoleic acid, both of which not only benefit the heart but also help protect from premature ageing and degeneration. They have anti-cancer and anti-ageing potential thanks to their beta-carotene content and they support the adrenals, enhancing your ability to deal with stress. Eating only 30 grams of sunflower seeds a day will double most people's vitamin E intake.

Buy nuts and seeds raw, preferably from stores where they are kept refrigerated, since the essential fatty acids they contain are highly prone to rancidity. Once you get them home, make sure you put them in your refrigerator. I find the best way to use nuts and seeds is to mix two or three types together. I often grind mine in the coffee grinder – since you can do a very small quantity at a time. You can keep ground nuts and seeds for a week or two at a time in a tightly covered jar in the refrigerator.

TUMMY SOOTHER

Basil has some pretty remarkable healing properties. It calms the stomach and brings a soothing quality to the whole body. Basil is also rich in monoterpenes. These are phytonutrients with powerful antioxidant properties. It contains other plant chemicals, which soothe stomach cramps and calm upset stomachs, including eugenol – known for its ability to ease muscle spasms. Finally, basil is antiseptic and mildly sedative.

Chillies for Pain

Most people think of chillies in terms of herbs and spices, not of health. But chillies are a great addition to a health-enhancing diet, even in the smallest doses. One small chilli boasts 100 per cent of the daily recommended dose of the antioxidant beta-carotene plus as much as 200 per cent of that of vitamin C. Both these nutrients help fight free radicals and therefore help protect against heart disease, cancer and early ageing. They also strengthen immunity. In addition, chillies contain a plant chemical called capsaicin, which not only creates their fibre but also prevents high LDL cholesterol in the blood.

Throughout history, chillies have been used to relieve pain. Recent research shows capsaicin has the ability to temporarily block chemically transmitted pain signals in the body. That is why you find it in natural ointments used to relieve arthritis and nerve pain. You will even find it in nose sprays helpful in clearing headaches. There is good evidence that capsaicin may even soothe pains of the mind and soul since it appears to trigger the release of mood-enhancing endorphins in the brain.

Fenugreek for Hormones

Fenugreek is rich in diosgenin, a phytochemical from which chemists in the laboratory derive nature-identical progesterone. As a result, fenugreek is now also widely grown for the pharmaceutical industry. It enhances libido and helps clear premature ejaculation in men. Fenugreek also improves digestion and is one of the best deep cleansers for the body that you can find in nature. It has a slightly spicy and bitter taste. When the leaves are very young and fresh, they are a bit like curry. I generally use the seeds to make tea.

Garlic for Everything

Garlic has been prescribed for thousands of years as a cure for just about everything. But just in case this information has you running out for garlic pills, don't. It is much better to eat a couple of cloves of garlic a day in your food, either raw or lightly cooked. Garlic has much more powerful antibiotic properties when you eat it raw than when you cook it.

Here are some of its benefits:
- ❏ Lowers overall cholesterol while increasing HDL (the good) cholesterol and reducing the susceptibility of LDL (the so-called bad) cholesterol to oxidise. This oxidation process is the first step to the arterial walls becoming damaged. One study showed that even half to one clove of garlic a day can lower cholesterol on average by nine per cent.
- ❏ Lowers blood pressure. Garlic mimics the action of hypertensive drugs but has none of the side-effects.
- ❏ Blocks the ability of carcinogenic compounds to affect normal

cells. This may be the means by which garlic inhibits the growth of cancer cells within the body.

❏ Stimulates immune function. Garlic fights off many of the bacteria and fungi that medicine believes to be responsible for illness in humans. It also boosts the number of natural cure cells. Many epidemiological studies show a link between eating garlic frequently – as well as spring onions, chives and onions – and a significant reduction in the risk of stomach cancer within a population.

❏ Protects the cells against free-radical damage and therefore the body against premature ageing and degeneration.

❏ Reduces the tendency of blood to clot and even helps dissolve existing clots once they've formed.

No wonder garlic has such a good reputation.

Glorious Ginger

The spicy-sweet ginger root is one of the greatest of all the natural health enhancers of the vegetable kingdom. It is not only well known for its ability to calm an upset stomach and banish travel sickness: it is also brilliant at alleviating the symptoms of colds and flu by increasing circulation and calming fevers. It even helps PMS and headaches, and has heart-protecting properties thanks to its ability to discourage the clumping of blood cells.

BANISH NAUSEA

To help prevent nausea all you need to take is half a teaspoon of dried ginger or a tiny piece of fresh ginger. It relieves indigestion and flatulence, stimulates circulation and is used in natural medicine to counter rheumatism. In a study done in Denmark in 1992, researchers confirmed what Ayurvedic practitioners have long insisted, that ginger relieves the pain of arthritis and rheumatism without side-effects. Many scientists studying this amazing root believe that ginger works its wonders thanks to an ability to block inflammatory tendencies in the body.

Rosemary Revives

Rosemary has a natural ability to soften the skin. When used in a carrier cream and rubbed on the body, its essential oils are a great help in relieving muscular soreness. But what I like best about rosemary is the way it revitalises the senses through its pungent odour and taste.

Go Fish

It is not only specific fruits and vegetables that carry healing power – so do animal foods. Many are rich in *zoochemicals* – special nutraceuticals of animal origin. Zoochemicals were first discussed by Anthony Almada, a nutritional biochemist. He used the word to describe compounds in fish, dairy products, eggs, meat and poultry that are particularly health enhancing to the human body. Part of the reason why fish is so wonderful is that it is rich in polyunsaturated omega-3 fatty acids. A high level of these essential fatty acids in the diet is associated with very low levels of stroke as well as a decreased risk of every sort of heart disease. In part, this is because EFAs make the blood less likely to clot. They also help lower blood pressure, reduce triglycerides – the fats that circulate in the blood – and decrease the levels of the low-density lipoproteins (BLDL) and cholesterol, which in turn reduces the tendency that blood platelets have to clump and build up on artery walls. Omega-3 fatty acids also inhibit the progress of breast cancer and help prevent tumours in general. The best sources of omega-3 fatty acids are cold-water fish such as anchovies, sardines, swordfish, bass, mackerel and wild salmon. Even oysters and squid are high in omega-3. Unless you are vegetarian, meat and fish are going to make up most of the cooked proportion of your Powerhouse diet. Eat your fish raw if you like, but even if you are going to cook it, make sure it is from a clean source and as fresh as you can get it. I would never touch uncooked meat unless I was absolutely sure it was organic and from superbly healthy animals.

Get More Omega-3s

In the average diet, the ratio of omega-3 to omega-6 fatty acids tends to be about 1:10, a ratio which most nutritional experts believe is undermining our health. When the level of omega-6 is much higher in the body than omega-3, this triggers an increase in some prostaglandins and leucotrines – substances like hormones which can undermine immune function, encourage the formation of blood clots and produce irregular heart rhythms. Much better for health is the balance of 1:2 or 1:3 omega-3 and omega-6 which our hunter-gatherer ancestors got.

Flax oil provides a good balance of omega-3 and omega-6 fatty acids. The omega-3s it contains are not taken from fish, but from cold-pressed vegetable oils. You can buy it in the best health-food stores. It must be kept chilled in the refrigerator at all times, and you need to use it within a few weeks, as all the essential fatty acids are prone to degeneration. One thing more: never heat it. Use it for salad dressings.

There is more to the fish oil story too. Two omega-3 compounds found in fish oil, eicosapentaenoic acid (EPA) and docosahexaenoic acid (DHA), are known to help prevent the build-up of plaque on the walls of the arteries. They even help mitigate the destructive effects of a diet high in fat. Both EPA and DHA also help to relieve the pain of rheumatoid arthritis and decrease the number of headaches in migraine sufferers.

TUMOUR PROTECTION

Anchovies (even the tinned variety) are a great source of omega-3 fatty acids. These fatty acids, which are virtually impossible to come by on a diet of convenience foods, have been shown to inhibit the growth of cancer tumours and may also help lower soaring cholesterol levels. Anchovies are also rich in the nucleic acids DNA and RNA, which some experts in human biochemistry believe may help prevent premature ageing. They appear to help the body create healthy and long-lived cells.

Mussels Have Muscle

With their beautiful blue-green shells, when harvested from unpolluted water, these sea gems are not only a highly nutritious form of protein, they are rich in vitamins and trace minerals. In addition, mussels are an excellent source of mucopolysaccharides and of the free radical-scavenging enzyme, superoxide dismutase. Extracts of green-lipped mussel have been used successfully to treat inflammatory diseases from rheumatoid arthritis to osteoarthritis, eczema and emphysema. Recently, mussels have even taken their place in the growing arsenal of natural cancer treatments. Always eat them cooked.

PRAWNS FOR SKIN BEAUTY

Prawn shells are filled with chitin – a protein substance that cosmetic manufacturers now use to strengthen skin from both within and without. Like most shellfish, prawns are rich in iodine and in the antioxidants zinc and selenium. Prawns are excellent for people who eat very little, thanks to their being an easily digested form of top-quality protein. They are also a good source of calcium and the important omega-3 fatty acids, which offer not only protection for the heart but good support for hormonal health and skin health and beauty too. Delicious grilled, especially on a teppenyaki grill.

Cleansing Seaweeds

All seaweeds are marine algae – the oldest form of life on the planet. Most of them have something in common: they are filled with soothing mucilaginous gels such as algin, agar and carrageen, and they alkalinise the blood. They help clear liver stagnation and therefore, from the point of view of Oriental medicine, help activate the *chi* – the body's life energy – when we eat them. Seaweeds are excellent lymphatic cleansers. Even in small quantities, they supply biologically available minerals and trace elements as almost no other food can. Just five to 15 grams of sea plants a day (measured before soaking or cooking) will supply you with a broad range of minerals – so broad that it's unlikely you will need to take any mineral supplements unless you have a specific high requirement for particular minerals.

Orientals make the best use of seaweeds in their foods. However, in peasant traditions in Europe and the United States, you also find many seaweeds. Bladderwrack, for instance, sea lettuce and kelp make good soups. The only problem with seaweeds – and it's a big one – is that you need to make sure the sea plants you eat come from seas that are relatively unpolluted, particularly by heavy metals, since wherever seaweeds grow they tend to accumulate whatever metals and minerals are in the waters. When you first introduce seaweeds to your diet, it's a good idea to do it slowly as it sometimes takes a week or two for the body to get used to digesting sea vegetables. Their flavour is also unique, and for a few people it takes a bit of getting used to.

Sea Gelatine

The sea vegetable derivative, agar agar, is made out of the mucilaginous fibre from several seaweeds, many of which grow to great size. In the Orient it is used to promote weight loss and to improve digestion. It's a great source of both iron and calcium, and it makes wonderful fruit jellies. The Japanese call it *kanten,* and it has a particular ability to gel. The seaweeds from which agar agar are made are known collectively as agarophytes, the most important of which is a seaweed called gelidium, which grows as deep as 60 metres, waving its huge leaves in the sea. Perhaps 1,000 years ago the Japanese discovered how to dehydrate the fronds so that they became transparent and could be made into kanten bars and used as easily as gelatine. These are available in good Japanese supermarkets.

CLEAR INFLAMMATION

In many ways, agar agar is far superior to gelatine. However, it has a much firmer texture and does not melt easily. It is also calorie-free and ideal for vegetarians, as it is a completely natural vegetable product. Not only that, but this wonderful gift from the sea with a slightly sweet flavour benefits the body in many ways – by reducing inflammation, strengthening the heart and lungs and through its mildly laxative action. Finally, it is an excellent dietary source of both calcium and iron.

Bring Back the Egg

Eggs are a great food – a superb source of top-quality protein among other things. It is a pity that for so long they were wrongly accused of raising cholesterol levels. The protein they offer is just about the best you can get, apart, maybe, from fresh raw fish or raw organic liver (and not many people are drawn to raw organic liver). Rich in the sulphur-based amino acids, eggs have excellent antioxidant properties to help protect you from free-radical damage that leads to degeneration and early ageing. Such sulphur amino acids need to be available for the body to make its own natural free-radical-fighting enzymes such as glutathione peroxidase. Eggs are also full of antioxidant vitamins A and E as well as vitamins D and B$_{12}$ and lecithin. An emulsifier essential to good brain functioning, lecithin has been shown to enhance memory, mood and concentration. Finally, eggs are truly satisfying. They 'stick to your ribs', and their protein-based energy is released slowly into the bloodstream. This makes them great for breakfast. They help guard against the blood sugar ups and downs that have you reaching for a cup of coffee and a packet of biscuits mid-morning.

Soya Guards

Populations who regularly consume soya products have reduced rates of breast cancer, colon cancer and prostate cancer. Why? The soya bean is rich in phytohormones – plant-based oestrogens such as the isoflavones genistein and daedzein. Unlike the dangerous xenoestrogen chemicals from petrochemically derived herbicides, pesticides and plastics in our environment – which lower male sperm count and wreak havoc with women's reproductive systems – soya's plant hormones are gentle.

When we eat foods rich in phyto-oestrogens, like soya, these weak plant hormones are taken up by the oestrogen receptor sites in our body, where they help to protect us from the uptake of dangerous cancer-inducing xenoestrogens all around us. This is important for men as well as women. In effect, if you eat a good quantity of phyto-oestrogens you go a long way towards protecting yourself from the reproductive damage and the higher susceptibility to cancer and degeneration that has resulted in recent years from rising environmental pollution.

CARE FOR BONES

There are many other health claims now being made about soya products. Most of them are proving to be true. The isoflavone daedzein, for example, is a metabolite which helps prevent the decrease in bone mass that leads to osteoporosis. Along with the isoflavones, soya is rich in saponins and other phytosterols, which help lower cholesterol levels, either by blocking cholesterol absorption or by enhancing the body's ability to get rid of any excess. This is probably why soya is often credited with an ability to reduce the risk of cardiovascular disease in people who eat it frequently.

Long-term consumption of a mere 30 to 50mg a day of isoflavones has been shown to lower the risk of heart disease. As in the case of other health-enhancing phytochemicals such as the carotenoids, flavonoids and antioxidants, there is a powerful synergistic effect in getting the protection of isoflavones, saponins and other plant chemicals all together as nature packaged them in soya beans. They work synergistically: when it comes to the good effects they bring, the whole is greater than the sum of the parts. There is simply no way to create in a nutritional supplement the fine synergy that natural soya bean foods offer. Just one serving of soya a day is a great strategy for lowering your risk of degenerative diseases and protecting yourself from the carcinogenic effects of environmental chemicals. A serving of soya is 250ml (9fl oz) of soya milk or 50g (2oz) of soya beans, tofu or tempeh.

One word of warning, however. Soya beans, like corn and tomato products, have been highly genetically engineered in recent years, and there is a powerful argument against eating any genetically engineered products. We have no idea what the long-term effects of eating artificially manipulated products will be. But in most countries, provided you choose organic foods, you should be safe from any genetically engineered products – another good reason to eat organic.

Meet Good Meat

All forms of meat contain high levels of protein and an abundance of minerals and trace minerals. Wild game is low in fat – much lower than pork, lamb or beef – and the fat itself is highly unsaturated, very much like fish fat. Partridge, venison, grouse and quail are all higher in iron than any other meat except for offal, such as liver and heart. They are also extremely rich in zinc as well as vitamins B_6, B_{12} and B_2, niacin and pantothenic acid.

EAT ORGANIC

The problem with domestic meats is that in many countries most of them are laden with hormones, toxins and antibiotics. When you routinely eat large quantities of meat, you can end up not only with a high level of uric acid in your body, but also a tendency to form a lot of mucus and to build up toxicity. This is why, when I eat meat – and I prefer fish or game – I eat certified organic meat. The difference in flavour is remarkable and I know that the animals I am eating have been carefully raised and are free of both excess fat and the toxicity that most domestic farm animals carry these days.

I was a vegetarian for 20 years and I still believe that a vegetarian diet is ideal for many people. I discovered in my mid-30s, however, that vegetarianism was not ideal for me – probably because my ancestors, being Nordic, spent most of their lives living on fish, salted meat and whatever vegetables they could dig up from the frozen tundra. Our genetic makeup determines to a great extent what works for us and what doesn't. When I added fish and game to my meals, my energy levels soared and I looked and felt better.

Each one of us is unique. This not only determines what kind of foods we thrive on, it also determines the foods that are best for us at any particular time of our life. Many women at menopause, for instance, find they do better by cutting meat out of their diet. Others discover just the opposite – that they need more protein. It's a question of 'suck it and see'. Don't hesitate to shift from eating more fruit at one time of your life to more vegetables at another, and more fish at another. The human body is always changing, as are our needs for various foods. The magnificent variety of health-enhancing foods we have to choose from makes the process of finding which foods serve us best a great pleasure.

SPROUT FOR LIFE

A seed has more power for generating life than any other part of a plant. Little wonder, since seeds are designed to grow new plants. Although the needs of a growing plant are not identical to our own, seeds come packed with the superb balance of protein, carbohydrates, fats, vitamins, minerals and plant factors necessary to launch a new plant. As such, they are the finest natural food that 'home farming' can provide.

Sprouted seeds and grains, grown in a bowl in a kitchen window or airing cupboard, are the richest source of naturally occurring vitamins known. A mere tablespoon of tiny seeds can produce up to a kilo of sprouts. Sprouts come in all shapes and colours, from the tiny curlicue forms of mustard to the round yellow spheres of chickpeas. Common seeds for sprouting are mung beans, aduki beans, wheat, barley, fenugreek, lentils, mustard, oats, pumpkin seeds, sesame seeds, sunflower seeds and soya beans.

Energy and Order
The Chinese invented living sprout foods centuries ago. They carried mung beans on their ships, sprouting these seeds to provide vitamin C and prevent scurvy in sailors. In their dormant state, chickpeas, mung beans and lentils are filled with enzyme inhibitors. This makes them hard to digest even when cooked, and is one of the reasons why eating beans and lentils creates so many digestive troubles. Our bodies are not very well designed to handle them in this form.

Enzyme inhibitors can interfere with our ability to absorb minerals present in a food. But, when you sprout a seed, all this changes. Its content of B-vitamins and vitamin C soars, and enzyme inhibitors get neutralised. Meanwhile, the enzymes dormant in these embryonic plants spring into life to improve the way your own body's enzymes function. Sprouted seeds of mung beans, chickpeas, unshelled sesame seeds, lentils, adzuki beans and buckwheat are delicious in salads, as snacks, or used to create live muesli for breakfast. You can buy them already growing or sprout them yourself in bowls on the kitchen windowsill. Because they are young plants and eaten raw, they also convey the highest level of biophoton order to your living matrix.

PERFECT FOODS

'A vegetable which will grow in any climate, will rival meat in nutritive value, will mature in three to five days, may be planted any day of the year, will require neither soil nor sunshine, will rival tomatoes in vitamin C, and will be free of waste in preparation . . .' Clive McCay, professor of nutrition at Cornell University, praising sprouted soya beans. They are, he declared, 'an almost perfect food'.

Because they contain an almost perfect balance of amino acids, fatty acids and natural sugars, plus a high content of minerals and enzymes, sprouts are capable of sustaining life on their own – provided you eat several kinds together. They are also one of the cheapest forms of food around. A few years ago, one American enthusiast calculated that he could live healthily and well on an all-sprout diet for a mere 25 cents a day (18p). Double that to allow for inflation and it is still a pretty dazzling claim. Amazing as this is, I would not endorse a diet of all raw foods of any sort except for short periods for healing, under the wise guidance of a skilled practitioner.

Cheap and Cheerful
Basic seeds and grains are cheap ounce for ounce. These days, many sprouted seeds are readily available in supermarkets and health-food stores. When you sprout seeds yourself with nothing but clean water, they become an easily accessible source of organically grown fresh vegetables, even for city dwellers. In an age when most fruit and vegetables are grown in artificially fertilised soils and treated with hormones, fungicides, insecticides, preservatives and all manner of other chemicals, the home-grown-in-a-jar sprouted seeds emerge as a pristine blessing – fresh, unpolluted and ready to eat in a minute by popping them into salads or just eating them as a snack.

In many ways sprouts are the perfect compromise between the agriculture of years gone by and the 'just add water' mentality of recent times. All one needs is flat glass trays, or a jam jar, some fresh water and a few seeds, and in three to five days you have a marvellous miniforest of the sprout. For full instructions on sprouting, see Sprout it Yourself on page 189.

ANCIENT TREASURES

Far from being the new-fangled invention of food faddists and quasi-hippies, sprouts have been recognised as high-quality food for almost 5,000 years. They are mentioned in Chinese writings dated around 2939 BC. Szekely, co-founder of the international Biogenic Society, found references to them in documents written at the time of Jesus. Sprouted seeds are an important part of the diet of the long-lived Hunza people of the Himalayas. In the late 18th century, Charles Curtis, a surgeon in the British Royal Navy, recorded the fact that sprouted seeds could be used to prevent scurvy, but that ungerminated seeds had no anti-scorbutic virtues. Some rather marvellous things happen to seeds when they start to germinate.

Little Dynamos

A seed is a treasure chest of latent energy in the form of proteins, fats, carbohydrates, vitamins and minerals. When it is soaked in water some remarkable changes occur. Enzymes which until then have lain dormant become active; they begin to break down stored starch into simple sugars like glucose and fructose, they split long-chain proteins into free amino acids, and they convert saturated fats into free fatty acids. The tendency that some seeds have to produce flatulence when we eat them unsprouted disappears as these dormant vegetables spring into life. In fact, enzyme activity in plants is never so intense as at this early sprouting stage. Physicians who use freshly grown sprouts as part of healing diets claim that it is this high level of enzyme activity that stimulates the body's own enzymes into greater activity.

Protein levels rise with germination, and as germination proceeds, the ratio of essential to non-essential amino acids increases, providing more of those that the body needs. When maize seeds germinate, the concentration of lysine and tryptophan (two essential amino acids whose low levels in unsprouted corn make it a poor-quality protein food if eaten on its own) rise, while the concentration of other amino acids not absolutely necessary for human nutrition decreases.

QUANTUM NUTRITION

The vitamin content of seeds soars when they germinate. The vitamin B_2 content of oats, for example, rises by 1,300 per cent soon after germination begins. By the time the tiny leaves form it has risen by 2,000 per cent. Other B-vitamins increase drastically too: biotin increases by 50 per cent, pantothenic acid by 200 per cent, pyridoxine by 500 per cent and folic acid by 600 per cent. The vitamin C in soya beans multiplies five times within three days of germination. A mere tablespoon of soya beansprouts contains half the recommended daily adult requirement of vitamin C. In sprouted wheat the vitamin content multiplies six times; thiamine increases by 30 per cent, B_2 by 200 per cent, niacin by 90 per cent, pantothenic acid by 80 per cent and biotin and pyridoxine by 100 per cent. Nowhere else in nature does one find such high-quality nutrition at such an infinitesimal cost.

Nitriloside Protection

Many years ago, when he was studying the dietary patterns of various 'primitive' cultures amongst whom cancer was virtually unknown, Weston A. Price discovered that many of their foods – millet, passion fruit and apricots, for example – were rich in a group of compounds called nitrilosides. Their cattle and sheep fed on grasses rich in nitrilosides, and so the meat and milk they produced were rich in them too.

Nitrilosides are water-soluble compounds that occur in large quantities in the growing tips of seeds and young shoots and to a lesser degree in the body of mature plants. They were first isolated by Californian physician Ernst T. Krebs and his biochemist son Ernst T. Krebs Jr. The controversy over whether or not nitrilosides can be used to treat cancer still rages, with many biologically oriented physicians claiming that they cause remission, and their more orthodox colleagues dismissing such claims as absurd. Nevertheless, it is a fact that nitrilosides figure heavily in the diets of primitive people who suffer not at all from cancer or degenerative diseases. British physician Dr Alex Forbes was one of the many physicians who used nitriloside-rich sprouts in anti-cancer regimes. Sprouted grains are rich in nitrilosides. Mung beans, aduki beans and lentils increase their nitriloside content by 50 per cent when they sprout.

CANCER FIGHTERS

Why may sprouts be effective against cancer? Ernst T. Krebs Jr explains: '. . . when they are broken down in the body they release two chemicals . . . cyanide and benzaldehyde. Body cells – the normal cells of the body – can protect themselves from such released chemicals; but cancer cells are incapable of doing this . . . both these chemicals kill unprotected cancer cells . . . consider quickly just the nitriloside content of the diet of primitive man. He relied heavily upon the fresh succulent sprouts of the grasses, the wild legumes, millet, vetch, the lupins, wild beans and the like. Vitamin content of these plants at the sprouting stage often exceeds by 20 times or more that of the mature plant. Indeed the nitrilosides and other accessory food factors that occur in prodigious quantities in the sprouting stage of the plant may be completely absent in the mature plant.'

Another major ingredient of sprouts is chlorophyll (*see page 118*). This too is known to have health-enhancing and anti-cancer properties. Dr Chiu-Nan Lai at the University of Texas Systems Cancer Center discovered this when he exposed bacteria to carcinogenic chemicals in the presence of chlorophyll extracts taken from wheat, mung beans and lentil sprouts. Cancer development was 99 per cent inhibited.

Free Minerals
The body can only assimilate minerals effectively if they are part of organic molecules. Unfortunately, the calcium, zinc and iron in peas, beans and some grains tend to be bound by phytic acid, which makes them unavailable for absorption. This is why nutritionists sometimes warn against a diet too rich in beans and seeds. Sprouting greatly lowers the phytic acid content of seeds, making the minerals bound to it available to us. At the same time it increases the content of desirable phosphorus compounds such as lecithin, which is necessary for healthy nerves and for the brain to function. Lecithin does a lot of other useful things too. It helps to break up and transport fats and fatty acids around the body; it prevents too many acid or alkaline substances accumulating in the tissues; it encourages the transport of nutrients through cell walls; and enhances hormone secretion. Many studies have demonstrated that sprouted diets have serious rejuvenating powers.

Leave Alfalfa Alone

Ironically, the only sprouted seeds it may be wise to avoid are the most widely available: alfalfa sprouts. Research shows that alfalfa embryos may inhibit some of our immune functions. In some people they may also contribute to inflammatory conditions like lupus or arthritis. This is because alfalfa contains an unusual amino acid – *canavanine* – which can actually be toxic to humans when eaten in large quantities. As the alfalfa plant grows to maturity, this amino acid is metabolised so it is no longer present in the mature grass.

Cereal Grasses – Great Support

Properly processed with low heat and freeze-dried – so that the enzymes in raw sprouts remain intact – sprouted seeds and grasses like wheat and barley make superb nutritional supplements when stirred into a glass of water or vegetable juice. Professor Takauki Shibamoto, chairman of the Environmental Toxicity Division, University of California at Davis, spent many years studying an antioxidant compound contained in young green barley leaves called 2-0-GIV. He discovered that this flavonoid inhibits lipid peroxidation at least as effectively as any other antioxidant, including the vitamins and carotenoids. In addition to its antioxidant action, green barley extract taken as a supplement reduces inflammation, swelling and heat as well as pain. Its enzymes are capable of inactivating and breaking down carcinogens as well. So, like many of the other green grasses, it acts as a cancer fighter.

GRASS SPROUTS – THEN AND NOW

The green tips of sprouted wheat plants and other grain plants were eaten as a delicacy in the Holy Land 2,000 years ago. King Nebuchadnezzar of ancient Babylon reportedly lived on nothing but young seed grasses for seven years in order to regain his health and mental clarity. Then, in the 1920s and 30s in the United States – before vitamin and mineral pills were in existence – bottled dehydrated cereal grass become a popular food supplement.

Living Foods

When rice, wheat, corn, oats, barley, rye or millet are planted, either in good healthy soil or grown in jars on your kitchen windowsill, and are harvested at just the right moment – a few days after they begin to sprout – they are unbelievably rich in growth hormones as well as vitamins, minerals and plant factors. They are quite literally living foods – and carry a quality of energy that goes beyond anything we are able as yet to measure in chemical terms. The ungerminated seed is a little miracle of nature. When it opens up and produces tiny leaves, photosynthesis makes simple sugars which are transformed into proteins, fatty acids, nucleic acid such as DNA and RNA, as well as complex carbohydrate through the action of enzymes and substrates produced from minerals in the water or soil. The peak of nutritional bounty in all cereal grasses – the moment when chlorophyll, protein and most of the vitamins and minerals reach their zenith – occurs just before *jointing*. This is the moment at which the young inter-nodal tissues in the grass leaf start to elongate to form a stem. This is when cereal grasses are best harvested – usually between five and 12 days after planting. Afterwards, the chlorophyll, protein and vitamin content drops dramatically.

BLOOD BUILDERS

It was back in the late 1920s when the power of cereal grasses came to the fore. The American chemist Charles Schnabel had been searching for material that could be added to poultry feeds to improve egg production and lower chicken mortality. He wanted what he described as a 'blood building material'. By then scientists had identified chlorophyll – the green substance in plants – and noticed that it had a remarkable similarity in its chemical structure to haemoglobin, the oxygen-carrying element in our blood. Schnabel figured that 'green leaves should be the best source of blood'. So he began to feed all sorts of green things to chickens, in combinations of up to 20 green vegetables. He found them all wanting. Then he tried giving hens a green mixture which 'just happened to contain a large amount of immature wheat and oat sprouts'. Animals who got a mere 20 per cent of this cereal grass feed responded amazingly. Winter egg production shot up from an average of 38 per cent to 94 per cent of summer levels, and the eggs that were produced had stronger shells and hatched healthier chicks.

Food for All

Intrigued by his success with chickens, Schnabel began to investigate every aspect of cereal grasses, from the soils that produced the most nutritionally rich grasses, to the effect that eating dehydrated grasses had on the health of humans. He fed his own family of seven on them and was known to boast that none of them ever had a serious illness or decayed teeth. He even developed a vision of how to feed the hungry of the world on the extremely high-quality protein from cereal grasses. In the decades that followed, other scientists found that green cereal grass feeds – which contain natural plant steroid hormones – enhance fertility and improve lactation in many kinds of animals, including humans.

SPROUT AND DRINK

There are three ways to go when it comes to making use of the wonderful properties of sprouted seeds and grasses. First, you can sprout the seeds themselves and use them in salads, snacks and stir-fries. Second, you can buy extracts of seeds such as wheat and barley in powdered form. Third, you can drink their fresh juices.

Better than Malt Whisky

Wheat grass juice is one of my favourite foods, and the best I have ever had was freshly extracted at the organic market held twice a week in Union Square in New York. You drink wheat juice by the shot glass and there are certain parallels between the experience of drinking it and the experience of drinking a shot of the best malt whisky. Not that the grass juices will make you drunk – far from it – but a glass of wheat grass juice has a similar ability to go right to your head the moment you drink it. So powerful is wheat grass juice that many people whose bodies are slightly toxic will actually be made ill by it. It is a good idea to mix it with other vegetable juices in small quantities and gradually work your way up until your system detoxifies and you get used to its power.

These days most people prefer to get their sprouted grass seeds in the form of tablets or powders. These products often contain other healthful ingredients such as chlorella or herbal extracts. They vary tremendously in quality. Just because something is green and contains wheat grass does not mean that it is high quality, so choose your supplements carefully and they will serve you well.

FOUR

MAKE THE LEAP

In India the best foods are often those you buy in the cheapest cafés because they have been made with love and joy (sometimes humour too). The word 'café' is a euphemism, for these places are little more than a few stone slabs over a fire. Yet the foods they sell are infinitely better tasting, more nourishing and 'safe' (less likely to cause Delhi belly) than all the fancy foods you get in India's expensive restaurants. It doesn't matter how skilful, knowledgeable or important a cook is either, so long as the food is cooked with affection.

Have you noticed how much better food tastes when it's cooked by someone who actually likes cooking? This is not because they know what they are doing – often they don't. But they do manage to impart fun and life into the foods they make, even when they 'go wrong'. Anyone who only 'does their duty' in the kitchen drains energy from themselves and from the poor souls who have to eat the food they prepare. The key to Powerhouse eating is to enjoy the whole experience – from shopping for ingredients to eating the results.

A POWERHOUSE LIFE

Now you have all the savvy you need about the remarkable payoffs of Powerhouse eating, it is time to put it into practice. You are about to enter a whole new world of radiance, vitality and good looks. Let's get started.

Quick Guide to Powerhouse Eating and Living
- ❑ Eat 50–75 per cent of your foods raw.
- ❑ Choose your foods for two reasons. First, because they are irresistibly delicious, and second, because they can supply your body with the highest possible support biochemically (through the nutrients and plant factors they contain) and energetically (because they offer optimal biophoton order).
- ❑ Eliminate wheat and other grain-based carbohydrates (except for small quantities of rice and oats).
- ❑ Eat as much buckwheat (actually a seed, not a grain) as you like, since it does not have the detrimental effect of grains like wheat and maize.
- ❑ Turn away from starchy vegetables like potato, yams and sweet potato (except very occasionally as a condiment, for example croutons), and from sugar and other sweeteners in favour of fresh, raw, non-starchy fare.
- ❑ Eat masses of natural, fresh, organic, non-starchy vegetables and fruits.
- ❑ Eat two salads a day – one of them a huge Power Salad complete with protein. Power Salads are not the usual thing made from lettuce and tomatoes plus the odd cucumber. They are medleys of nutritional and energetic order complete with sprouted seeds and a great variety of fresh herbs, not to mention crunchy peppers, carrots, apples and beetroot, as well as anything else beautiful you can lay your hands on or grow on your kitchen windowsill.
- ❑ Stay away from soft drinks, packaged fruit juices, alcohol (a glass or two of wine a day if you must) and all processed drinks.
- ❑ Use cold-pressed, extra-virgin olive oil, walnut oil and flaxseed oil on salads, and coconut oil or olive oil for cooking. Never heat flaxseed oil.
- ❑ Stay away from margarine and other processed oils or any sauces or salad dressings which contain them.

❑ Enrich your diet with omega-3 fatty acids by eating fish at least three times a week.
❑ Eat plenty of good-quality protein like fish, free-range chicken, eggs, game, organic meat and low-carbohydrate soya products at lunch and dinner.
❑ Eliminate coffee or at the very most have only one cup a day. It dehydrates and contributes to toxicity in the system.
❑ Stay away from processed foods.
❑ Walk briskly for 20 to 30 minutes each day to counter insulin resistance, enhance energy, bring radiance to the body, and maintain good emotional balance.

Now let's get down to making it happen.

Powerhouse Meals and Menus

Let's look at some typical Powerhouse breakfasts, lunches and dinners and good snacks too, if you want them. The menus that follow are great for getting you started on this new way of eating. They help you grasp what Powerhouse living is all about. But they are only suggestions to lead you to trust your own creative impulses. You will be forging for yourself a whole new way of eating and thinking about food. Spend a day or two cleaning out your cupboards and refilling the fridge with Powerhouse-supporting foods, then launch into the programme with unbridled passion. Your meals can be as simple as a piece of grilled fish, liver or steak with a lovely salad, or as complex and indulgent as you wish to make them. It's fun and you will be delighted with the changes you experience. Some of the suggestions listed below refer directly to recipes supplied. Others, like 'grilled fish', leave you to your own devices.

START RAW

Begin a meal with something raw – just a glass of fresh-pressed vegetable juice, perhaps. This helps avoid *digestive leucocytosis* – an immune reaction which has white blood cells rushing to the lining of the stomach when we eat cooked foods before raw (*see Cooking May Damage Your Health*). Have a few mouthfuls of salad or a slice of melon before moving on to the fish. You could even start with raw oysters if you are lucky enough to find really fresh ones.

QUICK-START BREAKFASTS AND BRUNCHES

Breakfasts come in two varieties – instant meals for when you are dashing out the door and hearty fare when you have the time and inclination to indulge. They are equally good nutritionally and equally delicious.

- ❑ **Macaroon Surprise** (*see page 210*) made from fresh coconut, almond extract and sparkling orange juice.
- ❑ **Berry Bliss Smoothie** (*see page 210*) made with 20 to 30 grams of microfiltered whey protein powder, a teaspoon of flaxseed oil, and an apple, pear or a handful of berries blended with a few ice cubes. It will have you out the door in a New York minute. Serve with a cup of herb tea or green tea.
- ❑ **Instant Cranberry Porridge** (*see page 218*) made with steel-cut oats and cinnamon, topped with fresh cream, oat milk, soya milk or rice milk.
- ❑ **Omelette Made Easy** (*see page 219*) with fresh sprouts. Cook your omelette in olive oil, toss in chopped tomatoes, peppers, spinach – whatever you have. Serve with a slice of melon and a cup of herb tea or green tea if you wish.
- ❑ **Live Muesli** (*see page 215*) made with coconut oil and soaked or sprouted raw buckwheat, apples, pears or berries. Serve with a cup of herb tea or green tea.
- ❑ **Sweet Nothing Soufflé** (*see page 220*) made with shredded coconut, plus a glass of fresh carrot and apple juice.
- ❑ **Grilled Fish** – wild salmon is especially good with garlic and sweet onions – plus a bowl of mixed berries. Serve with a cup of herb tea or green tea.
- ❑ **Blueberry Curds and Whey** a delicious new twist on an old-fashioned dish. Serve with a cup of herb tea or green tea.
- ❑ **Hand-made Sausages** (*see page 222*) – make ahead of time for a lazy morning in bed. Accompany with finely grated raw apples, carrots and beetroot dressed with the juice of an orange and some curry powder. Serve with a cup of herb tea or green tea.

❑ **Vanilla Nutmeg Smoothie** (*see page 211*) – another instant blender meal, rich and creamy with a spicy overtone. Serve with a cup of herb tea or green tea.

POWER SALAD MEALS

Make one meal a day a huge raw salad complete with top-quality protein food. It is the fastest way to experience just how quickly this new way of eating can raise your energy and make you look and feel great.

❑ **Crudités** (*see page 270*) served with **Aïoli** (*see page 281*) or **Raw Pesto** (*see page 285*) or **Fish Dip** (*see page 285*). Half a rock melon.
❑ **Spinach, Egg and Mushroom Salad** (*see page 229*) dressed with **Basil and More Basil Dressing** (*see page 264*).
❑ **Grilled Prawns and Rocket Salad** (*see page 231*) sprinkled with hand-ground black pepper and drizzled with olive oil and lemon dressing.
❑ **Wild Salmon Salad** (*see page 235*) with celery, fresh coriander, onions and fresh ginger dressed with **Orange Zest Mayonnaise** (*see page 259*).
❑ **Caesar Salad with Potato Croutons** (*see page 231*), slivered Parmesan and anchovies, dressed with fresh free-range egg dressing and seasoned with Cajun seasoning.
❑ **Salad Niçoise** (*see page 236*) with fresh or tinned tuna, mangetout, fine green beans, olives and cherry tomatoes.
❑ **Chef's Salad** (*see page 230*) with ham, chicken, shaved Parmesan, basil and coriander.
❑ **Sprout Salad** (*see page 233*) with mangetout, chickpea sprouts, mung sprouts, radish and mustard sprouts, cherry tomatoes and **Teppenyaki Tofu** (*see page 316*).
❑ **Scallop Salad with Ginger and Lime** (*see page 234*) with endive, lamb's lettuce and fennel toped with fresh coriander dressing.
❑ **Big Greek Salad** (*see page 234*) with leftover chicken or lamb made with lettuce, cucumber, tomato wedges, sprinkled with sunflower seeds and a teaspoon of pumpkin seeds, Greek olives and two teaspoons of feta cheese – olive oil and lemon dressing.

POWERHOUSE MEALS

Traditional meals – not meat and two veg but protein and many raw vegetables – are a joy to prepare and to devour. They are loved even by salad-haters at lunch or dinner.

❑ **Nut-crusted Tuna** (*see page 297*) on a bed of rocket with black olives and herbs smothered in **Curried Avocado Dip** (*see page 281*) and served with **Fresh Citrus Salad** (*see page 340*).

❑ **Chicken Curry** (*see page 311*) served on a bed of fresh raw salad vegetables, brown rice or **Kasha** (*see page 312*), accompanied with **Blood-apple Slaw Salad** (*see page 255*) and **Mulled Stuffed Apple** (*see page 342*).

❑ **Herbed Lamb Shanks** (*see page 310*) with **Crunchy Broccoli Salad** (*see page 253*) and **Redcurrant and Pear Fruit Freeze** (*see page 355*).

❑ **Mussels Straight Up** (*see page 301*) with **Mesclun and Flower Salad** (*see page 244*) and **Tropical Fruit Salad** (*see page 339*).

❑ **Coriander Tofu** (*see page 318*), **Wakame Salad** (*see page 239*) and **Sesame Sticks** (*see page 353*).

❑ **Fresh fish** cooked on a Teppenyaki grill (*see page 307*) with **Wild Herb Salad** (*see page 245*) and **Stuffed Pineapple** (*see page 343*).

❑ **Mackerel** sautéed with garlic, fresh tomatoes, slivered olives and fresh garlic and **All Melon Salad** (*see page 341*).

❑ **La Bourride Pacifica** (*see page 298*) with **Chicory, Apple and Pecan Salad** (*see page 241*) and **Raspberry Chocolate Mousse** (*see page 345*).

❑ **Sandstone Loaf** (*see page 319*), **Iguana Salad** (*see page 249*) and **Lemon Cream Pie** (*see page 348*).

❑ **Chicken and Water Chestnut Wraps with Thai Peanut and Ginger Sauce** (*see page 313*), **Confetti Sprout Salad** (*see page 250*) and **Carob and Honey Ice Cream** (*see page 356*).

SNACKS

Eat snacks only if you feel the need. Judge for yourself whether or not snacks work for you. For some people they are terrific; for others eating more often than every four to five hours increases insulin resistance and leads to food cravings. You need to play it by ear and find out which works best for you. Most people find they feel better simply eating three meals a day. Many feel so good they find themselves eating less and less food, yet feeling satisfied. But if you love snacks, here are some suggestions.

❑ Half a chicken breast
❑ An apple, an orange, a pear or a few strawberries
❑ Half a cup of unsalted walnuts, cashews, almonds or brazils
❑ A few crudités dipped in salsa

❏ A handful of sunflower seeds
❏ A hard-boiled egg

Out and About
Navigating your way through high-raw, low-grain eating when you're away from home is not as difficult as you might imagine. There are a few tricks for negotiating the complex world of foods and snacks once you walk out the front door which can be really helpful. If you usually drink a cup of coffee and munch biscuits at 11 a.m. and 3 p.m., the habit is easier to kick when you have a good breakfast of, say, a protein drink, scrambled eggs or live muesli to hold you over.

RESTAURANT FARE
Restaurants are the easiest away-from-home eating situations because you can choose what you want. The better the restaurant, the more obliging they will be. The best restaurants for Powerhouse eating are invariably those that cook their food to order in contrast to fast-food restaurants where foods are all pre-packaged and come whatever way they happen to be served. In a restaurant where foods are cooked to order, you can pretty much write your own ticket. You might have green beans or asparagus with a spinach side salad to go with sea bass steamed or grilled with a little butter and garlic, instead of served (as it states on the menu) smothered in a questionable sauce. Don't be afraid to ask for a 'doggy bag' to take any extra foods you don't eat in the restaurant home. These leftovers can make good snacks for the next day.

SIMPLE IS BEST

The toughest restaurants, apart from fast-food chains, are those known as 'health-food restaurants'. This means their dishes are chock-full of flour, honey and raw sugar. If you get stuck in one of these it's generally best to go for a salad and see if they have some tofu you can eat with it.

JAPANESE DELIGHTS
I love eating in Japanese restaurants, first because I find the food so good in general, and second because it is one of the easiest places in

the world to get simple foods. Order sashimi if you like it, plus a beautiful Japanese sprout salad with umibushi vinegar, but make sure the raw fish is very fresh. Most of the fish the Japanese serve are rich in precious omega-3 fatty acids. If you have any doubts about the fish being served in a restaurant, never eat it raw as there is always the risk of parasite contamination. This makes me very careful about the Japanese restaurants I choose, particularly when in the northern hemisphere. In the southern hemisphere, the fish is often so fresh that I don't need to worry about it. Teppenyaki is an ideal dish. So is teriyaki chicken, or beef and salad (always ask for sauces to be made without any sugar), seaweed broth, miso soup and tofu. Stay away from tempura since it is battered and fried.

MEXICO IS HOT

Mexican food tends to be a bit of a hotchpotch. There are some excellent ways to go, however. You can order a tostada or taco salad, but don't eat the shell beneath. Grilled fish, beef, pork medallions, chicken, as well as shredded beef, chicken or pork are great, served with an *insalata mista* – a tossed salad. Mexican restaurants often have a good selection of fish served Vera Cruz style, foods with tomatoes, peppers and onions. I adore red snapper prepared this way. Stay away from high-fat cheeses and too much sour cream, and ask for a salsa or guacamole made with olive oil on the side – since much guacamole tends to be made with cheap vegetable oils. Gazpacho is a great soup to start.

FRENCH CONNECTIONS

French restaurants are easy. You can always go for their gorgeous salads (ask for extra large) as well as grilled or poached fish, or any kind of roasted game. Make sure that any of the sauces that come with your main course are not made from flour (fewer and fewer are these days).

WHEN IN ROME

Italian restaurants are easy as well. I go for a calamari salad to start or an antipasto plate followed by chicken piccata, grilled fish and one of those wonderful Italian salads brimming with herbs, radicchio and rucola smothered in extra-virgin olive oil and spiked with fat Italian olives.

GREEK AND GREAT

Souvlaki – skewered lamb, beef, chicken or prawn kebabs – with vegetables is great. What you have to steer clear of in these restaurants are the pasties, the breads and the pastas that garnish many Middle Eastern and Greek dishes. Their salads are wonderful, particularly those full of feta cheese with olive oil and red wine vinegar dressing. Even their tzatziki sauce, which they pour on top, is delicious.

BOXED LUNCH

Airlines are still a big hassle. You would think that none of the catering directors of any of the airlines (despite their dozen or more 'special meals' including kosher, vegetarian, vegan and the lot) had ever heard of high-raw, low-grain eating. Since I travel a great deal and many of my trips are long-haul flights, some of which take more than 24 hours, I plan this part of my life pretty carefully.

Some of the food on airlines, of course, you can eat. The simpler it is the better. Things like steamed fish and cheese are manageable. If you order a 'kosher meal' in advance, you are less likely to get some silly sauce poured over your fish or meat. Often you can explain to the cabin crew (if you are not sitting in business or first class) that you are on a special diet and unfortunately the airline was not able to fulfil your needs, then ask if it is possible for them to gather together some fish, meat, salads and other high-raw, low-grain foods from the first-class menu for you. Most airlines are willing to do this.

INSTANT FIX

The other thing I do whenever I'm travelling by plane, in the car or simply out for the day, is carry a plastic shaker and a couple of little plastic bags with me, into which I put a good dose of microfiltered whey protein, plus something green like powdered wheat grass or barley or Pure Synergy (*see Nature's Supplements*) – my favourite. Then all I need to do is pour clean water into the shaker, add my protein/green powder mix, shake it up and drink it. This is a special backup that I carry with me all the time, even in meetings, so that I am never forced to eat food I don't want. Whatever else happens, I know at the very least that microfiltered whey protein plus green powder will carry me through to the next decent meal.

TRAVELLER'S TRIALS

Travelling anywhere, especially long plane journeys, is likely to upset your normal routine. Often just the excitement of going somewhere on holiday or the pressure of an important business trip is enough to derail your digestion. It is best not to eat too much when travelling – you are usually sitting still for several hours on end and not burning up calories.

❑ Travelling on planes is also a perfect time to go on a juice or fruit fast. Not only is lots of liquid a good antidote to the dehydrating effects of cabin air but the presence of aeroplane 'unmentionables' gives you the instant willpower to see a fast through! Fasting also relieves a lot of jet lag when your internal clocks are operating hours behind or ahead of clock time at your destination. One of the things that slows down recovery from jet lag is eating meals at strange times. On west–east transatlantic flights, for example, you can be served breakfast at 4 a.m. body time. By fasting and drinking lots of water or juices you avoid this problem and arrive at your destination feeling lighter and livelier instead of tired and suffering from indigestion. Make your first meal at your destination (be it breakfast, lunch or dinner) a light fruit or vegetable salad with some good lean protein if you feel really hungry.

❑ If you feel that you cannot possibly last the flight without something to eat, you can also put together a bag of fresh fruit, vegetables, sprouts and seeds and a Thermos of juice or herb tea or a bottle of spring water to take with you. A juicy apple or orange way up above the clouds comes like a welcome breath of fresh air.

Make Way for Radiance

Powerhouse eating can not only make your body healthier and more dynamic, it may also be the beginning of a delicious new way of living. You become more alert and more active. You may sleep less – yet far better than ever before because your body clears itself of toxic build-up. You can deal with stress better than before and feel calmer, yet stronger. Three weeks on Powerhouse eating can bring an inner light and outer beauty together, creating your own brand of unmistakable charisma and authenticity. Meanwhile, your body glows and your vitality radiates. It's what I call deep beauty of the highest order. Enjoy it and all around you will delight as well.

EQUIP YOURSELF

Every kitchen – big or small – should be like an artist's atelier – a place in which you can lose yourself in creative games. The kitchen has always been the centre of a home. In the past it was the place of fire, of inspiration, warmth and imagination. I remember as a child sitting in front of an old Stanley stove gazing into the flames – filled with delightful visions – while my grandmother canned pears, peaches and green beans for winter.

My own kitchen, out of which the Powerhouse food style has developed, is more like a sculptor's studio than a food preparation station. It is a place where I can get together with my friends, workmates and family to laugh and talk about both serious and trivial stuff while we prepare meals together.

A kitchen should have the atmosphere of freedom in it. Hang quirky things from the ceiling if that inspires you. Put a potted plant where you wouldn't expect one. Paint cupboard doors in wild colours. No matter how simple, your kitchen should reflect things that delight and amuse you. Ten years ago I bought a gigantic soup ladle, which has hung above my sink ever since. It is so big I think I have only used it four or five times. It would be ideal for a Salvation Army soup kitchen. Practical? Not at all. But it makes me laugh. I like its beautiful shape and am continually amused by the absurdity of its size.

Mandolin Magic

With a well-organised, well-equipped kitchen, Powerhouse foods are a pleasure to prepare. But there is nothing more annoying than setting out to make a meal in someone else's kitchen and spending ages looking for a brush to scrub vegetables only to find that the one you used was the floor brush! Let's look at some of the tools which are most useful for the raw-food gourmet.

AN ABSOLUTE MUST

The one piece of equipment I would never be without is a mandolin. I prefer the simple plastic ones that sell for a fifth of the price of the expensive stainless steel variety. They have a 'v'-shaped blade into which plastic inserts fit, each of which has different-size knives so you can julienne, make chip-size chunks, slice thin or thick. Unlike the conventional grater which mashes vegetables and fruits when you use it, a mandolin slices them clean and sharp. Be sure to use the hand-protecting device that comes with either model. If you don't – and I know from experience – what you will end up with is shredded fingers instead of shredded cabbage.

Power Tools

Although it is nice to return to nature wherever possible, you have to draw the line somewhere. Using electric equipment takes the tediousness out of chopping vegetables, gives you a greater choice of textures, allows you to make splendid desserts, nut loaves, sauces, soups and whips, and cuts down enormously on preparation time. I find a few simple machines give full rein to my imagination. These are the raw chef's equivalent of the oven or the microwave. For those who like an 'all manual' kitchen I suggest alternatives, but they really are second best.

Apart from a mandolin, the three machines I consider useful are a food processor, a juicer and a blender – in that order. You can get by without a blender because a food processor does many of the same things, but it is useful nonetheless. You can buy appliances which combine the functions of all three, but keeping them separate lets you work on several recipes at the same time and encourages helpers. Choose good strong machines that will stand up to heavy use. If you have a large family it can be worth investing in catering or industrial models which are sturdier and can cope with larger quantities.

A Smooth Process

A good food processor is a blessing to the raw food chef as there are so many remarkable attachments to choose from – a blade, several coarse-to-fine graters, various slicers and shredders. The blade attachment is excellent for grinding nuts and seeds, wheat and other sprouts, homogenising vegetables for soups and loaves, and making dressings, dips and desserts such as ice cream. You can do most of these things with a blender, but if your ingredients are gooey they tend to stick around the blade and you spend ages scraping with very little to show for it. The blade in a food processor is removable and easy to scrape, so you lose very little. The grater, slicer and shredder attachments are terrific for making salads. With their help you can prepare a splendid whole meal salad for four people and have it on the table in 10 minutes. Do experiment with all these attachments because, believe it or not, vegetables actually taste different depending on how they are cut up.

Juice Extractor

The most important considerations when buying a juicer are power, capacity and ease of cleaning. The fewer fiddly parts to wash up the better. Some have a removable strip of plastic gauze in the pulp basket which is helpful in cleaning.

There are basically three types of juicer: the hydraulic press type, the rotating blade type and the centrifugal type. Some hydraulic presses are hand-operated and therefore less convenient than the electric kind, but some doctors who prescribe raw juices prefer them on the grounds that they reduce the amount of oxidation that takes place when juices are exposed to air. I have all three myself. Centrifugal juicers are best to start with and come in two types: either they are separators, which operate without needing to be constantly cleaned out, or they are batch operators, which have to be cleaned out after every 2lb (roughly a kilo) of material has been juiced. That gives the separator kind the edge when it comes to convenience; they expel leftover pulp rather than fill up with it. But they tend not to extract juice as efficiently as the batch operator kind. If you decide on a batch juicer, look for a large-capacity model which does not require emptying too often. It can be infuriating working with a machine that insists on being cleaned out after juicing only two glasses when you are juicing for six people. One other thing to check before buying a juicer is the size of the hole through which you feed your vegetables and fruits. Some are really too small and it can be a real drag to have to cut carrots and beet-roots lengthwise.

Power Blenders

There is not much to choose between blenders except their power. You will need one of at least 400 watts (anything less will be unable to cope). My favourite has attachments for grating, chopping, kneading, etc., which are very useful. Glass models are preferable to plastic, as plastic tends to stain and look tatty very quickly. Look for one that has a removable blade (the base unscrews) for ease of cleaning.

Other Gadgets

Two other devices I find useful are an electric citrus fruit juicer and a lettuce spin-drier. The citrus juicer has a central rotating cone onto which you press your halved grapefruits, oranges and lemons. Very quick and easy. There is nothing to stop you juicing citrus fruits in a centrifuge juicer, but you need to peel them first. The lettuce spin-drier is a great invention. There are several types but my favourite is a basket which fits into a container with holes in the bottom and has a lid with a spinning cord. You put the whole contraption in the sink, put your lettuce or greens into the basket, put the lid on, run water slowly through the hole in the lid and pull the spinning cord. This spins the basket and expels the water, in theory cleaning and drying the greens. In practice they need to be rinsed before you put them in the basket, but by spinning you get beautifully crisp, non-watery leaves very quickly.

Back to Basics

A few other gadgets can be helpful if you cannot afford or have basic objections to electrical equipment. But you will be more limited in the number of textures and recipes you can prepare.

A sturdy grater – the box type with a fine, medium and coarse face, and a face for grating nutmeg and ginger.
Hand coffee grinder – for rendering down nuts, seeds and spices.
Meat mincer – the sort you screw to the table, with coarse and fine cutters; good for grinding grains, seeds, nuts and sprouts.
A strong stainless steel sieve – for rubbing soft fruits through or extracting the juice from finely grated vegetables.
Hand hydraulic juicer
A stainless steel 'mouli' rotary grinder – with coarse and fine grater inserts; quite effective for juicing finely grated fruit or vegetables.
Pestle and mortar – for grinding herbs, spices, flowers, etc.
A lemon squeezer
Wire salad basket – the sort you swing maniacally round your head in the garden.

Cutting Edge

Of primary importance to raw food preparation are good knives and a good chopping board. At least two knives are essential: a large one for tackling spinach leaves, onions, carrot sticks and so on, and a smaller one for more delicate jobs. The best knives are made from carbon steel. Some enthusiasts disapprove of carbon steel because, unlike stainless steel, it encourages oxidation of cut surfaces, but I prefer them; for although stainless steel knives look nice they do not keep their edges as well and a sharp edge is important for creating beautiful salads. If none of your knives will cut a tomato without squashing it, then they need sharpening! A good sharpener is worth investing in.

Chopping Block

Good chopping boards are hard to find. Either they lose their pretty patterns with repeated chopping, or they warp when they get wet, or they are not large enough to slice an orange on without most of the juice running over the edge. Find a decent-sized wooden chopping board if you can, with runnels around the edge. Look in a professional chef's shop for the biggest you can find. Here is my solution to the problem. When I had a new kitchen installed I kept some big leftover pieces of Formica-covered board. You can prepare a salad, or leave the chopped vegetables, on one end and the peelings on the other. If it's big enough, it can fit over the sink so you can drop the peelings into a waste bowl underneath.

Earthy Vessels

All told, the high-raw chef uses very few utensils – there are no enormous pots and pans to go in and out of the oven or to wash up. Choose dishes and platters made of inert or natural substances – glass, earthenware and wood rather than plastic and metal. Avoid all things made of aluminium, which is highly active. When it comes into contact with the acids in some raw foods, such as tomatoes, it can be bleached out and end up in the food, producing heavy-metal poisoning over time.

Here are some other things to be found in my own kitchen:

A special 'vegetables only' scrubbing brush
A large colander, with feet so that it can stand in the sink to drain
Bread pans (preferably glass) for making vegetable loaves
Flat boards or trays for making sweet treats
Ice cube trays

A garlic chopper – achieves much better and quicker results than a pestle and mortar or a garlic press
Scissors for cutting up fresh herbs such as chives, parsley, mint and so on
Salad bowls of different shapes and sizes
Soup plates, fairly wide and deep, for individual 'dish salads'
Salad platters – you can create attractive banquet-like effects by serving crudités arranged on a large platter, perhaps one with several compartments for dips
Several pairs of salad servers
A large pitcher for drinks, and a strainer

Germination Time

Although you can buy commercial sprouters, I find home-made ones simpler and less hassle. This is what you will need.

Glass jars – the bigger the better
Or trays – glass baker's trays or the kind of trays gardeners use for sowing seeds
Cheesecloth or metal gauze, and some rubber bands
Strainer
Dish strainer to stand sprouting jars on (optional)
Water purifier, because some sprouts insist on pure water before they will germinate. So might you if you were a city dweller and afflicted with bad tap water. A water purifier can provide you with untainted drinking water, and water to use in sauces, soups and herb teas. This can be as simple as those in a pitcher form with a replaceable filter which needs to be changed every few months. You regularly top it up with tap water so that you have a constant supply of pure water. Even better is a reverse osmosis filter plumbed into your water supply.

Preserving Life

It is important to store living foods carefully so they stay alive. I keep my seeds, pulses and grains in sealed polythene bags or airtight glass jars. Empty sweet jars make useful storage containers, as do the plastic tubs. But glass is always best. Always cover salads as soon as you have prepared them, even if it is only for 10 minutes while you prepare the rest of the meal, to protect from wilting.

YOUR HIGH-RAW, LOW-GRAIN PANTRY

'Cooking' – since there is no other word in the English language to describe food preparation – starts at the shopping stage. It is when you are in the market surrounded by mounds of lettuces, avocados, fresh peppers, parsley and squid that you get your inspiration. Never set out to buy food with too fixed an idea of what you want. Look for what is particularly cheap and good. Some of the very best dishes can be made from the commonest vegetables like carrots, turnips and watercress. Often the cheapest fish is the most tasty, provided you know how to prepare it. You may come across something which, although you have not thought of it, is beautiful. It draws you to it. Buy it.

Forget what you thought you were after. A good menu is created while you shop. Why seek something which is not there or is out of season? Fresh foods bought in season offer the highest complements of vitamins and minerals you can get. Even better, they are rich in the phytonutrients – plant factors such as lycopene, co-enzyme Q10 and the remarkable flavonoids. These plant factors are so effective in enhancing health and good looks that if they are missing from your diet (as they are from the diet of all who rely on convenience foods) then you are quite simply missing out on vitality at the highest level. Let yourself be tempted by all the gorgeous vegetables and fruits you find. Make them the focus of your menu. Always seek temptation. To enjoy food fully, to celebrate the beauty of your food, your senses need to be heightened.

LIVING FOODS

In Powerhouse eating, half to three-quarters of your foods will be fresh and raw. As many as possible will be living foods –

sprouted seeds and legumes with all the health-enhancing biophoton order they impart to your body. That is why raw and living foods are used throughout the world at the most famous natural clinics and spas for beauty as well as for healing chronic and acute illness. Such foods improve cellular functioning, enhance the energy and biochemistry of your body's living matrix, and provide high levels of antioxidant and immune-enhancing plant factors. A high percentage of raw foods increases overall energy and stamina too, and makes you look and feel radiant.

Variety is the Secret

Making raw food a part of your life means making changes. They begin with what you choose to put in your larder. Take a look at the contents of your kitchen shelves and cupboards and ask yourself, 'Do I really feel *good* about putting those things into my body?' Variety is the secret of a really useful raw-food pantry because at certain times of the year you may be limited by the fresh fruits and vegetables available. The foods which provide this precious variety and make raw foods exciting at any time of the year are: seeds and pulses for sprouting; seeds; nuts; dried fruit for those times when fresh fruit is hard to come by; herbs, seasonings and spices. A high-raw, low-grain diet heightens your senses, which is especially important in appreciating good food. You begin to notice and delight in the hundreds of delicate aromas and taste sensations which exist in foods in their natural state but which are lost in cooking.

A Clean Break

Before you head for the supermarket, delicatessen, whole-food emporium or local farm store, clear out your cupboards of all the convenience foods, ice creams and breakfast cereals you have been collecting. Jams and jellies, rice cakes, popcorn, flour, grains, pasta, pretzels, low-fat salad dressings, fruit-flavoured yoghurt and icing sugar can all go. What you will want to keep around is some ordinary granulated sugar to serve to friends who drink sweetened drinks. Most people find the process of clearing out their pantry and refrigerator a salutary experience. It gives you the sense that you're starting a new life, as indeed you are.

BUY ORGANIC

Whenever possible, go organic. Not only do organic vegetables taste better, the organic matter in healthy soil is nature's factory for biological activity and biophoton order. Organic brings your body a superb balance of minerals, trace elements, vitamins and phytonutrients you cannot get any other way. The organic matter in soil is built up as a result of the breakdown of vegetable and animal matter by the soil's natural residents – worms, bacteria and other microorganisms. The presence of these creatures in the right quantity and type – which you never find in factory farming – gives rise to physical, chemical and biological properties which create fertility in our soils and make plants grown on them highly resistant to disease. This resistance to illness and degeneration is then passed on to us when we eat the foods. Destroy the soil's organic matter through chemical farming and, slowly but inexorably, you destroy the health of the people and animals living on the foods grown on it. Natural-food emporiums are great places to find good organic vegetables and other produce, as well as eggs, meat, dairy products and fish, from animals that have not been stuffed full of antibiotics, dipped in chemicals or treated with hormones. Try to shop as much as possible in stores that offer organic produce and untreated food.

The most important foods you can eat are the non-starchy vegetables, low-sugar fruits, and proteins like meat, seafood, eggs and game, as well as maybe a little unprocessed cheese and soya proteins like tofu, if you're a vegetarian. The healthiest, freshest and the most natural foods such as these are found around the edge in a supermarket. On the inside rows you find all the packaged convenience foods riddled with refined grains and sugar, junk fats and chemicals, which play no part in Powerhouse eating.

Natural, wholesome foods are perishable. They have to be replaced often, unlike ready-in-a-minute pre-made stuff that you find in the inner aisles. You will be shopping 'at the edge' in another way too: you'll be looking for foods as close as possible to those our ancestors ate. Choose a wide variety of vegetables and fruits which you can eat raw. Here are some shopping lists and suggestions to take with you when you go:

CHOOSE THE BEST

❑ Go for natural whole foods.

❑ Buy foods as fresh as possible and eat them as soon as you can. This allows little time for the deterioration which occurs as a result of oxidation.

❑ Choose foods that are non-toxic and non-polluting to your body. They should contain no synthetic flavours, colours, preservatives or other additives used to commercially 'enhance' them.

❑ Try to vary the foods you choose from day to day and week to week. Down through evolution the human body has adapted to a wide range of foods offering a broad spectrum of nutrients. You need variety.

❑ Use fresh garlic and herbs often. They bring high-level support for body regeneration.

❑ Eat what you enjoy and enjoy what you eat.

❑ You can say goodbye to addictive eating forever. Once your body clears itself of the residues of starchy grain-based foods, sugar, chemicals and junk fats, all those cravings that can make you feel you have no willpower will vanish.

Powerhouse Vegetables and Fruits

There is no better way of raising vitality and improving health than eating phytonutrient-rich foods – lots of them. You will find these in fresh vegetables and fruits. They provide powerful antioxidant and immune-enhancing plant chemicals, which nobody can afford to be without. Our Paleolithic ancestors took in as much as 300 times the phytonutrients that we do today. So we have some catching up to do.

These powerhouses for health and energy – phytonutrients or nutriceuticals – play a vital health and anti-ageing role. A good supply of phytonutrients brings protection from degenerative conditions associated with ageing, such as inflammation of the joints, loss of memory and concentration. Many now believe they help slow the ageing process altogether. Full of biophoton order and phytonutrient power, and just plain delicious, these fresh living foods are the best you can get.

CHOOSE FROM:

Vegetables
avocado
bean sprouts
beet greens
beetroot
broccoli
cabbage
carrots
cauliflower
celery
chickpea sprouts
chicory
collards
courgettes
cucumber
endive
escarole and other
   dark-green lettuces
garlic
kale
lettuce
mushrooms
mustard greens
onions
pepper
radishes
rocket
romaine lettuce
spinach
Swiss chard
watercress

Fruits
apples
apricots (fresh)
berries – blackberries, blueberries,
   raspberries, strawberries
cantaloupe
citrus fruits – lemons, mandarins,
   oranges, tangerines, grapefruit
honeydew melon
kiwi fruit
peaches
pears
plums
rhubarb
tomatoes

VIBRATE WITH COLOUR

The more vibrant and beautiful the colours of your vegetables and fruits are, the greater the immune-enhancing and phytonutrient antioxidant protection they carry. Bright blueberries or strawberries, and deep-green leafy vegetables such as spinach and rocket, tell us that the food we are about to eat is brimming with polyphenols, helpful in preventing diseases including cancer and heart disease, as well as countering Syndrome X (*see page 11*) and protecting the body from early ageing.

Simply the Best

When selecting fish, there are two major considerations: make sure it's fresh and in as unprocessed a form as possible. Fresh is far better than smoked fish, crab cakes or breaded fish. There's no harm in having the odd slice of smoked salmon, especially if it is naturally smoked. But the more a fish is processed, the less quality it brings you in terms of high-level health. (And these days, sadly, most smoked salmon has sugar added to it.)

MORE OMEGA-3s

Eat oily fish at least three times a week, but every day if you can. Preformed omega-3 fatty acids DHA and EPA are fantastic for the body. The omega-3s in wild salmon, mackerel, sardines, tuna and herrings can be absorbed by your body without conversion to make it usable. Omega-3s help balance hormones, protect from degeneration, and have powerful anti-inflammatory properties. Flaxseed oil is also a good source of omega-3 fatty acids. It is great used on its own or with extra-virgin olive oil to dress your salads, but it differs from fresh fish oil in a couple of significant ways. Flaxseed contains a lot of linolenic acid, which is the precursor to DHA and EPA, but the problem is that your body needs to convert the linolenic acid to DHA and EPA.

Some people can't make this conversion, especially if they have eaten a lot of trans-fatty acids and an overabundance of omega-6 fats in the past.

Ask Questions

Always ask the person serving you which fish is the freshest and what days of the week different kinds of fish arrive in the shop. You can tell a lot about the freshness of fish just by its smell and its look. Really fresh fish does not smell like fish at all. It smells more like the salty bite of a sea breeze. If it's a whole fish you are looking at, pull back the gills. They should be bright red. The moment they go pale pink or grey, you know the fish has been sitting in the shop too long. Try poking the flesh of the fish with your finger as well. If it springs back instead of forming an indentation then you're likely to have a piece of fresh fish. Check out the eye of the fish. It should be dome-shaped and clear and not sunken and murky. Because I live a fair way from the centre of the city where I buy my fish, I always protect it when I buy in quantity by taking a chill-box with me. That way it stays ultra fresh until I can get it home, bag it and freeze whatever I am not going to use immediately.

HEALTHY MEATS

The meats we get today are a far cry from those our palaeolithic ancestors ate. Probably the closest you can get to those is by buying wild boar, rabbit, buffalo, venison or kangaroo. These meats are higher in protein and lower in fat. That being said, all organic red meats like beef and lamb are excellent sources of zinc, a mineral enormously important not only for insulin balance and weight loss but also for the reproductive system and many other functions. Organic meats are the best, free of antibiotics, steroids, herbicides and pesticides.

One exciting development in some countries is that some farmers are beginning to feed their animals on foodstuffs rich in omega-3 fatty acids. Within a few years we may have meat available with a healthier fatty acid profile than the meats we have had to put up with. (It may well cost a fortune too!) Free-range and organic meat is far better than factory-farmed in every way, including the protection it offers from BSE.

When choosing dairy foods, it is good to remember that although butter is not a source of essential fatty acids, it is a perfectly respectable food – far better than margarines, no matter how fancy or sophisticated their formulation. When choosing other dairy foods, try to go low-fat. Look for low-fat cottage cheese, ricotta, mascarpone and unsweetened yoghurt. Eat a bit of cream or sour cream as a special treat now and then. Stay away from flavoured cottage cheeses, yoghurts and other dairy products which are almost always chock-full of sugar or other kinds of sweetener, as well as questionable flavourings.

Age-slowing Immune Power

The most bioavailable protein in the world, microfiltered whey, is the best and easiest way to take in quality proteins with ease – in drinks for instance. Make a great snack or quick liquid meal by mixing it with pure water and maybe a handful of berries. Use it regularly and it is a superb way to help bring about cell renewal and new tissue growth. It improves skin, strengthens arteries and restructures the musculature of your whole body. Whey protein does wonderful things for the immune system too, thanks to some of its active ingredients known as subfractions.

These subfractions, as well as other ingredients, mean that whey protein has the remarkable ability to increase your body's level of age-slowing glutathione – by providing your body with the building blocks it needs to produce glutathione itself. This is hot stuff when it comes to preventing and reversing ageing as well as protecting you from illness. Glutathione is an antioxidant. It neutralises toxicity in the body from pesticides and herbicides in our environment, from cancer-causing substances and from heavy metals and peroxides. It helps protect many physiological processes related to immune functions. It also enhances enzyme activities and protein synthesis and helps protect your DNA. Using microfiltered whey protein, which is available in health-food stores and gyms, enables you to increase the levels of glutathione and therefore your protection from free radicals in a manner that's virtually impossible any other way. You cannot rely on taking oral supplements of glutathione since your body breaks it down before it can be used.

Powerhouse Proteins

FISH AND SHELLFISH
bass
trout*
sole
sardines*
herring*
mackerel*
wild salmon*
tuna, fresh*
tuna, tinned in water
tarakihi
dory
cod*
haddock
halibut
snapper
swordfish
green-lipped mussels
calamari
oysters
clams
crayfish
lobster
crab
scallops

* rich in omega-3 essential fatty acids

MEATS
organic beef
organic pork, bacon and ham
organic lamb

GAME AND POULTRY
organic or free-range chicken
turkey
wild duck*
pheasant
quail
rabbit*
venison*
wild boar*

* rich in omega-3 essential fatty acids

EGGS

If possible, buy organic. If not, at least free-range. Eat them any way you like: soft and hard boiled, in omelettes, poached, scrambled or fried.

CHEESE

Occasional treats:

- ❏ Parmesan
- ❏ Camembert
- ❏ feta
- ❏ cottage cheese
- ❏ ricotta
- ❏ mozzarella
- ❏ mascarpone

VEGETARIAN OPTIONS

- ❏ tofu, tempeh, miso and other soya products
- ❏ microfiltered whey protein

A Good Balance of Essential Fatty Acids

OMEGA-6 – found in avocados, nuts and seeds.

OMEGA-3 – found in good supply from eating wild fish, game, flax seeds, flaxseed oil and walnuts.

The ideal ratio of one group to the other is two parts omega-6 to one part omega-3. This is what our palaeolithic ancestors got. Most of us these days get 22 parts omega-6 to one part omega-3. This is a long way from what we need for the best possible gene expression for beautiful skin. In short supply in most people's diet, the omega-3s are vitally important to skin beauty and body health. They increase the body's metabolic rate – great for fat burning. They have powerful anti-inflammatory properties – great for skin. They heighten your ability to deal with stress and increase your insulin sensitivity, helping to protect you from Syndrome X (*see page 11*).

OMEGA-9 – these fats are found in good supply in extra-virgin olive oil. Olive oil is rich in oleic acid, a monounsaturated fat which is resistant to the damaging effects of heat and light – far more than any polyunsaturated oil. Great for salads, olive oil can also be gently heated without turning into a trans fat.

COCONUT OIL – What? But isn't this a saturated fat? It is indeed. So is butter, which you can eat on the Powerhouse diet too. The fats in coconut oil, however, are something special. Far from contributing to heart disease and other degenerative processes, medium-chain triglycerides (MCTs) found in coconut actually help lower cholesterol. In Sri Lanka, where coconut oil is the main source of dietary fat, you will find the lowest death rate from heart disease in the world. Coconut also encourages your body to shed its fat stores and offers great help to sugar babies wanting to become lean machines. Years ago, farmers figured a good way to fatten cattle for market would be to feed them coconut oil. After all, it was cheap, widely available and high in calories. Their experiment failed dismally. The animals only grew leaner and more muscular. Over 50 per cent of the fat in coconut consists of MCTs. Great for skin and your whole body, coconut also fills you up and provides energy when you need it, helping to eliminate cravings for sugar and muffins.

POWERHOUSE FATS

The fats you'll be eating are the healthiest available. Most can be used in salad dressings or for cooking proteins. Eat at least a tablespoon or so per meal from the list below. In addition to the fat you get from food, use 2 teaspoons of flaxseed oil every day on your salads and, if you are over 35, consider taking a good supplement of omega-3 EPA and DHA fish oils.

- ❑ almonds and almond butter
- ❑ avocados (and guacamole)
- ❑ butter
- ❑ coconut oil
- ❑ extra-virgin olive oil
- ❑ flaxseed oil (never cook with it)

❑ macadamia nuts and macadamia butter
❑ olives
❑ tahini

Powerhouse Drinks

As far as drinks are concerned, the best you can find is pure water. Buy it plain, sparkling or even flavoured, so long as there are no artificial sweeteners in the product. These days you can find a huge selection of good herbal teas, as well as organic green tea. Rich in antioxidants, green tea is the best drink around for the body. Coffee is a major contributor to body inflammation and blood sugar disorders. It also dries out your body – even an oily body – making it age more rapidly. Avoid it altogether if you can. If not, limit yourself to one cup a day.

Water plays the major part in digesting your food and absorbing nutrients, thanks to its role in helping your body create enzymes needed for digestion. When you don't drink enough water between meals your mouth becomes low in saliva and the body shows it. Water is the medium through which wastes are eliminated from your body. Each time you exhale, you release highly humidified air – about two big glasses' worth a day – and metabolic wastes carried on it. Your kidneys and intestines eliminate another six or so glasses of water and waste every 24 hours, while another two glasses' worth are released through the pores in your body. That makes 10 glasses a day – and this is on a cool day. When it gets hot, when you are exercising or working hard, the usual 10 glasses lost in this way can triple.

POWERFUL WATER

On average, in a temperate climate – when you are not sweating from exertion or heat – you need about 3.5 litres or 6 pints of water a day for optimal health, although few of us consume as much as one-third of that. The important thing to remember is that how thirsty you are is not a reliable indication of how much water you need to drink. Do as French women have done for decades. Keep a large bottle or two of pure, fresh mineral water within easy reach and make sure you consume your quota of this clear, delicious, health-giving drink.

Here are some tips for Powerhouse drinking:

❑ Use filtered or spring water.
❑ Choose herbal teas, flavoured mineral water (only those with no sweeteners or calories) and organic vegetable bouillon or broth.
❑ Make vegetable broth with broccoli, cabbage, cauliflower, bean sprouts, asparagus, mustard greens, spinach, watercress, ginger, garlic in any combination. Bring to the boil and simmer for 15 minutes. Season with herbs and sea salt and store in the fridge, reheating as necessary.
❑ Go easy on alcohol. A glass of good wine a day – two at the very most – is great to aim for.

GO EASY ON ALCOHOL

Alcohol is another substance you want to go easy on. Not only is it high in empty calories and pretty useless in terms of nutrients, alcohol causes your liver to produce one of the most potent cross-linkers known for the body – acetaldehyde. The more acetaldehyde in your body, the faster your body ages. Spirits like whisky, gin and vodka raise insulin levels so are best avoided. A glass of dry white or red wine with one of your meals does most people no harm. It may even have a beneficial effect. A number of studies indicate that red wine, in particular, increases the body's sensitivity to insulin and carries some antioxidant power too. If you choose to have a glass or two, make sure you only drink *good* wine. Run of the mill *vin de table* is full of toxic substances your body can do without.

Powerhouse Extras

SEEDS FOR SPROUTING
These make great sprouts. Grow them in bowls on your kitchen worktop (*see Free, Wild and Cautious*). Always buy organic if you can:

- ❑ mung beans
- ❑ chickpeas
- ❑ marrow fat peas
- ❑ adzuki beans
- ❑ black lentils
- ❑ brown lentils
- ❑ raw buckwheat

SALAD DRESSINGS AND SAUCES
You can make these with walnut oil, extra-virgin olive oil or flaxseed oil together with lemon juice, Champagne vinegar, red wine, balsamic or apple cider vinegar (*see Dress It Up*).

FIBRE
The raw fruits and vegetables you will be eating in your salads are full of wonderful fibre. So is sprouted buckwheat. You can also add some whole or ground flax seeds to salads and mueslis for extra fibre if you ever feel you need it.

NUTS
When buying nuts make sure they are really fresh. The rancid oils in old nuts are harmful to the stomach, retard the secretion of pancreatic enzymes and destroy vitamins. If nuts are fresh and still in their shells you can buy them in largish quantities and keep them in an airtight container in a cool, dry place (preferably your refrigerator) for up to several months. Shelled nuts should be bought in much smaller quantities and they too should be refrigerated. It is a good idea to buy several different kinds and mix them in your recipes so that you get a good balance of essential amino acids. These are some of the nuts I regularly stock up with: almonds, brazils, cashews, coconut (fresh or desiccated), hazelnuts, macadamia nuts, peanuts (strictly speaking a legume), pecans (similar to walnuts but less bitter), pine kernels, pistachios, tiger nuts and walnuts.

SWEETENERS

The best natural sweetener in the world is stevia. Sadly it is not available in the EU for rather silly regulatory reasons to do with the lobbying power of the big chemical companies which sell artificial sweeteners like aspartame and saccharine. Artificial sweeteners are foreign chemicals and are not good to use at any time. Many studies show that they can have a dangerous effect on living organisms when used regularly. If you can get stevia, use it. It is 300 times sweeter than sugar itself and good for you. It comes in many varieties. The best is the organic Stevita Spoonable Stevia which can be used just as you would use ordinary sugar, although you will need a great deal less of it.

Maple syrup and Manuka honey are two alternatives for sweetening which carry some nutritional value apart from calories. Used in moderate amounts, Manuka honey does not have the same insulin-unbalancing effect that other honeys, sugars, malt extracts and the rest do. Manuka honey has a far greater molecular density than any other form of honey. It is this that makes it behave differently in the body. It also has remarkable anti-bacterial and anti-viral properties.

A WINNING DUO

Following these guidelines will automatically provide you with body transformation of the highest order. Powerhouse eating is rich in nutrients as well as in the biophoton order necessary to maintain a high degree of resistance to body reactions and degeneration. Provided your foods are fresh enough, and provided you eat at least half of them raw, you will also benefit from all the phytonutrients they bring your body.

HERBS AND SPICES

Buy spices and dried herbs in small quantities from shops that sell a lot of them, as they soon lose their freshness. The most flavourful herbs are freeze-dried, but these can be hard to find. Vacuum-sealed herbs are a good bet. Herbs and spices should be stored in the dark as the light affects their potency. So much for herb and spice racks! For the sake of flavour, it is best to buy whole spices and grind them as needed in a coffee grinder or with a mortar and pestle. If you have never ground your own spices, you will be amazed at the exhilarating aromas and tastes. With fresh herbs, wash and dry them well, then store in sealed polythene bags in the salad compartment of your fridge.

GENTLE HELPERS

Make good use of whatever fresh culinary herbs you have available: caraway, fennel, dill, chervil, parsley, lovage – the Umbelliferae family; summer savory, marjoram, the mints, rosemary and thyme – the Labiatae which have a strong aroma and are particularly useful for seasoning; the Liliaceae such as garlic, onions, chives and leeks. These three are my favourites: basil, tarragon and horseradish.

Herbs have a special role to play in Powerhouse eating. They contain pharmacologically active substances such as volatile oils, tannins, bitter factors, secretins, balsams, resins, mucilages, glycosides and organic vegetable acids, each of which contributes to overall health in a different way. The *tannins* in common kitchen herbs are astringent. They exert an anti-inflammatory action on the digestive system. They help inhibit fermentation and decomposition. The *secretins* stimulate the secretion of the pancreatic enzymes – particularly important for the complete breakdown of proteins in foods to make them available for bodily use. *Organic acids* in herbs have an antibiotic action and are helpful in the digestion of fats. So are the *bitter factors* – found in good-quality rosemary, marjoram and fennel. They also act as a tonic to soothe gut muscles and boost secretion of digestive enzymes. Use herbs lavishly in your meals and you will find you can create the most remarkable combinations of subtle flavours and aromas.

SAVOURY SEASONING POWDERS

I find the following seasonings useful in those moments of panic when a dish is lacking in that vital 'something': Cajun seasoning and Mexican chilli seasoning. One rescue remedy I wouldn't be without is good vegetable bouillon powder or cubes. I use it in dressings, sauces, ferments and soups, and in seed and nut dishes. Buy your seasonings from health-food stores as the ones you get in supermarkets tend to have been irradiated.

You can of course make your own seasoning powder. A recipe I am particularly fond of is made up as follows:

50g (2oz) onion powder
15g (½oz) garlic powder
70g (2½oz) comfrey leaf/powder

1 tsp cayenne pepper
1 tbsp kelp
15g (½oz) ginger powder

You can also make your own spice mixture for drinks and desserts by combining powdered allspice, coriander seeds, cinnamon, cloves, ginger, nutmeg and mace to taste.

FREE, WILD AND CAUTIOUS

The annual parade of fruits and vegetables in the average greengrocer's shop gives you a very poor idea of the amazing variety of edible plants. The cooks of past centuries relied heavily on herbs, salad greens, nuts, fruits, seeds, spices, flowers and seaweeds gathered from the countryside. You can find many of these wild plants growing locally. You can also sprout your own power vegetables in the kitchen. They are cheap, easy and fun.

Food for Free
Plenty of wild plants are edible, in small quantities. They tend to be filled with much higher levels of important phytonutrients than those we grow ourselves. Make use of them – they are wild, wonderful and free. A few are poisonous. Take a look at a wild plant encyclopaedia before you start foraging – one that gives all the fascinating culinary and medicinal uses of our native plants.

By their very nature, 'weeds' possess an incredible strength and resistance to all that weather, poor soil, parasites and disease can throw at them, and they have remarkable reproductive capacities. They have strong, foraging roots which penetrate the soil to great depths, and growing shoots that can struggle up to the light even through concrete. They are full of vitamins and minerals. Most should be used in moderation as they have sharply individual tastes.

Here are a few wild plants you might like to try:

❑ *Young dandelion leaves:* These contain lots of nutrients including calcium, potassium, sodium, silicon, phosphorus, iron, oxalic acid (cleanses the gall bladder and kidneys), vitamins A and C, and choline (essential to the efficient conduction of nerve impulses). The youngest leaves are delicious in salads. Be sure to pick real dandelions (there are many frauds): they have no hairs, the leaves have deeply toothed edges, are soft and not glossy, and the flowers are borne on a single stem. Dandelions are notably alkaline and therefore good for arthritis sufferers and anyone addicted to alcohol or white bread! They are digested very quickly and have a tonic action on the liver and kidneys.

❏ *Dock and Sorrel:* These have a good mineral balance and are particularly high in sulphur. They are good body cleansers, and have a tonic effect on the blood. Due to their vitamin A content they are good for an overworked liver. Sorrel is especially delicious in salads and soups, giving a very fresh, lemony taste.

❏ *Horehound:* This is high in vitamin C. Chopped and mixed with a little honey, it is a good cold remedy.

❏ *Plantain:* A very common weed this, noted for its blood-cleansing properties. It is high in chlorophyll and can be juiced with other vegetables to give a blood-boosting, chlorophyll-rich drink.

❏ *Chickweed:* After bindweed, the intruder most hated by gardeners. Chickweed has tiny starry white flowers and grows straggling across the ground. Its pale stems and small soft green leaves make it a nice addition to green and herb salads. Don't confuse it with milkweed or mouse-ear chickweed.

❏ *Couch grass:* A good diuretic this, particularly for women who retain water at the beginning of their periods. The runners can be chopped into salads.

❏ *Purslane:* Highly alkaline, purslane has a soothing effect, especially on over-acid stomachs. Its bright-green fleshy leaves, borne on purplish stems, can be shredded and added to salads.

Just to give you an idea of the variety awaiting the discerning rambler, here are some other palatable and flavourful free foods:

SALADS FOR FREE

SALADS: Salad burnet, watercress (usually an escapee), very young lime, beech and hawthorn leaves, fat hen, burdock, marsh samphire, common mallow leaves, chicory, wild cabbage

HERBS: Water mint, spearmint, apple mint, pennyroyal, wild marjoram and thyme, bay, jack by the hedge, ramsons (wild garlic), lovage, chervil, borage

SEEDS: Fennel, coriander, juniper

AS FLAVOURINGS OR INFUSIONS: Tansy, sweet cicely, galingale

ROOTS: Horseradish, pignuts, wild parsnip
SEAWEEDS: Kelp, dulse, laver, carragheen
FLOWERS AS FLAVOURINGS OR SALAD ADDITIONS:
Sweet violets, honeysuckle, wild rose petals, red clover,
chamomile, nasturtiums, broom buds, elder flowers,
meadowsweet
NUTS: Hazelnuts (filberts), sweet chestnuts, beechnuts
FRUITS: Blackberries, wild pears, crab apples, rose hips, sloes,
elderberries
FUNGI: Field mushrooms, ceps, boletus, horn of plenty, shaggy
inkcaps, blewits, chanterelles

It is interesting that weeds growing in areas where the atmosphere is polluted seem to be unaffected by their unhealthy environment. This is because most weeds have two root systems, one superficial in contact with the air and soil surface, and the other deep underground where all the nutrients are. The nutrients absorbed by deep tap roots pass up into the main body of the plant for synthesis into compounds which the plant needs. Pollution of ground water is different. The less cultivated the area where you pick your weeds the better, as it is less likely to contain pesticide residues, artificial fertilisers or dissolved detergents.

I am not advocating a return to a hunter-gatherer existence or that you ransack the countryside for these plants. However, you can grow many of these things in your own garden, and many of them grow wild there anyway. Eating them can make weeding a lot more interesting! Wild greens and herbs are generally more nutritious and healthy than the cultivated varieties you buy in shops. They also make you realise to what extent cultivation and mass-production techniques have muted the taste experiences available to us. I feel, quite simply, that some curiosity about wild plants, and a respect for them, is part of a Powerhouse life.

Sprout it Yourself
The beauty of sprouts is in their simplicity. They are one of the most fascinating natural phenomena – they release exceptionally nutritious vitamins and enzymes, and are delicious as well.

WHAT YOU NEED
Seeds – e.g. mung beans, chick peas, marrow fat peas, adzuki beans, black lentils, brown lentils, radish, mustard.

METHOD ONE:
Jar or bowl to soak seeds
Nylon sieve
Cheesecloth or stainless-steel sprouting screen

Place two handfuls of seeds or beans in the bottom of a jar or bowl and cover with plenty of water – use one part seed to at least three parts water. Leave to soak overnight. Pour the seeds into a sieve and rinse well with water. Be sure to remove any dead or broken seeds or pieces of debris. If you are using glass jars then return the soaked seeds to the jar after rinsing well and cover with the cheesecloth or sprouting screen, secure with a rubber band, drain well and keep in a warm dark place (18°C/65°F is ideal). They can even be covered with a bag or a cloth to create the darkness. Rinse thoroughly twice a day and be sure to drain them well or you will find they may draw mould.

or

METHOD TWO (MY FAVOURITE):
Rectangular glass dishes with 5-cm/2-inch sides and top
A terry cloth towel

Place seeds in rectangular glass dish and cover with 5 cm/2 inches of water. Let soak for 24 hours. Pour off water and rinse thoroughly two or three times. Drain. Cover with a damp terry cloth to hold moisture in, yet let the growing plants breathe. Rinse thoroughly once a day in cool weather, twice a day in hot weather.

Some sprouts, such as radish or mustard, are zesty and add fire to any dish. They mix well with milder sprouts such as mung beans. While they are sprouting, the hulls of some seeds come off – usually while you are rinsing them. Discard the hulls as they tend to rot easily. You can do this by placing the sprouts in a big bowl of water and shaking it gently to separate the hulls from the sprouts themselves. Usually the hulls sink to the bottom.

After about three days, place the seeds in sunlight for several hours to develop the chlorophyll in them. Rinse in a sieve, drain well and put in a polythene bag in the refrigerator to use in salads, stir-fries, etc. There are many different seeds you can sprout, each with its own particular flavour and texture. Use the chart as a guide to the variety of sprouts you can try.

HOW TO SPROUT

Seed and soak time	To yield 1 litre (1¾ pints)	Ready to eat in	Length of shoot	Growing tips and notes
Red clover (6–8 hrs)	3 tbsp	5–6 days	3.5cm (1½in)	Rich in organic vitamins and minerals, and natural oestrogens.
Fenugreek (6–8 hrs)	120g (4oz)	3–4 days	12mm (½in)	Have quite a strong 'curry' taste. Good for ridding the body of toxins.
Adzuki beans (10–15 hrs)	350g (12oz)	3–5 days	2.5–3.5 cm (1–1½ in)	Have a nutty flavour. Especially good for the kidneys.
Chickpeas (10–15 hrs)	200g (7oz)	3–4 days	2.5cm (1in)	May need to soak for 18 hrs to swell to their full size. Replace the water during this time.
Marrow Fat Peas (10–15 hrs)	200g (7oz)	3–4 days	2.5cm (1in)	Have an interesting 'grainy' texture.
Lentils (8 hrs)	120g (4oz)	3–5 days	5mm–2.5cm (¼–1in)	Try all different kinds of lentils. They are good eaten young or up to 6 days old.
Mung beans (15 hrs)	120g (4oz)	3–5 days	1–6cm (½–2½in)	Keep in the dark for a sweet sprout.

Seed and soak time	To yield 1 litre (1¾ pints)	Ready to eat in	Length of shoot	Growing tips and notes
Radish or mustard (6–8 hrs)	40g (1½oz)	5–6 days	1–6cm (½–2½ in)	Beautifully spicy and mix well with everything.
Wheat (12–15 hrs)	225g (8oz)	2–3 days	Same length as grain	An excellent source of the B-vitamins. The soak water can be drunk straight or added to soups and vegetable juices.

Sprouting Cereal Grasses

Cereal grasses can be grown all year round wherever you live and regardless of whether you have a garden. Use organic seed, which should be available from good health-food stores. Cereal grasses can only be juiced using a machine specifically designed for this purpose. Alternatively, they can be put into a powerful blender with 100ml (4fl oz) of raw fresh juice or spring water and blended for 10 to 20 seconds to pulverise them. Then you need to strain away the indigestible cellulose before serving.

WHAT YOU NEED

A seed-tray (a kitchen tray will do)
Organic compost
Plant spray or water mister
8–10 layers of newspaper
A sheet of plastic to cover the tray
Seed – hard red winter wheat or buckwheat, barley, etc.

HERE'S HOW

Soak approximately 225g (8oz) of seed for 12 hours in water (cover well), pour off the water and allow to drain for 12 hours. Half-fill the seed tray with compost (so that the compost comes halfway up the sides of the tray), level the surface and spray with a fine mist. Make sure you do not soak the compost. Place the soaked seeds on the wet soil so that they are evenly spread and not on top of each other. Soak the newspaper thoroughly, cut to the size of the seed tray and cover the seeds. Place the plastic on top of the newspaper. Leave the tray in a well-ventilated, not over-warm room for three days. At the end of three days, remove the plastic and newspaper and put the trays somewhere they will get plenty of light – a sunny windowsill, for instance – and water once a day, making sure you do not soak the soil. In about five to eight days, the plants should be 6–8 centimetres high, standing upright and nicely green. They are then ready to cut. Cut the greens close to the soil with a sharp knife. They can be kept in the fridge in plastic bags for several days.

Powerhouse Cautions

Some raw foods, especially the pulses, have a rather chequered image among health-food enthusiasts. Much depends on whether you eat them raw, cooked or sprouted, and on complementary nutrients in your diet.

Some of the beans, for instance, have certain negative attributes. Soya beans, broad beans and red kidney beans have a trypsin inhibitor, a substance which blocks the action of some of the enzymes in the body which break down protein. This means that a proportion of the valuable amino acids they contain cannot be used. Many years ago, researchers discovered that soya beans could not support life unless they were cooked for several hours. Cooking and sprouting neutralise the trypsin inhibitor.

In fact, sprouting greatly improves the safety and nutritional quality of all pulses, seeds and grains. The enzymes which go into action during germination not only neutralise trypsin-inhibiting factors but also destroy harmful substances such as phytic acid, an important constituent of seeds and grains, which tends to bind minerals, making them unavailable to the body. Sprouting, by destroying phytic acid, releases minerals for us.

Sprout Them

Chickpeas also contain a trypsin inhibitor, rendered harmless by sprouting but not by cooking. Green peas contain a hemaggluten which resists cooking (hemagglutins inhibit growth by combining with the cells lining the intestine and blocking nutrient absorption) – but in such small quantities that one would have to eat virtually nothing but peas, raw or cooked, to experience any adverse effects. Eating raw lima beans has been known to cause death.

Rhubarb leaves are widely known to be poisonous. This is because they contain massive amounts of oxalic acid. The stems contain much less. Swiss chard, beet greens, turnip and mustard greens, collards, kale, spinach and French sorrel also contain oxalic acid. If eaten to excess the acid in them can block calcium absorption and cause kidney damage as acid crystals deposit themselves in the urinary system. Although oxalic acid is not destroyed by cooking, it appears qualitatively different from the oxalic acid in raw foods. Norman W. Walker, the American raw-food expert, insists that the oxalic acid in raw foods has no harmful effect. On the contrary, it stimulates peristalsis (rhythmic squeezing of food through the gut). He and others often recommend adding spinach juice to other fresh vegetable juices for its oxalic acid content.

Thyroid Cautions

Another group of vegetables, the brassicas, has been blamed for suppressing thyroid activity. Cabbage, Chinese leaves, watercress, kale, turnips, Brussels sprouts and mustard all belong to the genus *Brassica*. They contain compounds called thioglucosides which can disrupt the function of the thyroid gland, and have been shown to contribute to the development of goitre. Drinking the milk of animals who have been grazing on these plants can also disrupt thyroid function. But you are unlikely to experience the undesirable effects of thioglucosides if you take in adequate iodine (from fish or seaweed) in the diet. It is only people deficient in iodine who suffer.

The Raw Egg Question

People are often cautioned against eating raw eggs. Raw egg yolks are fine, provided they are organic and free range. Egg whites do contain avidin, a substance which combines with the B-vitamin biotin and prevents its absorption into the blood. One young man who ate lots of raw egg whites developed scaly skin, anaemia, anorexia, nausea and muscle pains because of biotin deficiency. This is, of course, an extreme case. Raw egg whites are less likely to cause such symptoms if eaten with the yolks. Also, the albumen in egg whites can easily enter the bloodstream undigested and can cause allergies. I generally only use yolks in my cuisine. However, I don't think twice about preparing delicious eggnog occasionally, using the yolks and the whites. It is all a question of moderation.

NATURE'S SUPPLEMENTS

No matter how much we 'enrich' foods with specific nutraceutical compounds, we can never create the health-enhancing synergy of whole foods themselves. Only Nature can do that. That's why most of the optional supplements I use to complement Powerhouse eating, like green barley, MSM, wheat grass and Pure Synergy, are derived from Nature itself.

Sulphur is the most important element in your body. There is a high level of physiological sulphur in the healthy body. It helps regulate the sodium/potassium balance, bringing nutrients and oxygen to cells and neutralising wastes. A unique form of sulphur, MSM – *methyl-sulphonyl-methane* – is a superb free-radical scavenger. MSM is found in rain water, the sea and all living organisms. It exists in especially high concentrations in raw vegetables, fruits and seafood. Unless your diet is composed primarily of raw foods it is highly unlikely that you are getting enough MSM for optimal health.

POTENT HEALER

'MSM, an odourless, essentially tasteless, white crystalline chemical, demonstrates usefulness as a dietary supplement in man and lower animals. Our research suggests that a minimum concentration in the body may be critical to both normal function and structure. Limited studies suggest that the systemic concentration of MSM drops in mammals with increasing age. This may be due to dietary habits where one ingests food with lower MSM potential with maturity, or possibly, there is a change in the renal threshold.'

Dr Stanley Jacob

MSM – physiological sulphur – is important for clearing toxic build-up on a cellular level and in the body as a whole. It is safe as well as highly effective. Even people who are 'allergic' to sulphur and sulphur-based food additives thrive on it.

MSM Magic

As a prime free-radical scavenger, physiological sulphur also helps rid the body of allergies. It even protects the lining of the digestive tract from parasites and pathogens. This is important for skin, for when leaky gut or dysbiosis occurs in the digestive tract, skin suffers. If you have a tendency to acne, you can break out. If your skin tends to be dry, this can make it drier and give the face a colourless, lifeless look. Sulphur is also essential for cartilage strength and to build keratin – the fibrous protein out of which hair and nails are made – as well as to virtually every function of the skin. With extra MSM your nails grow faster and stronger. Your hair gets thicker and shinier.

A good dose of MSM is 2,000mg for each 60 kilos (130 pounds) of weight a day. Start with 500mg per 60 kilos of weight and work up. Use together with half that amount of vitamin C, preferably in the form of calcium or magnesium ascorbate (so if you take 2g of MSM, take 1g of vitamin C).

Potentiated Pollen

When it comes to brain power and using a natural supplement to protect your body from stress, you can't do better than bee pollen. It enhances immunity, improves digestion and is in many ways considered a complete food all on its own, boasting 22 elements essential to the human body as well as 27 vitamins and amino acids, 28 minerals, enzymes, RNA, DNA, micronutrients and hormones – all in synergy and balance. This superfood is something I never do without. It is great to mix into drinks or take from a spoon – a teaspoon two or three times a day.

Pollen must never be heated as heat destroys much of its value. A microscopic seed, pollen protects its nutrients with a hard cell wall which can resist even temperatures of 3,000 degrees during forest fires. This gives a grain of pollen the ability to lie dormant for a few thousand years and still retain its reproductive power. Special low-heat processes, which act as the reverse of decompression used to protect deep sea divers from the bends, are used to blow open the cell walls of pollen, releasing its nutritional bounty. It is important always to choose a pollen that has been 'potentiated' for you to get the full value of what it has to offer and, if you can find one, an organic pollen. You can take pollen in capsules or, as I prefer, from a spoon. It's great to keep you going on long-haul flights when you don't want to have to cope with the airline meals. Very occasionally someone might be allergic to bee pollen so it is a good plan to try only a little to start with and check this out before taking larger quantities.

Phytonutrient Scavenger Radicals

'Antioxidants' and 'free radicals' have become buzz words. Go into any pharmacy or health-food store and half of the products on the shelf have these terms written all over their labels. Yet most people are not clear about what they mean. Simply put, a free radical is a highly reactive oxygen molecule which can destroy tissues – particularly cell membranes and genetic materials. Electrons in molecules usually come in pairs. When oxygen is burnt in the body – a process absolutely necessary for life – one member of an electron pair can get stripped away, turning the molecule into a free radical and making it highly unstable. So it rushes about frantically looking for another electron to mate with. It desperately grabs on to any electron available, often destroying the molecule it has stolen it from, creating a chain reaction. These beastie molecules can tear through cell membranes and mitochondria membranes, shredding them, screwing up the cell's functions and even threatening its life.

PLANT PROTECTION

Natural antioxidants occur together in fresh raw foods. The leaves or the flesh of a plant or a mushroom can contain many different antioxidant immune-enhancing phytochemicals. Antioxidants work together and empower each other. The essential antioxidants carry the ability to deactivate free radicals, rendering them harmless. Vitamin C's overall talents as a vitamin, for instance, are quite distinct from its antioxidant properties. Some antioxidants, such as the bright-coloured carotenoids in vegetables, and tocopherols – forms of vitamin E, are also involved in cellular signalling. Others can play a role in gene expression or in guiding and regulating the actions of enzymes.

The best source of antioxidant support for your body comes through a diet high in fresh organic fruits, vegetables, sprouted seeds and herbs plus first-rate protein foods and plenty of essential fats. Such a diet supplies an almost perfect balance of essential antioxidant vitamins A,

C and E, and the antioxidant minerals zinc and selenium, all of which bring significant anti-ageing help. This way of eating also provides the body with a high complement of potent plant-based antioxidants which have proven to be of value. If you want to use phytonutrient supplements, it is best to buy a wide-spectrum, plant-based, antioxidant formula which includes most of the best phytonutrients, since they work in synergy. You can also find formulas based on plant-factor antioxidant vitamins and minerals. When it comes to combining nutraceuticals, the whole is far greater than the sum of its parts.

A WINNING FORMULA

When choosing a plant-based antioxidant, supplement or multiple vitamin and mineral, look for one that includes these phytonutrients:

❑ **Carotenoids** give vibrant fruits and vegetables their colour. More than 600 varieties have been identified. Fat soluble, they seek out the lipids in cell membranes where they protect from free-radical damage, look after the integrity of DNA, improve cell communication necessary for growth and reproduction and support immune functions.

❑ **Lycopene,** a red carotenoid found in tomatoes, pink grapefruit and watermelon, is the most efficient quencher of single oxygen free radicals. It protects against degeneration and cancer.

❑ **Flavonoids** and other **phenolics** belong to a large group of organic plant molecules produced by plants to protect themselves from attack by disease and insects, and from damage by intense UV light. Some, such as the anthocyanins found in wine, are deep red, some purple, others bright blue. They often have an astringent or slightly bitter taste. Green tea is rich in these flavonoid antioxidants, which is one of the reasons it is an excellent drink for skin. You will also find them in onions, apples and citrus fruits. They mop up free radicals, help fight off viruses, calm inflammation and help protect from allergies.

Go Green for Oxygen

Green foods are superfoods. Not only do they help clean up your body and continue to detoxify, they also help protect it from future damage by offering a high level of synergistic nutrients, immune enhancers and specific phytochemicals which together work their magic.

GREEN INHERITANCE

Some three billion years ago, algae began to fix nitrogen and sugars and, in the process, to release oxygen. If it had not been for the algae on the earth and the oxidation they produced, we would not have come into being. Nor would all the other animals who depend upon oxygen-based metabolism to survive. It is the algae that created the oxygen-rich atmosphere on which the rest of life was able to develop, and the whole process took over one billion years to complete. Blue-green algae are microscopic organisms that are harvested from freshwater lakes, ponds and man-made tanks. Using them as superfood supplements renews the body in no small part because they supply living cells with the oxygen they need to thrive.

Primordial Bounty

Spirulina is a near-microscopic form of blue-green algae made up of translucent bubble-thin cells stacked end to end to form an incredibly beautiful, deep-green helix. It is the most well known of the blue-green algae, of which there are more than 1,500 species. The chemical makeup of each species is unique. All are rich in beta-carotene and other antioxidants, B-complex vitamins, iron and trace minerals, chlorophyll, enzymes and various other plant factors. Some species are also rich in gammalinolenic acid (GLA), an omega-6 fatty acid that helps counter inflammation, lower cholesterol, and may even help protect against heart disease.

Spirulina, like many of the algae, is also rich in an unusual quality of protein which is alkaline rather than acid forming. It can play an important part in detoxifying the body and also in helping you deal with high levels of stress. Rich in vitamins E, B_{12}, B_1, B_5 and B_6 as well as beta-carotene, spirulina also contains good quantities of the minerals zinc, copper, manganese and selenium as well as other anti-ageing phytonutrients including *phycocyanin*, a blue pigment structurally similar to beta-carotene. The World Health Organisation, in attempting to deal with blindness due to vitamin A deficiency amongst malnourished children in India, found that when one gram of spirulina was added to their diet, there was a significant improvement. Recently, too, a report from the *Journal of the American Neutraceutical Association* indicated that a particular type of blue-green algae, *Aphanizoomenom flos-aquae* (AFA), has the ability to increase the surveillance activities of important immune cells. Researchers concluded that AFA may help prevent cancers by boosting immunity amongst mutant cells that can lead to the disease.

LIQUID LIFE

Adding between a teaspoon and a tablespoon of organic spirulina to a glass of water, juice or protein drink each day is a good way to reap the benefits it carries. As with all algae, however, it is important to use only organically grown varieties for some wild algae products may be contaminated by environmental toxins, bacteria, animal wastes or other potentially harmful substances.

Full-spectrum Radiance

Chlorella, another important green algae, is sometimes called the emerald food. It too can spike up protein drinks and juices. Chlorella gets its name from its high chlorophyll content – the highest of any known plant. In addition, chlorella is high in minerals, vitamins, fibre, nucleic acids, ammonia acids, enzymes and something called CGF – chlorella growth factor.

Chlorella contains the full spectrum of the carotenoids important for defending the cells against oxidation damage while other phytochemicals strengthen the immune system, encouraging the production of interferon. Because chlorella enhances the growth of beneficial bacteria in the intestines, it is also soothing and healing to the gastro-intestinal tract. It is used to advantage by people with *Candida albicans*, diverticulitis, Crohn's disease and ulcers.

Protein Detox

Chlorella has been cultivated in developing countries as an inexpensive substitute for animal proteins, for it is over 60 per cent protein. But chlorella offers some other important properties as well. Its high concentration of chlorophyll makes it a powerful detoxifier and allows it to play an important role in any purification programme. It helps eliminate many toxic wastes from the body, including cadmium and even uranium.

DETOX HELPER

Chlorella helps protect the liver from toxic injury. Some practitioners claim it can even help prevent hangovers by promoting the removal of alcohol from the body. Even half a teaspoon of chlorella a day, stirred into a glass of juice or other cold drink, can be of benefit. Many vegans rely on chlorella as well as seaweeds and algae as a source of vitamin B_{12}, since it has been shown to elevate blood levels of this vitamin. Chlorella also contains more pantothenic acid than any other natural source plus many of the other important B-vitamins, magnesium and other trace elements.

Green Lightning

Green barley and wheat grass are freeze-dried forms of the natural juice taken from young leaves. They need to be organically grown and pesticide free. Rich in proteins, flavonoids, minerals including iron, vitamins such as K and B_{15}, as well as chlorophyll and other nutrients, both are also rich in thousands of enzymes, not all of which are destroyed in the digestive process and many of which can play important roles in supporting metabolic processes. And they also contain a high concentration of superoxide dismutase (SOD), an antioxidant enzyme, as well as MSM. Both of these powdered grass juices help cleanse the tissues of toxic wastes, including heavy metals like lead, cadmium and aluminium. Sprinkle from half to one teaspoon of green barley on to salads, or mix into juices, miso broth or water.

Because all green superfoods are full of life, they degrade easily. This makes it essential to choose your green supplements carefully. The best are made from organic plants, processed at ultra-low heat to preserve their enzymes and integrity, and packed in glass to prevent the leaking of oxygen through plastics that cause oxidation. You can take supergreen foods as capsules, tablets or in powder form. Often you will find them mixed together, but the quality of the mixes varies tremendously from one manufacturer to another.

PURE SYNERGY – THE BEST

The best green superfood I have ever found is a supplement called Pure Synergy™. It is a combination of 62 of Nature's most potent and nourishing components including organic green juices, herbs, wild-crafted algae, and many other natural ingredients, all of them either wild or organically grown and carefully formulated in a synergistic way so that the energies of each balance those of the other. I begin each day with a drink of microfiltered whey protein, to which I add a little stevia and a teaspoon or two of Pure Synergy™, as well as some psyllium husks and organic flax seeds for extra fibre. This makes a quick breakfast or a wonderful meal or snack on the run during the day.

Each of us is biochemically unique. Ideally, if you want to design a concentrated programme of nutritional supplements, it is a good idea to consult a good nutritionally oriented doctor or health practitioner who can help you develop one tailored to your specific needs.

FIVE

GET INTO PLEASURE

Powerhouse 'cooking' is based on creative play, excitement, experimentation and sensuous enjoyment of fresh foods which enhance health in medically measurable ways. Pick foods that excite you, inspire you and delight you. Never follow a recipe by rote. To me that would be boring – the kind of 'sheep' mentality that went out with the 20th century. The recipes you find here are in no way meant to be imprisoning. I want them to be inspirational – to encourage you to explore the infinite possibilities of creating wonderful meals for all occasions with minimum effort and maximum fun. In Powerhouse cookery it is not rules that matter. What's important is a kind of passion for the foods themselves which is reflected in an affection for the earth and for all life.

DRINK YOUR BREAKFAST

Who, these days, has time for breakfast? Yet breakfast is an important meal. Not that you need to stuff yourself with food you don't want, for energy. That is an old wives' tale. You might be surprised at just how simple it can be to make a delicious morning meal. I'm not into breakfasts that take a long time to prepare – there are more interesting things to do at the beginning of the day.

There is a quick-start breakfast that is just right for you. You may be someone who thrives on a sense of emptiness, in which case reach for a glass of fresh vegetable and fruit juice which will let your body continue the process of inner cleansing that takes place each night through to lunch. You may crave something more substantial. Try a smoothie based on microfiltered whey – the best protein around. If you are someone who never gains weight no matter what you eat – the only class of people in the world whom I passionately envy – you are probably better off going for an instant whole porridge meal. Experiment. Find out what works best for you. Don't be afraid to change with the seasons either. Your body and psyche are always evolving, so let how you eat evolve with them. Whatever way you go, breakfast should be not only delicious, but instantaneous too.

Get Juiced

A glass of fresh juice can give you a terrific lift in the morning. You will feel almost immediately refreshed, alert and eager to see what another day has in store.

SPICY CARROT
Vegan
Serves 2

This juice is a great source of minerals such as magnesium, potassium, calcium, iron, sulphur, copper, phosphorus and iodine, as well as anti-oxidants beta-carotene, vitamins A, C, E and niacin, vitamins D and K. It will also soothe a slightly delicate stomach. Braeburn and Cox's apples are ideal for this juice, but any sweet apple will do.

WHAT YOU NEED
4 carrots
2 spears of pineapple
1 Braeburn or Cox's apple
pinch of ground cinnamon
pinch of ground nutmeg

HERE'S HOW
Juice all ingredients except the cinnamon and nutmeg. Pineapples vary considerably in size. You'll need half a small one or a quarter of a large one. Remove the fibrous skin with a sharp knife and cut into long spears that will fit into your juicer. The cinnamon and nutmeg can be sprinkled on top of the freshly-extracted juice or stirred in as you prefer.

SPROUT SPECIAL
Vegan
Serves 3

This juice is rich in natural phytohormones that help protect the body from the damage caused by petrochemically derived pesticides and herbicides. It is also enormously rich in life-enhancing enzymes.

WHAT YOU NEED
4 carrots
1 whole apple
225g (8oz) sprouted seeds (mung beans, chickpeas, adzuki beans, etc.)

HERE'S HOW
Juice all the ingredients. Sprinkle with some grated ginger or a little cinnamon and serve over ice.

RAW ENERGY
Vegan
Serves 2

Carrot and apple juice is the basis for this health-packed cocktail, which is devised to promote all-round health with the addition of celery and cucumber. As you become more adventurous with your juicing, try reducing the apple content and adding green leaves of cabbage, spinach or dandelion to increase the green energy content.

WHAT YOU NEED
1 apple
4 carrots
1 or 2 stalks of celery
5-cm (2-inch) section of cucumber
1-cm (½-inch) cube of fresh ginger (optional)

HERE'S HOW
Juice all the ingredients. The addition of a cube or two of ginger gives the Raw Energy mix a real zing.

Fruitful Ventures
There is little more wonderful for breakfast than fresh fruit. First, it is easy to digest. Eaten first thing in the morning, fruit helps your body continue the night-time detoxificatic process right through the morning. Your liver – the body's organ for cleansing itself – is most active between midnight and midday. If you can manage a breakfast of fruit or vegetable juice or a mixture of the two, and this is enough for you, more power to you. Your body will just keep on cleansing itself. If not, don't worry. Everybody is unique in their needs for breakfast. Whatever you choose (provided you don't suffer from *Candida albicans*) make fruit a part of it. The more colourful the fruit you choose, the better.

Go for Colour
Red, orange and yellow fruits, including raspberries, strawberries, red grapes, apricots, peaches, watermelons, cantaloupes, mangoes, guavas and papayas, contain a wealth of phytochemical compounds – the carotenoids. These not only foster health, but also prevent premature ageing. Each of the carotenoids has a slightly different protective ability. They tend to work best together, the way they are found in nature. No amount of pill popping will ever replace what you can get from eating fresh fruits as part of your diet.

Eat it Whole
As often as possible, eat fruits with the skin left on. The skin of fruits is an excellent source of pectin – the soluble fibre which helps balance blood lipids, stabilise blood sugar and reduce LDL cholesterol levels.

Pectin also encourages the elimination of bile acids in the intestines and reduces toxicity in the body.

Fruits are also rich in vitamin C as well as phenolic acids and flavonoids, all of which have been shown to help prevent premature ageing and heart disease. Raspberries, strawberries and grapes also contain ellagic acid, another ally in keeping your skin firm and unlined and in preventing illness.

Apart from the fact that they are incredibly beautiful, a bowl of sliced peaches, a fruit smoothie or a freshly made fruit juice pack a good punch when it comes to looking good and feeling great.

Quick-fix Drinks

These instant breakfasts are a favourite of mine to which I often add a tablespoon of Pure Synergy (*see Nature's Supplements*) or organic bee pollen. They are made either from microfiltered whey protein or from GM-free soya milk. They are fast, easy and get you ready to face the day ahead with ease.

PAPAYA BANANA SMOOTHIE
Vegan
Serves 1

Papaya, mango, guava, pineapple, banana . . . tropical fruits conjure up visions of the tropics, lazing by bright azure water. Bring this feeling into dark winter days with a Papaya Banana Smoothie for breakfast. It's quick to make, to drink – even to digest. Raw papaya contains a protein-digesting enzyme called papain. Some enthusiasts believe that regularly eating fresh papaya helps to clear out necrotic proteins, detoxifying the body and helping prevent ageing. So powerful is this enzyme that you can even use fresh papaya to tenderise meat and make it easier to digest. This luscious fruit supplies some 60mg of vitamin C and more than 800mg of carotenoids. Always use papaya ripe and, if you have time after peeling the fruit, rub the inside of the peel over your face. It is a natural exfoliator – one used for centuries before cosmetic companies discovered fruit acids and began to charge a fortune for them.

WHAT YOU NEED
1 small papaya
½ to 1 ripe banana (preferably organic)
2 ice cubes, crushed (50ml (2fl oz) crushed ice)

HERE'S HOW

Peel and seed the papaya and cut it into chunks. Peel and slice the banana. Purée together in a blender or food processor, add the ice and purée until smooth. Pour into a chilled glass and serve at once with small bowls of nuts and seeds if you want to nibble as well. Add Manuka honey if you feel the drink needs sweetening.

OTHER WAYS TO GO

Yellow Delight: Try a mango–pineapple combination.
Secrets of the Orange: Use pineapple and the juice of a fresh orange with a squeeze of lemon.
Protein Power: For a more sustaining drink, add a raw free-range organic egg and some freshly grated nutmeg.
Winter Treat: Fresh is best, but dried fruit soaked overnight is an easy option in winter when you can't get the real thing. Try cranberries with sun-dried apricots, figs, prunes or peaches with a banana. Use some of the soak water as it is delicious and filled with minerals.

ORANGE CASHEW NECTAR
Vegan
Serves 2

People avoid raw cashews because they are high in fat, but the fat they contain is good quality – mostly monounsaturated – and easy to digest. Because it digests slowly, it helps keep you from feeling hungry through the morning. These luscious, creamy nuts are also rich in magnesium for the nervous system, selenium for free-radical protection and vitamin B_1. Mix with a little fresh coconut or coconut milk and fresh orange juice and you turn an instant breakfast into nectar for the gods.

WHAT YOU NEED

450ml (16fl oz) fresh orange juice or, even better, 225ml (8fl oz) orange juice and the flesh of a seeded and peeled orange
30g (1oz) raw cashew nuts
2 tbsp fresh coconut, unsweetened coconut cream or dried shredded unsweetened coconut
maple syrup or Manuka honey to taste (optional)

HERE'S HOW
Place ingredients in a blender or food processor and blend until creamy smooth.

OTHER WAYS TO GO
Nuts to Go: Replace the cashews with almonds or hazelnuts, pecans or black walnuts.
Raisins: Replace the coconut with a handful of raisins.
Dates: Replace the Manuka honey or maple syrup with a few fresh dates.

BERRY BLISS SMOOTHIE
Vegetarian
Serves 1

WHAT YOU NEED
50g (2oz) fresh or frozen raspberries, strawberries, blackberries, logan-
    berries or a mixture
5 teaspoons cold filtered or spring water
2–3 scoops microfiltered whey protein or whey protein isolate powder
stevia or Manuka honey to taste
2 tbsp flax seeds (optional)
3 ice cubes (optional)
1 tsp lemon zest (optional)

HERE'S HOW
Put all the ingredients into a blender and blend well, but not for more than 20 seconds. You can add more or less water if you want a slightly thicker or thinner shake. Serve immediately.

MACAROON SURPRISE
Vegan
Serves 2

I adore coconut – the smell, the flavour, even the oil itself. This recipe makes a filling breakfast in a glass – one I especially like on hot summer's days. The oranges must be ripe, or you'll need to add a little Manuka honey. The coconut cream makes the drink rich and delicious. Coconut is a rich unsaturated fat but there is some evidence that it has unusual protective properties. I like using fresh coconut whenever possible. I look for heavy coconuts, shake them, and listen for lots of liquid. I also check to make sure they have no soft or mouldy spots. You can buy commercially shredded coconut, but lots of manufacturers add extra sugar to it and propylene glycol to keep it moist. If you don't have fresh coconut, look for unsweetened shredded or flaked coconut without additives (250g/9oz of shredded coconut equals about 700ml (23fl oz).

WHAT YOU NEED
225ml (8fl oz) freshly squeezed orange juice
75g (3oz) fresh coconut with both shell and inner brown skin removed
or 40g (1½oz) shredded unsweetened coconut
½ tsp almond extract
225ml (8fl oz) crushed ice

HERE'S HOW
Place everything but the ice in the blender and blend to mix. Now add the ice and continue to blend but not so much that you destroy the slushiness of the crushed ice. Serve immediately topped with a slice of orange and a sprig of mint.

VANILLA NUTMEG SMOOTHIE
Vegetarian
Serves 1

This breakfast-in-an-instant is based on the traditional eggnog that people used to drink at Christmas. In fact, the egg is optional. If you decide to put the egg in – I like to do this because it adds flavour – make sure your egg is free-range or organic. You don't want to mess around with battery-laid eggs eaten raw.

WHAT YOU NEED
200ml (7fl oz) cold filtered or spring water
6 ice cubes
1 to 2 scoops natural or vanilla-flavoured microfiltered whey protein
   or whey protein isolate powder
1 egg (optional)
1 tsp vanilla essence or several drops natural vanilla oil
pinch of freshly grated nutmeg to taste

stevia, Manuka honey or maple syrup to taste
1 heaped tsp psyllium husks (optional)
1 tbsp flax seeds (optional)

HERE'S HOW
Place all the ingredients in a blender and blend vigorously until combined. Be careful not to blend for more than 20 seconds, however, since this can change the nature of the microfiltered whey protein. Sprinkle a little extra grated nutmeg on top and serve immediately.

SPICED MANGO LASSI
Vegan
Serves 2

I fell in love with lassis in India where they cool a curry and refresh the palate. I once travelled from the middle of India to Calcutta by car. The food *en route* was wonderful – absolutely fresh and simple. When at last I reached the city – after pushing the car across bridges too rough to drive over – what I wanted most in the world was a spiced lassi. Lassis are traditionally made with milk or buttermilk, but I prefer to make mine with organic soya milk which is creamy and rich, or even rice or oat milk.

WHAT YOU NEED
1 small handful organic raw cashews (optional)
225ml (8fl oz) soya milk
2 ripe mangoes, chilled and chopped
1 tsp ground cinnamon
½ tsp ground cardamom
¼ tsp freshly ground nutmeg
Manuka honey to taste

HERE'S HOW
Place the cashews, if using, in a blender with 100ml (4fl oz) of soya milk and blend until creamy. Add the mangoes, the rest of the milk, cinnamon, cardamom, nutmeg and Manuka honey, and blend until smooth.

OTHER WAYS TO GO
Peach: Substitute three ripe peaches for the mangoes.
Blueberry: 225g (8oz) of blueberries instead of mangoes.

Apples: Two apples, increase the cinnamon.
Salt: Leave out the Manuka honey and add ½ tsp Maldon sea salt.

PEACH AND DATE DELIGHT
Vegetarian
Serves 1

This is a great protein drink, with all the brilliance of fresh, ripe fruit to it. Dates are one of the most nourishing forms of natural sweetness you can find – rich in fibre and ultra-high in potassium and niacin, they even boast easily-absorbed iron.

WHAT YOU NEED
2 ripe peaces, sliced – don't peel if organic, but do peel if not
25g (1oz) soya milk powder or 50g (2oz) vanilla microfiltered whey powder
½ tsp vanilla extract
4 pitted dates
4 ice cubes

HERE'S HOW
Combine all the ingredients in a blender and process until smooth. You can substitute any manner of fruit in this recipe, such as blueberries, blackberries, loganberries, strawberries, apricots, apples (in which case add some extra water as well as cinnamon). You can also use oranges or even figs, but you will need a little extra water if the fruit is dry. Drink immediately.

STRAWBERRY PROTECTOR
Vegan
Serves 2

This instant breakfast is full of vitamins and minerals. High in fibre and low in fat, it is also rich in potassium. All you need to make it is a blender. It has many variations, all of them delicious. I use whatever fruits I happen to have available. It is particularly good made with soya milk, since soya is full of isoflavones which help counter the damaging effects to the reproductive system of herbicides and pesticides. Most important of all, it is delicious, especially in summer with some chopped ice added.

WHAT YOU NEED
225–350ml (8–12fl oz) soya milk
100g (4oz) fresh or frozen strawberries
1 ripe medium banana, peeled and sliced
2 tbsp oat bran
1 tbsp vanilla extract
shake of nutmeg

HERE'S HOW
Put everything into a blender, except the nutmeg, and mix until thick and smooth. Sprinkle with a little nutmeg before serving.

OTHER WAYS TO GO
Applejack: Replace the strawberries with two fresh apples and add cinnamon to the top.
Pineapple delight: Replace the strawberries with fresh pineapple and blend together with three or four leaves of fresh mint.
Blueberry Shake: Use a large handful of blueberries in place of the strawberries. Top with chopped almonds.

GET BRUNCHED

The smell of oranges and the crunch of fresh linen as light slips through the window. It happens seldom, but I love having the time to make a leisurely brunch. Lazy Sunday mornings are the best – sharing a luscious, languid meal with friends, or getting up late and taking an enormous plate of something delicious back to bed. This sort of leisurely brunch needs to be spiked with surprises: omelette topped with Mexican salsa served with fresh vegetable juice, or perhaps the sweet innocence of Live Muesli made with strawberries or fresh mangoes. Here are some of my favourites.

Mighty Mueslis

My favourite breakfasts in the world are mueslis. Here you will find two: traditional Bircher Muesli made with steel-cut oats soaked overnight, and Live Muesli made with sprouted buckwheat and coconut oil. They also make great evening meals when you want something light and different.

LIVE MUESLI
Vegetarian
Serves 1

This is my own invention and my favourite muesli. It takes advantage of the health-enhancing properties of coconut oil (*see Foods that Heal*). Everybody loves live buckwheat muesli – even children raised on sugar-crunch convenience foods. Nothing carries revolutionary breakfast power to the body's living matrix quite like it. Not only are live mueslis higher in essential nutrients than their grain-based counterparts, the quality of the phytochemicals they contain is the best in the world. This recipe – my family's favourite breakfast – calls for an apple, but you can use almost any fruit – strawberries, peaches, apricots, cherries, pears – whatever is inexpensive and in season. It serves one, but can just as easily be made for 12. This particular form of muesli is dairy free. If you prefer, you can add a little plain low-fat yoghurt or soya milk to taste. The raw buckwheat has been soaked overnight so that enzymes break down the hard-to-digest starches, making them taste sweeter while being much easier to absorb. It is even better if you let it sprout for two or three days before you use it.

WHAT YOU NEED

2 dsp raw buckwheat, soaked overnight in water or sprouted
2 tsp coconut oil (it is firm when room temperature is below 24°C/76°F
    – this is the usual way I make use of it)
1 apple or any other fruit, chopped or grated
juice of 1 orange or tangerine
soya milk or low-fat plain yoghurt to taste (optional)
1–2 tsp Manuka honey (optional)
¼ tsp powdered cinnamon or nutmeg, or some fresh grated ginger

HERE'S HOW

Mix together the soaked buckwheat with the coconut fat using a fork to cream it all together. Combine with the fruit and juice, soya milk or yoghurt and sweeten with the honey if you like. Sprinkle with cinnamon or ginger. Serve immediately.

OTHER WAYS TO GO

Fruit Juice Muesli: Substitute some fresh fruit juice, such as apple, orange or grape, for the soya milk or yoghurt. To thicken the juice, blend with a little fresh fruit in season, such as pear or apple.
Summer Muesli: Add a handful of fresh or frozen strawberries, black-berries, loganberries, raspberries or pitted cherries to the basic muesli, or substitute a finely diced peach or nectarine for the apple.

BIRCHER MUESLI
Vegetarian
Serves 1

Bircher muesli was created by the great Swiss physician, Max Bircher-Benner, who first healed himself of what was apparently an incurable condition using a high-raw diet, and then went on to heal hundreds of thousands of others in the same way. Bircher Muesli is so delicious that even dyed-in-the-wool junk-food eaters fall for it. This recipe uses an apple, but you can use almost any fruit – strawberries, peaches, apricots, cherries, even unsulphured dried fruits. If you are using dried fruits, be sure to soak them overnight in spring water so that they plump up. The grains are soaked overnight so that enzymes break down the hard-to-digest starches in natural sugars, making them much sweeter and easier to absorb.

WHAT YOU NEED

2 tbsp steel-cut oat flakes, soaked overnight in a little spring water or fruit juice
handful of raisins, also soaked overnight
1 apple or any other fruit, chopped or grated
juice of ½ lemon
3 tbsp coconut milk or plain yoghurt
1 tbsp concentrated apple, pear or strawberry juice
¼ tsp powdered cinnamon or fresh grated ginger

HERE'S HOW

Mix together the soaked oat flakes and raisins and combine this mixture with the grated apple, lemon juice and the coconut milk or yoghurt. Drizzle with fruit juice and sprinkle with cinnamon or ginger. Serve immediately.

OTHER WAYS TO GO

Winter Muesli: Soak a selection of dried fruits such as apricots, sultanas, figs, dates or pears overnight in spring water. Dice into small pieces or cut up with scissors and add to the soaked grain flakes. Add the lemon juice, coconut milk or yoghurt and concentrated fruit juice. Spice with a little grated nutmeg.

Fruit Juice Muesli: Substitute some fresh fruit juice, such as apple, orange or grape, for the coconut milk or yoghurt. To thicken the juice, blend with a little fresh fruit in season, such as banana, pear or apple.

Banana Muesli: Add a banana sliced in quarters lengthways and then chopped across into small pieces, or mash a banana with a little soya milk, yoghurt or fruit juice and use it as a topping.

Summer Muesli: Add a handful of raisins, strawberries, blackcurrants or pitted cherries to the basic muesli, or substitute a finely diced peach or nectarine for the apple.

Grainless Muesli: Use two tablespoons sunflower seeds or sunflower and pumpkin seeds instead of the cereals and soak overnight in the same way.

Creamy Muesli: Use fresh cream instead of yoghurt or a little goat's milk blended with a tablespoon of ground cashew nuts. Goat's milk on its own gives a thinner muesli.

Dairyless Muesli: Use fruit juice (apple and grape are particularly good) instead of the yoghurt, and leave out the raisin soak water if the consistency is too thin.

Sprinkles: Try adding some sesame seeds or dried coconut.

Cook When You Wish

Everybody loves cooked breakfasts sometimes – lazy Sunday mornings for instance, or as a brunch when friends arrive. Here are some of my favourites:

INSTANT CRANBERRY PORRIDGE
Vegetarian
Serves 2

I like to make porridge before I go to bed, when I know I will want an instant breakfast the next day. Oat porridge is a great way to start the day, steadily releasing energy into your body throughout the morning. This breakfast is particularly good if you are someone who just does not function on juice or fruit alone. Add dried cranberries or dates, maybe a sliced banana or some dried figs to a good organic porridge, and you have a truly gourmet breakfast.

WHAT YOU NEED
30g (1oz) dried cranberries
30g (1oz) rolled oats
1 tsp Manuka honey or concentrated apple or pear juice
225–350ml (8–12fl oz) cups boiling water
¼ tsp cinnamon or freshly ground nutmeg
1 tsp butter to top (optional)

HERE'S HOW
Put all the ingredients except the cinnamon or nutmeg and the butter (if using) into a Thermos and close. Set aside until the morning. You can also use a Pyrex jar with a lid and place it in warm place, such as the warming oven of an Aga, through the night. Eat as is, or cover with soya milk, oat milk or rice milk. You can vary the porridge you make by using brown rice flakes instead of oats.

OTHER WAYS TO GO
Date Dream: Use 75g (3oz) of pitted and chopped dates instead of the cranberries.
Fruit on Hand: Make the porridge without fruit, then, just before eating it, top it off with a handful of fresh or defrosted berries, a sliced banana, a grated apple or whatever else you can find.

Get into Eggs

For years, eggs have been given a bad deal – mostly because of the false ideas that people once held about cholesterol. Eggs are a great food – a superb source of top-quality protein among other things. Rich in the sulphur-based amino acids, they have excellent antioxidant properties to help protect you from free-radical damage. Such sulphur amino acids need to be available for the body to make its own natural free radical-fighting enzymes such as glutathione peroxidase. Eggs are also full of antioxidant vitamins A and E as well as vitamins D and B_{12} and lecithin. An emulsifier essential to good brain functioning, lecithin has been shown to enhance memory, mood and concentration – all of which suffer if you don't get enough of it. Finally, eggs are truly satisfying. They stick to your ribs. Their protein-based energy is released slowly into the bloodstream, which makes them great for breakfast. They help guard against blood sugar ups and downs that cause mid-morning energy slumps.

OMELETTE MADE EASY
Vegetarian
Serves 1

I once thought making an omelette was hard work. The secret of omelette making is not to complicate the issue by adding milk and other ingredients, not to overbeat your eggs – or they go flat – and to serve the omelette the minute it is ready. You also need a good heavy non-stick pan. I often use my French crêpe pan, especially if the omelette is a small one. When making more than one, don't be tempted to make one big omelette. They are much, much better cooked individually.

WHAT YOU NEED
3 free-range organic eggs
1 tbsp butter or extra-virgin olive oil

handful of fresh herbs, chopped
Celtic or Maldon sea salt and coarse-ground pepper to taste

HERE'S HOW

Break the eggs into a good-sized bowl. Hand-beat them with either a beater or fork until they are just mixed and fluffy. Do not overbeat. Do not season now. Heat butter or olive oil in the pan over a high heat – just enough to melt the butter. Pour in the eggs and let them bubble, tilting the pan and using a wooden spatula to pull the cooking eggs away from the sides of the pan so the liquid eggs fill up the gaps and cook. Just as soon as the omelette goes opaque, flip it in half, sprinkle with fresh herbs, salt and pepper and serve immediately. Serve with Powerhouse Salsa (*see Salsas and Sauces*).

SWEET NOTHING SOUFFLÉ
Vegetarian
Serves 2

Soufflés usually take a long time to make and are a lot of trouble. This one is virtually instantaneous and is just as much fun for breakfast as it is as a sweet at the end of a meal.

WHAT YOU NEED

6 egg whites
3 egg yolks
1 tbsp microfiltered whey powder
3 tbsp shredded unsweetened coconut
several drops of stevia extract, Manuka honey or maple syrup to taste

HERE'S HOW

Put your egg whites in a mixing bowl and beat until thick peaks form. In a separate bowl, mix together egg yolks and whey powder, beating until smooth. Gently add the egg yolk mix to the beaten egg whites, at the same time folding in the shredded coconut. Pour into a soufflé dish or two individual ramekins and pop into a hot oven for about 25 minutes, until the soufflé rises and peaks on top. Be careful not to overcook this soufflé, otherwise it will lose its fine texture. Add the stevia, Manuka honey or maple syrup if you want a sweet soufflé, though I personally find that this soufflé is sweet enough. Sprinkle with cinnamon and serve immediately.

LIGHT-AS-AIR PANCAKES
Vegetarian
Serves 2

This is a recipe I developed for my family. I used to make masses of pancakes on Sunday morning, and my kids loved them. It makes very light and fluffy pancakes, rather like pancake soufflés. They need to be eaten immediately; the egg white gives them their fluff which quickly gets lost once they have been cooked. They can be served with a delicious raspberry or blueberry syrup or some butter.

WHAT YOU NEED
4 eggs
100g (4oz) creamed cottage cheese
30g (1oz) soya flour
pinch of Celtic or Maldon sea salt
½ tsp baking powder
2 tbsp soda water
½ tbsp coconut oil
stevia, Manuka honey or maple syrup to taste

HERE'S HOW
Separate the eggs and beat the whites until almost stiff. In another bowl, combine the egg yolks with the cottage cheese, soya flour, salt and baking powder. Blend thoroughly. Gently fold in the egg whites and soda water. Heat coconut oil in a frying pan or crêpe pan. Pour out individual dollops of the mixture and cook until the underside turns a light golden brown. Flip each pancake only once. Take off the heat and serve immediately topped with the stevia, honey or maple syrup, or some berry syrup (*see below*).

RASPBERRY SYRUP
Vegan
Serves 1

This you can also make with blueberries, strawberries, loganberries or blackberries – whatever happens to be in season. It's great on pancakes or cottage cheese for breakfast or over mascarpone as a dessert or snack.

WHAT YOU NEED
225g (8oz) raspberries or other berries
125ml (4fl oz) filtered or spring water
1 tsp grated orange or lime zest
stevia or Manuka honey to taste
pinch of nutmeg

HERE'S HOW
Bring the berries with a little water to the boil and gently simmer over a low heat. Add the other ingredients and cook very gently until the syrup thickens slightly. Then remove from the heat. You can either put this syrup into a blender or purée it, or you can leave it chunky and serve as is. The syrup will keep well in the fridge for a week.

HAND-MADE SAUSAGES
Serves 4

I adore sausage. Yet the sausages you buy are full of all sorts of artificial flavourings and colourings, not to mention 'stuffers' which you don't want to eat. This is an old-fashioned pattie sausage which you can vary, depending upon your taste and what herbs and meats you have available. You can make it with pork, venison, chicken, lamb, beef or wild boar. I mix the ingredients together the night before, then put them into the fridge to chill and absorb all the flavours. Eat within three days.

WHAT YOU NEED
350g (12oz) lean minced pork, chicken, beef, lamb, venison or wild
    boar
1 tsp Celtic or Maldon sea salt
2 tsp oat bran
4 garlic cloves (optional)
2 tbsp chopped fresh parsley, coriander or sage
½ large onion, finely chopped

HERE'S HOW
Combine all your ingredients in a big mixing bowl and mix thoroughly with your hands. Refrigerate until well chilled, then separate into four patties and cook in an oiled pan until crunchy on the surface and cooked through.

SCRAMBLED TOFU
Vegan
Serves 1

Lighter and more delicate in texture than scrambled eggs, tofu works well for breakfast provided you season it richly, for tofu has almost no flavour of its own. If you add a pinch of turmeric and omit the Parmesan, you will create a 'vegan scrambled egg' in a rich yellow colour, just like the real thing.

WHAT YOU NEED
1 tsp extra-virgin olive oil
2 spring onions, finely chopped
2 garlic cloves, crushed or chopped
200g (7oz) tofu
pinch of turmeric (optional)
Celtic or Maldon sea salt to taste
freshly ground black pepper to taste
Mexican chilli powder to taste
½ tsp curry powder
½ tsp cumin powder
4 tbsp grated Parmesan cheese (optional)

HERE'S HOW
Heat the oil in a heavy frying pan and sauté the spring onions and garlic until soft (2–3 minutes). Mash the tofu then stir it into the pan with the turmeric, if using. Add your other seasonings and any other herbs you want. Cook over high heat, turning frequently, until the tofu goes firm. This takes about 2–3 minutes. Sprinkle on the cheese if you are using it. Season with salt and pepper and serve immediately.

POWER SALADS – THE MAIN THING

Gorgeous salads begin at the shopping stage. Buy what is most beautiful and forget the rest. Bring home your vegetables, wash them thoroughly and dry them, then place them ready-to-use in vegetable bins in the refrigerator. When you do this a couple of times a week, you are all set not only for instant salads, but also for instant salad whole meals.

Salad making is far more an art than a science. I am always amused by people who say they love salads but just don't have time to make them. I can create a salad that is a whole meal for four people and have it on the table in 10 minutes.

Brimming with Life
The quickest and easiest way to change your life for the better is to make at least one meal a day a huge crunchy salad supported by good-quality protein – be it fish, chicken, eggs, tofu, seeds or nuts. Forget the limp lettuce leaf and tomato fare. We're talking rich green mesclun and brilliant flowers, wild herbs, fennel and orange with mangetout tendrils, bright peppers, brilliant Swiss chard and almonds – crisp, delicious and a snap to make. Salads brimming with biophoton order and phytonutrients to detoxify your body, protect from premature ageing and energise your life.

Buy Beautiful
The key to keeping your vegetables fresh for a whole week once they've been washed is always to store them in plastic trays in the fridge and cover with big plastic bags. This keeps things fresh and crisp for so long it surprises me. When it comes to fresh herbs such as basil, coriander and parsley, I place them in a bowl of cold water in the refrigerator. This way they too will last a week.

WASH AND BIN

It is important to have all your vegetables ready for use, for preparation is what takes time. Then when you come into the kitchen you can pull out two, three or four trays full of lovely, bright-coloured, fresh foods and dive into salad making. I love working with whatever is there. You can make a fabulous salad from a bunch of rocket and some gorgeous black olives, and fresh slivers of Parmesan cheese. Delicious and nutrient-rich salads are especially easy to make. Use shredded raw broccoli and cauliflower, red and yellow capsicums, chopped red onion and slivers of Chinese leaves, smothered in a creamy home-made mayonnaise made with extra-virgin olive oil or an irresistible curried avocado dressing.

Instrument of Torture

The one piece of kitchen equipment I never want to be without is a mandolin. These remarkable vegetable shredders are very different to the usual graters you find in most stores. Unlike the conventional grater which mashes vegetables and fruits, a mandolin slices clean and sharp. The tiny knives they contain make perfect slices of whatever vegetable you like (*see Equip Yourself*). You can julienne, make chip-size chunks, slice thin or thick.

Shred It

For a long time I was troubled by how to make salads tasty when using vegetables like broccoli and cauliflower which are particularly rich in phytonutrients. Then I discovered the way to do this: simply shred them very finely using a mandolin, so that you get small crunchy pieces. This adds texture and richness, while giving your salad great nutrient density. When I first began experimenting with this, I thought that no one but me would eat my offerings, but I soon discovered otherwise. My friends love these salads – especially when they are tossed with a rich home-made mayonnaise or avocado dressing. Now I shred broccoli and cauliflower into many of the salads I make day after day.

TWO-TO-FIVE MAGIC

I try to mix between two and five vegetables together to make a salad. Not only do I combine varieties of vegetables, I also mix textures, using fine-julienned celeriac, for instance, with a coarsely grated red cabbage plus slivered spring onions. It's the mixture of colours and textures that makes it all work. Let your imagination take over. Feel and taste the ingredients you are using. Treat the whole process of salad making as you would that of painting a picture or making a sculpture. Have fun. Make it a delightful experience and you can't miss.

Get Lazy

Lazy about salad dressings, I usually make my salad in a large, flat bowl. Then, instead of mixing the salad dressing separately, I dress the salad right there and then. A few tablespoons of extra-virgin olive oil, some chopped fresh herbs, crushed raw garlic, a dash of Worcestershire sauce, some Celtic or Maldon sea salt, the juice of a lemon and a couple of tablespoons of wine vinegar or balsamic vinegar, some home-made Cajun seasoning from the fridge or a dash of the powdered variety from the market. To top it off I use some freshly ground black pepper. I like to grind peppercorns with a mortar and pestle because the pepper tastes so much better that way. I sprinkle this on top and toss. Ready in an instant. Sometimes I top off salads with seeds like pumpkin, sesame or sunflower. Others, I scatter with chopped fresh garlic or shredded wild garlic leaves when they are growing down the path near where I live. When they are to be found in the garden, I even add some fresh edible flowers like marigold petals or heartsease.

UNLEASH YOUR CREATIVITY

What you need to turn a simple salad into a masterpiece is a child's sense of experimentation, plus plenty of love, for that is the ingredient which makes every meal a joy. It is not just what you make and how you make it that matters, but your attitude to what you are doing in the kitchen.

Delicious Salads

I love one-bowl eating. Maybe it is an atavistic regression to my peasant ancestors, but I love the idea of sitting down to a big salad, complete with top-quality protein – tofu, prawns or chicken – all in one big bowl. One-bowls in any form consist of colourful, simple, tasty food which is as good for you as it is delicious. They make a meal that is a pleasure to eat alone or share with others. The trouble is, once you get into creating one-bowl meals, you begin to wonder why you ever did anything else.

MAKE DO WITH WHAT YOU'VE GOT

The hardest part about making a salad is simply getting your vegetables ready to use. When all this is done in advance, putting together beautiful, bright-coloured gifts from Nature becomes a kind of blissful meditation. I love working with whatever is there. You can make a fabulous salad from a beetroot and a couple of apples grated using a mandolin, then topped with fresh orange juice, a handful of chopped herbs and some curry powder. It is that easy.

These salads are a meal in themselves and are quick and easy to prepare. They are made in individual dishes, one for each person. You can create a salad to suit the specifications of each member of the family just as easily as making one large salad. You simply put little piles of vegetables, fruits and sprouts in each dish and pour on the dressing or dip of your (or their) choice. Experiment by chopping, grating and slicing different vegetables. Usually the more finely cut a vegetable is, the more flavour it has and the more delicious the salad.

Salad Tips

❏ I often use finely shredded greens such as lettuce or Chinese leaves as the base of a salad; the dressing and juices run down into it so that it is especially tasty when you get to it.

❏ Carrots, cucumber and celery are nice chopped into sticks. Cut the celery twice lengthwise into three strips, then cut once crosswise and you have six sticks of even size. Leave the leaves on – they are attractive and tasty. Carrots take a bit more care. Cut them in half lengthwise, then lay a half side down and cut in half again, then cut each of the quarters in half lengthwise, so you have eight sticks. As with all kinds of vegetable sticks, the thinner they are, the better they taste. If you take a little bundle of sticks and chop them across, you get neatly diced vegetables.

❑ Courgettes, aubergines and some cucumbers have a bitter flavour which can be removed by slicing them and soaking in a little cider vinegar. Leave for about minutes so the bitter juices are drawn out. Then wash the slices thoroughly under a cold tap to rinse away the vinegar and pat dry. Using this method, or the salt-sprinkling method, means you lose some vitamins and minerals.

❑ Tomatoes are nice chopped or sliced into salads, but don't forget to remove the hard green stem area. Their skins can be removed for special dishes by dropping them in boiling water for half a minute, or spitting them with a fork and turning quickly over a naked flame. The skins split and shrink with the heat and can easily be pulled off.

❑ Grate an apple into any salad and it makes it special – this often appeals to meat and potato lovers who ordinarily would not touch anything fresh.

❑ Half an avocado chopped into a salad gives a pleasant smooth-ness that contrasts with the crunchiness of most other vegetables. To dice an avocado quickly, cut it in half and remove the stone, then hold one half in your hand and make several cuts first length-wise and then crosswise. Scoop the chopped flesh into your salad with a spoon.

❑ Spring onions, chives and other fresh herbs are nice chopped very finely. With spring onions, cut them two or three times length-wise first, then across.

❑ Use fruit in dish salads – sliced orange, apple or peach to add flavour and colour. A handful of seedless raisins is good too; try chilling them in the fridge first – they become quite chewy.

❑ Sprouts are a must – they really do make a dish special. Chickpea, mung, lentil, aduki and fenugreek sprouts combined together make a one-bowl salad on their own.

SPINACH, EGG AND MUSHROOM SALAD
Vegetarian
Serves 4

Spinach has been touted as a healthy food for generations, but there's a big irony here. When I was a kid, we were told to eat our spinach because it was iron-rich – what made Popeye strong. Yet this information came out of a mistake – somebody high up in officialdom in the United States misplaced a decimal point, which multiplied spinach's iron content by 10. Yet this became the official line. The irony is that spinach turns out to be even better for you than when it was believed to be rich in iron.

I buy spinach as fresh as possible because it actually tastes quite different once it's sat around for a while. I like to use red peppercorns in this recipe, as I do in many of my recipes, and to hand grind them using a mortar and pestle to release the finest flavour. Few people these days use red peppercorns, yet they have a completely different, unique flavour and add such colourful beauty to your dishes.

The combination of spinach with grated hard-boiled eggs and mushrooms is a surprising one. The crunchiness of the spinach is offset by the rich, creamy protein of the eggs. There is something very special about topping any salad with grated hard-boiled eggs. I discovered this years ago, and it always surprises me that more people don't know about it. I often grate hard-boiled eggs on a salad to create a rich, whole meal for four people in as little as 10 minutes.

This salad travels well, provided that you carry the dressing and the grated hard-boiled eggs in separate containers and add them just before serving.

WHAT YOU NEED
2 large handfuls baby spinach or very fresh full-grown spinach
100g (4oz) raw white button mushrooms, washed and sliced
2 garlic cloves, finely chopped (optional)
100ml (4fl oz) vinaigrette dressing (*see Dress It Up for suggestions*)
6 hard-boiled eggs, grated coarsely
½ tsp red peppercorns (you can use black peppercorns if you don't have red ones)

HERE'S HOW
Clear out any wilted bits or nasty stalks from the spinach and give it a really good wash, making sure to remove any sand. Spin it dry or

dry in a tea towel then pop it into the fridge for 15–20 minutes to crisp up. When you're ready to serve this salad, place the spinach leaves in a bowl, add the mushrooms and sprinkle garlic over the top (if using). Pour over your vinaigrette dressing, top with grated hard-boiled eggs and sprinkle with coarsely ground red pepper. Serve immediately.

CHEF'S SALAD
Serves 2

A chef's salad is one of those perfect meals you can not only order in a restaurant but also make yourself – provided you have plenty of left-overs.

WHAT YOU NEED
1 head of the most beautiful lettuce you can find (any kind), torn into
    bite-sized pieces
½ cucumber, cubed
1 small tomato, cubed
3 tbsp fresh parsley, basil or coriander, chopped
2 tbsp extra-virgin olive oil, or half olive oil and half flaxseed oil
2 tbsp lemon juice
1 tbsp balsamic vinegar
dash of Worcestershire sauce
4 hard-boiled eggs, halved
100g (4oz) cooked chicken, sliced in strips
100g (4oz) ham, sliced in strips
50g (2oz) Parmesan cheese, shaved (or more, if you like it as much as
    I do)
2 garlic cloves, crushed or finely chopped

HERE'S HOW
Arrange lettuce, cucumber and tomato in a big flat salad bowl and sprinkle on the fresh herbs. Pour the oil, lemon juice, vinegar and Worcestershire sauce over the top and season and toss. Arrange eggs, chicken, ham and cheese on the top of the salad and serve immediately.

GRILLED PRAWNS AND ROCKET SALAD
Meat free
Serves 4 generously

There is some magic about grilled prawns and rocket mixed together. The richness of prawns and the crunchiness of rocket – especially if you can get wild rocket – is worth any amount of effort to get. The lovely thing about this salad is that it's no effort to make. You can grill the prawns ahead of time and simply take them out of the refrigerator and add to the rocket, or you can grill them, as I tend to do, on a teppenyaki grill and serve them immediately on top of the rocket.

WHAT YOU NEED
400g (14oz) tiger prawns
2 tbsp extra-virgin olive oil
2 garlic cloves, chopped
zest and juice of ½ a lemon
Celtic or Maldon sea salt to taste
100g (4oz) rocket, washed and with any heavy stems removed
vinaigrette dressing (*see Dress It Up for suggestions*)
freshly ground red or black peppercorns

HERE'S HOW
Peel the prawns and run a knife down their backs to pull away any small black threads. Rinse and pat dry. Heat the pan or grill, coating with a little olive oil. Cook the prawns quickly at a high temperature for about 3 minutes until they start to go golden. While they're cooking, sprinkle with garlic, lemon zest, salt and pepper.

Line a flat salad bowl with the rocket. The moment the prawns are done, remove them from the heat. Add a garlicky vinaigrette to the rocket, place the prawns on top, sprinkle with lemon juice and coarsely ground black or red peppercorns and serve immediately.

CAESAR SALAD WITH POTATO CROUTONS
Meat free
Serves 4

Add something surprising to a salad or do it your own way. One day I hit upon the idea of making potato croutons for a wheat-free Caesar salad. This is one of the very few recipes I use potatoes for. Crispy, oven-baked gems with traditional Caesar dressing complete with raw, free-range, organic egg is great. To this Caesar salad you can also add slices of leftover chicken, turkey or fish to create a delicious whole meal in a bowl.

WHAT YOU NEED
2 heads of romaine lettuce
12 anchovy fillets, drained and cut into thirds
Celtic or Maldon sea salt to taste
freshly ground black pepper to taste
50g (2oz) Parmesan cheese, shaved, not grated

FOR THE CROUTONS
3 medium new potatoes
1 tbsp extra-virgin olive oil
freshly ground black pepper to taste
Celtic or Maldon sea salt to taste
3 tbsp finely grated Parmesan cheese
½ tsp dried Cajun seasoning or 1 tbsp of fresh
2 garlic cloves, finely chopped

FOR THE DRESSING
3 medium-sized lemons, juiced
¼ garlic clove, finely chopped or crushed
4 tbsp extra-virgin olive oil
several dashes of Worcestershire sauce
1 free-range organic egg

HERE'S HOW
To prepare the croutons, first preheat the oven to 220°C/425°F/Gas Mark 7. Spray a non-stick baking sheet with vegetable cooking spray or wipe with olive oil. Wash the potatoes leaving on their skins, drain, cut into wedges 15mm wide and then again to make cubes. Spread out on a double layer of paper towels to dry. Mix together the olive oil, pepper, salt, Parmesan, Cajun seasoning and garlic in a large bowl and drop the potato cubes into it, using your fingers to coat them. Add a bit more olive oil if you need it. Place the potato chunks on the baking sheet and bake for 15 to 20 minutes, turning occasionally so they brown evenly. Remove from the oven and drain on double layers of paper towels to cool.

To prepare the dressing, mix together the lemon juice, garlic, olive oil and Worcestershire sauce in a small bowl. Break the whole egg into a jar and whisk with a fork to blend well before adding to the other dressing ingredients. Pour over the salad just before serving.

Then, for the salad, wash and dry the romaine leaves. Tear into chunky morsels, wrap in a clean tea towel and chill in the refrigerator until needed. Place the romaine chunks in a large, flat salad bowl, add the cooled potato croutons and pour the freshly made salad dressing over all. Add the anchovies and season. Toss and serve topped with Parmesan cheese.

SPROUT SALAD
Vegan
Serves 6

The trick to making a great sprout salad is to mix these light-as-air vegetables with something richer and creamier such as a good mayonnaise or avocado dressing and then spike them with something larger and crunchier – say chicory or julienned carrots or even apples.

WHAT YOU NEED
50g (2oz) mangetout sprouts
50g (2oz) chickpea sprouts, marrow fat pea sprouts or mung bean sprouts
25g (1oz) radish or mustard sprouts
½ chicory or other lettuce in large pieces
½ bunch of watercress
8 slices of teppenyaki-grilled tofu
a few fresh edible flowers (optional, to garnish)
dressing of your choice

HERE'S HOW
Wash and dry the sprouts and wrap in a tea towel. Place in the refrigerator for 15 minutes or more to crisp up while you prepare the other ingredients. Then place everything but the tofu in a bowl, pour garlicky vinaigrette over the vegetables or try Cashew Mayonnaise, Creamy Lemon Dressing or Avocado Delight (*see Dress It Up*). Toss gently. Add the tofu slices on top and serve immediately, decorated with an edible flower or two if you have them in your garden.

BIG GREEK SALAD
Vegetarian
Serves 2

So simple, this salad is such a delight. Although it is pretty readily available in restaurants, I prefer to make my own.

WHAT YOU NEED
100g (4oz) dark lettuce leaves, spinach or rocket, torn into bite-sized pieces
1 small Spanish onion, sliced in rings
80g (3oz) feta cheese, cubed
handful of fresh, black olives, drained
1 small tomato, wedged
½ a green pepper, julienned
50ml (2fl oz) extra-virgin olive oil
50ml (2fl oz) balsamic vinegar
juice of ½ a lemon
Celtic or Maldon sea salt to taste
freshly ground black pepper to taste

HERE'S HOW
Lay all the ingredients in a large salad bowl and pour over the olive oil, vinegar and lemon juice. Season to taste, toss well and serve immediately.

SCALLOP SALAD WITH GINGER AND LIME
Meat free
Serves 4

The spicy-sweet ginger root, whose use dates back more than 5,000 years, is one of the greatest of all the natural health enhancers of the vegetable kingdom. Grating a little fresh ginger into soups and sauces, salads and sweets adds zing to anything you are cooking. Combine ginger with lime and add it to a scallop salad, and you have a real winner.

WHAT YOU NEED FOR THE SALAD
zest of 1 lime, finely shredded
18 king scallops

2 tbsp extra-virgin olive oil
a finger of fresh ginger, finely shredded
juice of 2 fresh limes
150g (5oz) lamb's lettuce
150g (5oz) curly endive
1 bulb of fennel, cut into spikes or shredded with the large knife of
  a mandolin
1 green chilli, seeded and chopped

FOR THE DRESSING
6 tbsp extra-virgin olive oil
3 tbsp balsamic vinegar
small bunch of fresh coriander, finely chopped (about 4 to 5 tbsp)
Celtic or Maldon sea salt to taste
freshly ground black pepper to taste

HERE'S HOW
Zest the lime. Remove the corals from the scallops and cut any large
parts of the white in two. Heat the oil in a pan or teppenyaki grill. Add
the shredded ginger and cook for a few seconds. Now throw in the
whites and corals and cook for 2 minutes. Turn over and cook for
another 2 minutes. Pour the lime juice on top, remove immediately
from the heat and let cool. Wash and dry the lamb's lettuce and curly
endive and tear into appropriately sized pieces. Add the shredded fennel
and chopped chilli, and place in a large, flat bowl.

Now make the dressing by adding all the ingredients except the
seasoning to a food processor or blender and pulsing, being careful
not to chop the coriander too fine. Taste your dressing and season.
Pour half of the dressing over the salad and toss. Add the corals and
whites of the scallops and spoon on the rest of the dressing. Garnish
with lime zest and serve immediately.

WILD SALMON SALAD
Meat free
Serves 4

I like to make whole-meal salads spontaneously. You choose your vegetables then add them to ready-cooked protein foods: tofu fried in
coconut oil and seasoned with Cajun seasoning; cooked salmon; flaked,
cooked chicken; small cubes of leftover lamb roast or wild duck; even

hard-boiled eggs. This salad is ready in a minute, easy to prepare and delicious.

WHAT YOU NEED
500g (18oz) cooked wild salmon, flaked
4 large stalks celery, sliced into thin, diagonal strips using a mandolin
3 tbsp fresh coriander, finely chopped
½ small red onion, finely chopped
small finger of fresh ginger, finely shredded
2 tbsp fresh lemon juice
100ml (4fl oz) mayonnaise (preferably home-made)
4 glorious lettuce leaves

HERE'S HOW
Combine the flaked salmon (or whatever else you're using) with the celery, coriander, onion and ginger. Drizzle with lemon juice and mix in the mayonnaise with a fork. Spoon on to a plate covered with four large lettuce leaves and chill for half an hour before serving.

SALAD NIÇOISE
Meat free
Serves 6 generously

The run-of-the-mill salad niçoise turns me off completely. Most of what is served in its name tastes like day-old tuna and limp vegetables in a gooey sauce. This recipe is completely different. It uses fresh swordfish or tuna – sliced almost paper thin and seared or grilled. Then you take crunchy vegetables and create double-decker sandwiches, using the slices of fish as the 'container'. The result makes a visually pleasing, light and surprising meal. You can make it as an appetiser or make more and serve as a main course with a light, ultra-chilled white wine.

WHAT YOU NEED
4 tbsp extra-virgin olive oil
500g (18oz) swordfish or tuna (get your fishmonger to slice them as thin as he can)
200g (7oz) mangetout, de-stringed if necessary, blanched and cut diagonally
200g (7oz) fine green beans, blanched and cut diagonally
1 large red onion, coarsely chopped

300g (10½oz) cherry tomatoes (either red or yellow)
150g (5oz) baby spinach
50g (2oz) fresh basil
50g (2oz) flat-leaved parsley
50g (2oz) black olives
1 tin of anchovies
4–6 quail eggs, hard-boiled (optional)

FOR THE DRESSING
2 tbsp extra-virgin olive oil
2 tbsp fresh lime or lemon juice
1 tsp seed mustard
1–2 garlic cloves, finely chopped
1 tbsp chopped chives
freshly ground black pepper to taste
Celtic or Maldon sea salt to taste

HERE'S HOW
Heat a heavy frying pan or a teppenyaki grill to very hot. Add the olive oil and sear the pieces of swordfish or tuna, allowing them to sit in the pan until they brown and being careful not to disturb them. Do only a few at a time, replacing the oil if necessary. Then turn them over and cook quickly on the other side so that both sides become crisp. Remove from the heat and drain well on paper towels. (You can also cook them on a baking sheet under the grill, which takes about 5 minutes for each side.)

Mix together the blanched and fresh vegetables in a bowl. Add the olives and the anchovies. Place the dressing ingredients in a closed jar and shake. Pour over the salad and toss. Then layer the swordfish slices with salad, decorate with quail eggs in their shells and serve.

SALAD ON THE SIDE

I never met a vegetable I didn't like, but it took me a while to realise this. Like a lot of people, I grew up with mushy Brussels sprouts, canned spinach, revolting beetroot salads and other nameless horrors served in school meals. It was only when I began to make vegetable juices and exuberant salads that I discovered just how delicious they can be in all their wonderful incarnations.

These are salads to stand beside a meal of fish, meat, vegetarian or game. Dress your salads with dips and dressings (*see Dress It Up and Dip It*) or just pour on extra-virgin olive oil with lemon. Nuts and seeds make great toppings for all-vegetable offerings (*see Vegetarian Gourmet*).

Neptune's Bounty

The sea is said to be the source of all life. In the plant kingdom, sea vegetables have unparalleled power to create high-level well-being. Our blood contains more than 100 minerals and trace elements found equally in the sea and in the plants that live there. Sea plants contain up to 20 times the minerals of land plants plus an abundance of vitamins and other phytochemicals that are useful for health. Much of the fibre in seaweeds is so powerful in its ability to help the body detoxify that it can even remove traces of radioactive and toxic metals.

The only problem with seaweeds – and it's a big one – is you need to make sure the sea plants you eat come from seas that are relatively unpolluted, particularly by heavy metals, since wherever seaweeds grow they tend to accumulate whatever metal and minerals are in the waters.

When you first introduce seaweeds to your diet, it's a good idea to do it slowly, as it sometimes takes a week or two for the body to get used to digesting sea vegetables. Their flavour is also quite unique. Once you get to like it you will never want to be without it, but a few people find it takes a bit of getting used to.

One of my favourite seaweeds is nori. This comes in long, thin sheets and is used to make sushi. It makes a great snack or can be added to a salad, and has a beautiful crisp flavour. I like to toast it quickly by putting it under a grill for no more than 10–15 seconds, then crumbling it on a salad or simply taking a sheet or two and eating as a snack. You can use nori to wrap around just about anything from a sprout salad to cooked grains. You can even make little pieces of sushi with it.

WAKAME SALAD
Meat free
Serves 3

Wakame (*Undaria poinnatifida*) is an olive-coloured seaweed that grows in wing-like fronds. It is extremely high in calcium and rich in the B-complex vitamins niacin and thiamine. In Japan, wakame is used to cleanse the mother's blood after giving birth.

Buy wakame in its dried form and you need to soak it in water for 5–15 minutes to reconstitute it for cooking or salad-making. Be sure to save the liquid for cooking as it's rich in minerals. You can use wakame like a green leafy vegetable in stews and salads and by adding it to baked vegetables. It can be added to sauces such as pesto, and it's great chopped and tossed into a big pot of brown rice that you're cooking.

This is a rather lovely one-bowl meal you can carry with you, as it doesn't matter if it's not refrigerated for a few hours. It's great also to eat in the garden. When I make it to be eaten three or four hours later, I generally use finely sliced fennel bulb instead of lamb's lettuce.

WHAT YOU NEED
100g (4oz) wakame seaweed, soaked in water for 15 minutes then drained and finely sliced
2 courgettes, julienned in medium-size pieces
a finger of fresh ginger, finely sliced
Celtic or Maldon sea salt to taste
200g (7oz) cooked shrimp, cooked scallops or cooked tofu (optional)
50–100g (2–4oz) lamb's lettuce, dried, and prepared by cutting off the tip that grows out of the earth (if it is to be served 3–4 hours later, substitute medium-sliced fennel for the lamb's lettuce)
2 tbsp tamari
4 tbsp rice vinegar
3 tbsp sesame oil
2 garlic cloves, finely chopped
2 tbsp sake or white wine
3–4 tbsp dried bonito flakes or katsuobushi as a garnish

HERE'S HOW

Put the slices of wakame into a salad bowl and add the courgettes and ginger, sprinkling with salt. Add the shrimp, scallop, or tofu if using, and the lamb's lettuce. Mix together in a jar the tamari, vinegar, sesame oil, garlic and sake, and shake up. Pour over the salad and toss. Spoon into three deep Oriental serving bowls and garnish with dried bonito flakes or katsuobushi. (If you are going to serve this salad a few hours after making it, carry the bonito flakes or katsuobushi in another container and sprinkle them on when serving.) I sometimes add an edible flower such as a nasturtium or a marigold to this salad – one per serving – just for colour.

SEAWEED SALAD
Vegan
Serves 4

Some of my favourite salads are made from seaweed. These salads are so unusual in look and flavour that most people would never think of making them. The key to making a beautiful one is to use more than one kind of seaweed. Hijiki is one I use frequently. I also like wakame and arami. You can, however, use some of the others such as dulce and even nori. When using nori in a salad it's best to toast it for just 15–20 seconds under a grill or in a frying pan. Then break it up into small pieces and sprinkle on top, otherwise it tends to go soggy.

WHAT YOU NEED

150g (5oz) dried mixed seaweeds
1 light-coloured lettuce e.g. curly endive or little gem (shredded)
2 large carrots, julienned
3 small turnips, julienned
40g (1½oz) sesame seeds

FOR THE DRESSING

1 tbsp cold-pressed sesame oil or cold-pressed flaxseed oil
2 tbsp umeboshi vinegar, rice vinegar or lemon juice
2 garlic cloves, chopped
Celtic or Maldon sea salt to taste
freshly ground black pepper to taste

HERE'S HOW

Soak the seaweed in water for 30 minutes and then drain. Wash the lettuce and then chill both for 15 minutes if possible, since this salad is more delicious chilled than at room temperature. However, you can serve it at room temperature as well. Line your salad bowl with the lettuce then, after draining the seaweeds, add the julienned carrots and turnips.

Now place all the dressing ingredients in a jar and shake well. Pour over the seaweed, carrot and turnip mixture and toss. Now toast the sesame seeds in an oil-free frying pan or under the grill and sprinkle over everything immediately before serving. This salad will keep in good condition for several hours if you want to take it on a picnic. Unlike most salads it does not go limp, especially if you choose a good, crisp, light-coloured lettuce.

Savoury Salads With Fruit

CHICORY, APPLE AND PECAN SALAD
Vegan
Serves 4

Whenever I serve mushrooms at brunch, I like to complement them either with a beautiful bowl of crunchy radishes or a nut and fruit salad – especially apples and chicory. There is something magical about adding an apple to a salad. I only discovered this three or four years ago when by accident – being low on vegetables at the time – I grated a large apple into a salad I was making, using the coarse grater of my mandolin. This produced beautiful, slim pieces of apple. I then served the salad to a man who, unbeknown to me, disliked salad tremendously. He ate it with glee and then told me that it was the only salad he'd ever had that tasted good. That's when I learned the secret of salad-making for those who hate salads: practically any salad can be enhanced and made sweeter by grating an apple into it. In the case of this salad, the apple forms the central part of the recipe, but don't hesitate to try it with other salads too. I think you'll be delighted by the response.

WHAT YOU NEED
150g (5oz) lamb's lettuce
150g (5oz) chicory
2–3 large crunchy apples

75g (3oz) fresh, whole pecans
Celtic or Maldon sea salt to taste
freshly ground black pepper to taste

FOR THE DRESSING
juice of 2 lemons
2 ripe tomatoes
1 garlic clove
13 chives, finely chopped
1 tsp powdered kelp (optional)
75ml (3fl oz) walnut oil or extra-virgin olive oil
1 tbsp tamari
¼ tsp of cayenne pepper
1 tbsp Dijon mustard
1 tsp vegetable bouillon powder

HERE'S HOW
Wash, drain and wrap the lamb's lettuce and chicory in paper towels or a tea towel to crisp up in the refrigerator. Tear these greens into bite-sized pieces. Grate the apples on the coarse grater of a mandolin. (Do not try to use an ordinary grater for this: it does not work and your apples will end up as mush. If you don't have a mandolin, then simply cut the apples in long, lean chunks about 6mm/a quarter of an inch thick.) Now add half the pecans and season to taste. Blend together the salad dressing by placing all the ingredients in a food processor or blender and mixing thoroughly. Now pour the dressing over the salad, mix well, sprinkle the remaining pecans on top and serve immediately. This dressing may be refrigerated and kept for up to four days.

FENNEL, ORANGE AND GRAPE SALAD
Vegan
Serves 4

The fresh, crunchy taste of fennel makes you feel as though it's good for you when you eat it, and indeed it is. Sodium and potassium are antagonists – they need to be taken in by the body in good balance in order to maintain health. Most of us eat too much salt – sodium chloride. Fennel, which is rich in potassium, helps redress the balance.

WHAT YOU NEED

2 medium-sized bulbs of fennel

2 large or 4 small ripe oranges

125g (4½oz) mangetout (get the tendrils as well if you can, as they are so beautiful)

175g (6oz) black and/or white grapes, removed from the stalk

FOR THE DRESSING

2 tbsp walnut oil

1 tsp Meaux mustard

1 tbsp chopped broad-leafed parsley

Celtic or Maldon sea salt to taste

freshly ground black pepper to taste

HERE'S HOW

Slice the fennel crosswise so that you end up with oval-shaped pieces. Peel the oranges and pull into segments. Add all of these to a flat bowl and garnish with the mangetout tendrils and grapes. For the dressing, put everything into a jar, shake it up and pour over the salad. Toss and serve immediately on separate plates.

ORANGE ORANGE SALAD
Vegan
Serves 2

A surprising combination, but it works.

WHAT YOU NEED

4 carrots

6 oranges

75–150g (3–6oz) white cabbage

2 handfuls of raisins or small seedless grapes

4 tsp sesame seeds

HERE'S HOW

Coarsely chop the carrots. Juice four of the oranges and mix with the carrots until you have a smooth mixture. Finely shred or grate the cabbage and put in a bowl with the raisins or grapes. Pour the carrot mixture over it and mix lightly with a fork. Sprinkle with the sesame seeds and garnish with the two remaining oranges, peeled and sliced.

Garden Delights

Flowers and wild herbs are the stuff of which magnificent side salads are created. I always keep my eye open for some wonderful offering from Nature – baby dandelion leaves, wild garlic, the autumn's first wild blackberries. I make them the centre around which a festival of texture, taste and colour can be created. Let the vegetables speak for themselves and you are sure to create one winning combination after another.

MESCLUN AND FLOWER SALAD
Vegan
Serves 4

A French Provençal word, 'mesclun' means a mixture of delicate salad leaves, including such things as curly endive, romaine, red radicchio, flat-leaved parsley, dandelions – even purslane. These leaves are very easy to grow, and most are harvested by cutting a few at a time and allowing the plants to go on producing yet more beautiful leaves. You can buy mesclun to grow in your own garden. It comes in packages of seeds called 'saladisi', or buy one of the 'cut-and-come-again' salad varieties.

WHAT YOU NEED
3 or 4 of any of the following mesclun leaves:
   curly endive
   dandelion leaves
   lamb's lettuce
   oak-leaf lettuce
   purslane
   red radicchio
   rocket
   romaine lettuce
10–12 brightly coloured nasturtium flowers

FOR THE DRESSING
2 garlic cloves, finely chopped
¼ tsp Dijon mustard
4 tbsp walnut oil
1 tbsp white wine vinegar
1 tbsp chervil, finely chopped
1 tbsp flat-leaved parsley, finely chopped

HERE'S HOW

Put all the mesclun leaves into a huge glass salad bowl – I use glass because the leaves are so beautiful that it's a shame to conceal them. Then, for the dressing, put all the ingredients in a screw-top jar and shake vigorously to blend. Sprinkle over the leaves, toss very lightly and serve immediately. This is a very delicate salad and needs careful handling to prevent bruising.

WILD HERB SALAD
Vegan
Serves 4

Herbs are powerfully health-enriching plants. They are even more valuable than fruits and vegetables in terms of their antioxidant and other health-giving properties. Herbs have to struggle hard to survive, and have learned to thrive over generations. We benefit from the strong life force they can bring to us.

I use herbs as often as I can when I cook, raw whenever possible. In fact, when I'm using a herb such as sage, thyme or rosemary in a cooked dish, I often add the herb right at the end. In this way it maintains all its wonderful nutritional and energetic properties – not to mention its brighter colour and stronger taste.

My favourite way of eating herbs is in a wild herb salad. You can make this salad, with almost anything, but the more wild herbs and dark-green vegetables you use, the better it works. Even the flavour of this salad is wild, and its nutritional value is superb.

You certainly don't need all the ingredients listed here. You can use as few as two or three different herbs. I love to sprinkle the whole lot with edible flowers, like marigold petals, just for colour. This is a recipe you can make a hundred ways and it works perfectly each time. Don't be afraid to omit ingredients such as olives or lovage if you don't happen to have any. Just one word of warning – when it comes to choosing your light-green lettuce, don't go for iceberg since the flavour does not work with the herbs, but you can use chicory. The salad needs little tossing. Some of its ingredients are very strong, but others are rather fragile, so it requires careful handling.

WHAT YOU NEED

1 large bunch of fresh organic rocket or 2 hearts of Cos lettuce, sliced
   or torn
1 light-green lettuce
18 sprigs of lamb's lettuce
12 leaves of purslane
18 leaves of fresh basil
1 small bunch of fresh tarragon
6 sprigs of lovage
12 leaves of broad-leafed parsley
1 small radicchio
1 red onion, chopped, or some fat red radishes, slivered
1 yellow pepper, sliced
1 red pepper, sliced
handful of fat black olives
handful of marigold petals, to garnish
few sprigs of fennel, to garnish
mint leaves (optional), to garnish

FOR THE DRESSING

6 tbsp extra-virgin olive oil
3 tbsp balsamic vinegar
Celtic or Maldon sea salt to taste
freshly ground pepper
dash of Cajun seasoning

HERE'S HOW

Wash the rocket and lettuce in a salad basket, then dry and shred diagonally in medium pieces or tear into bite-sized chunks. Place in a flat
salad bowl and chill in the refrigerator for half an hour. Wash the lamb's
lettuce, getting rid of the root ends, then whirl in a salad basket to dry
and wrap it in a tea towel to chill. Wash and prepare all the other
ingredients similarly and chill them for 15 minutes.

When you are ready to serve the salad, remove the salad bowl from
the refrigerator. Arrange the herbs and sprigs, including the lamb's
lettuce, in the bowl and incorporate whatever additions you wish, such
as the pepper, radishes or olives. Now add the dressing ingredients one
by one on top of the salad and toss lightly. Garnish with flower petals,
fennel and mint if you happen to have it, and serve on individual flat
dishes.

FLORENCE FENNEL SALAD
Vegetarian
Serves 4

In Italy, fennel is often eaten raw at the end of a meal as a digestive. It has a refreshing aniseed taste.

WHAT YOU NEED
2 fennel bulbs, cut into fine slices
1 romaine lettuce, torn into small pieces
225g (8oz) ricotta cheese or tofu
50g (2oz) coarsely chopped pecan nuts
Italian dressing (*see Dress It Up*)
1 tbsp chopped chives, to garnish
feathery fennel tops or seeds, to garnish

HERE'S HOW
Discard the outer leaves of the fennel if they are tough and either slice the whole bulbs crosswise or separate them into stalks and slice them. Mix with the torn lettuce leaves. Dice the cheese or tofu and add to the salad, along with the nuts. Dress with an Italian dressing and serve with a sprinkling of chives and fresh fennel tops or seeds.

WILD MUSHROOM SALAD
Vegetarian
Serves 4

Easy to make, delicious and health-enhancing, this salad is a winner at brunch, lunch or tea. I like to mix wild mushrooms with shiitake, reishi and maitake mushrooms, which I buy fresh if I can, though as often as not I am forced to use the dried ones instead. Dried mushrooms are easy to prepare. Pop them into a pot and cover with water then bring them to the boil and simmer for 15–20 minutes. Drain the mushrooms. Now they are ready for use in any recipe.

WHAT YOU NEED
250g (9oz) mixed salad leaves (whatever is in season)
300g (10½oz) wild mushrooms, washed and dried, or dried mushrooms
    prepared as above
25g (1oz) butter

2 tbsp extra-virgin olive oil
125ml (4fl oz) dry white wine
pinch of saffron threads
vinaigrette dressing
Celtic or Maldon sea salt to taste
freshly ground black pepper to taste
fresh coriander or other fresh herbs e.g. basil or broad-leafed parsley,
  to garnish

HERE'S HOW

Clean the salad leaves and dry either in a tea towel or in a basket. Pop
them into the refrigerator to crisp up. Slice the mushrooms and, if
you're going to cook them, fry very quickly in the butter and olive oil
over a gentle heat until they begin to look juicy. Then add the wine
and saffron to help the flavours combine. Remove from the heat and
cool. If you're going to use the mushrooms raw, wash and slice them
and, after reconstituting any dried mushrooms you are going to use,
you're ready to go. Put the salad leaves into a bowl and toss with a
light vinaigrette dressing, then add the mushrooms and pour on the
rest of the dressing. Season with salt and coarsely ground black pepper,
add the other herbs to garnish and serve.

SUMMER SYMPHONY
Vegan
Serves 4

This salad is an exciting play of colours and shapes.

WHAT YOU NEED

1 lettuce (Cos is a good choice)
100g (4oz) small cauliflower florets
2 celery stalks, finely chopped
2 carrots, finely grated or cut into matchsticks
6 cherry tomatoes
4 radishes, sliced
1 green pepper, cut into thin strips
mayonnaise
watercress, to garnish
fresh sweetcorn, to garnish (remove the kernels with a sharp knife or
  just pop them off with your fingers)

HERE'S HOW

Place the lettuce leaves, torn into bite-sized pieces or shredded, into a bowl. Prepare the vegetables and arrange in layers in the bowl, keeping the watercress for decoration. Dress with thinned mayonnaise – maybe blended with a tomato or two – and top with sweetcorn and sprigs of watercress.

ITALIAN SALAD
Vegan
Serves 2

If you can get hold of the ingredients, this salad is something special.

WHAT YOU NEED
1 Italian red lettuce (radicchio)
1 small Cos lettuce or 2 chicories
1 red pepper, cut into rings or diced
1 green pepper, cut into rings or diced
1 or 2 large Italian tomatoes, peeled and diced
4 radishes, cut into segments
1 red onion, cut into thin rings
button mushrooms, thinly sliced
Italian dressing (*see Dress It Up*)
fresh basil
fennel seeds or black pepper to taste

HERE'S HOW
Shred the lettuces and chicories finely and put them into a large bowl. Make a nest in the centre and put the other vegetables into it, sprinkling the onion and mushroom slices in last. Toss with spicy Italian dressing with lots of fresh basil and sprinkle with toasted fennel seeds or freshly ground black pepper.

IGUANA SALAD
Vegan
Serves 2

This is one of the many variations of guacamole, a favourite Mexican dish based on avocados. Used as a dip or eaten straight, Iguana Salad is a real treat whichever way you go. (To ripen hard avocados, put them in a brown paper bag in a warm spot for a couple of days.)

WHAT YOU NEED
2 juicy tomatoes
½ red pepper
1 small onion
2 or 3 really ripe avocados
juice of 1 lemon or lime
small garlic clove
Tabasco sauce and/or 1 fresh chilli, very finely chopped
extra-virgin olive oil
pepper and vegetable bouillon, to season

HERE'S HOW
Chop the tomatoes and red pepper into small pieces, grate the onion and mix them together. Take the stones out of the avocados, scoop out the flesh with a spoon and mash it with a fork or in the food processor, adding the lemon or lime juice to prevent it going brown. If you are using a food processor, leave the avocado in it and add the garlic (pressed first), a few drops of Tabasco sauce and other seasonings, including the chopped chilli pepper if using. Blend thoroughly. If you are not using a processor, beat the garlic and spices into a little olive oil and pour over the salad last of all. Mix the avocado mixture with the other vegetables and adjust the seasoning to your taste.

CONFETTI SPROUT SALAD
Vegetarian
Serves 4

The more variety of sprouts in this salad the better.

WHAT YOU NEED
75g (3oz) buckwheat or sunflower greens, or lettuce or other greens
225g (8oz) mung bean sprouts
225g (8oz) lentil sprouts (green and black lentils for a stunning colour effect)
100g (4oz) chickpea sprouts
100g (4oz) fenugreek or aduki sprouts
a few radish sprouts
mayonnaise dressing (*see Dress It Up*)

sunflower seeds (optional)
a little dulse or grated cheese and paprika, to serve

HERE'S HOW
Place the greens in a salad bowl to make a bed for the sprouts. Mix the sprouts together and dress with a mayonnaise dressing. Some sunflower seeds soaked overnight are a nice addition. Spoon the sprout mixture on to the bed of greens and sprinkle with a little dulse or some grated cheese and paprika.

ORIENTAL SPROUT SALAD
Vegan
Serves 4

This is good prepared an hour or two in advance and left to marinate in its own dressing.

WHAT YOU NEED
225g (8oz) mushrooms, thinly sliced
225g (8oz) mung bean sprouts
75g (3oz) white cabbage, finely shredded
bunch of watercress or chives, to garnish

FOR THE DRESSING
2 tbsp extra-virgin olive oil
2 tbsp tamari sauce
2 tbsp lemon juice and a little grated lemon rind
dash of vinegar
2 tsp Manuka honey or maple syrup
½ tsp finely grated ginger or powdered ginger

HERE'S HOW
Mix the mushrooms, sprouts and cabbage together. Place in a shallow dish and pour over the dressing. Garnish with watercress leaves or chopped chives.

Mainly-for-winter Salads
The disadvantage in wintertime is that the selection of fresh vegetables is limited. Nevertheless, with a little ingenuity one can prepare some delicious winter salads.

KING OF HADES' SALAD
Vegan
Serves 4

This salad is dedicated to Pluto, god of the underworld, because its main ingredients are grown underground.

WHAT YOU NEED
350g (12oz) grated carrots
75g (3oz) finely grated beetroot
75g (3oz) finely grated turnip, parsnip, Jerusalem artichoke, kohlrabi, white radish (choose the three that most appeal to you)
raisins or diced onion, a handful or to taste
mayonnaise dressing (*see Dress It Up*)
nutmeg

HERE'S HOW
Mix all your root vegetables together and add the raisins or diced onion. Pour a mayonnaise dressing over the top and dust with nutmeg. Nutmeg is very warming and said to make one merry. Add a tub of plain cottage cheese and you have a very substantial main dish.

PERSEPHONE'S TEMPTATIONS
Vegan
Serves 4

Zeus proclaimed that Persephone, abducted by Pluto, the King of Hades, could only return to the bright world above if she refused to eat all food served to her in the underworld. She held out for a while, but finally succumbed to the temptation of a few succulent ruby-red pomegranate seeds. Little wonder!

WHAT YOU NEED
10–12 young Brussels sprouts
5–6 sticks of celery
2 pomegranates
2 or 3 seedless satsumas
Sweet Ginger or Cashew Mayonnaise (*see Dress It Up*)
sunflower seeds, to garnish

HERE'S HOW

Discard the outer leaves of the Brussels sprouts and grate the rest finely. Finely chop the celery. Remove the pomegranate seeds (don't use the pith as it is extremely bitter). Peel and slice the satsumas crossways as you would oranges, then separate the sliced segments. Mix all the ingredients together and dress with Sweet Ginger or Cashew Mayonnaise. Sprinkle sunflower seeds (toasted if you wish) over the top.

CRUNCHY BROCCOLI SALAD
Vegetarian
Serves 6

You can make this salad either with fresh, raw broccoli – the way I prefer it – or by trimming the stalks and florets and steaming the broccoli until tender but still crunchy. If you are using fresh broccoli, grate it finely on a mandolin. If you are using steamed broccoli, rinse it in cold water after cooking and drain.

WHAT YOU NEED
455g (1lb) fresh broccoli
50ml (2fl oz) mayonnaise (preferably home made)
50ml (2fl oz) soured cream (optional)
3 tbsp fresh lemon juice
¼ tsp dried tarragon, crushed
1 tbsp mild American mustard
2 tbsp finely chopped spring onions
Celtic or Maldon sea salt to taste
freshly ground black pepper to taste

HERE'S HOW

Steam the broccoli, if required, then chill. Place broccoli, either raw or cooked, in a bowl. Add mayonnaise, soured cream if using, lemon juice, tarragon, mustard, spring onions and season. Toss your salad until everything is evenly combined.

Slaws to Die for

Coleslaws are great winter salad favourites in my family, but of course the ingredients can be bought all year round. The principal ingredient of coleslaws – cabbage – has many health-giving properties. High in vitamin C, raw cabbage juice is used to treat stomach ulcers. It is also a good blood tonic for people with an iron deficiency and cleanses the mucous membranes of the stomach and intestines. In the past, cabbage leaves were warmed and crushed and either laid on the skin to cure such ailments as eczema or used as bandages for wounds and sores.

When choosing a cabbage, make sure its leaves are tightly packed, that the head is heavy and firm and that it still has its outer leaves on. To keep it fresh, put it in a plastic bag and keep it in the fridge.

ROYAL SLAW
Vegan
Serves 4

A slaw fit for a king. This recipe includes caraway seeds, useful for dispelling painful stomach wind. Some people chew a small handful before a meal to prevent flatulence and stimulate digestion (dill seeds have similar uses).

WHAT YOU NEED
75–150g (3–6oz) grated red cabbage
75–150g (3–6oz) grated white cabbage, plus a few outer leaves of either cabbage
75g (3oz) grated carrots
1 stalk of celery, finely sliced
½ red pepper, grated
1 small onion (optional)
raisins, to garnish
½ tsp celery seeds
1 tsp caraway seeds
1 tsp dill seeds
mayonnaise dressing (*see Dress It Up*)

HERE'S HOW
This salad can be made very quickly in a food processor. Use a medium-sized grater, rather than a small one that makes a mushy slaw that swims in its own juices. Grate the ingredients one by one, omitting the onion if you like. Line a bowl with cabbage leaves and put all the grated ingredients, mixed together, inside them. Scatter with raisins and seeds. Use a mayonnaise dressing with cayenne in it for bite.

BLOOD-APPLE SLAW
Vegan
Serves 4

This was my introduction to eating raw beetroot – until I tried it I wasn't at all convinced. Now this is one of my favourite salads. Beetroot is an excellent liver cleanser.

WHAT YOU NEED
6 sweet eating apples, grated
orange juice
2 small beetroots
cinnamon or nutmeg
fresh mint, to garnish

HERE'S HOW
Grate the apples and sprinkle with orange juice to stop them going brown. Finely grate the beetroots (no need to peel them, just scrub thoroughly), drain off any excess juice and add to the apples. This salad does not really need a dressing. Serve it with a dusting of cinnamon or nutmeg and garnish with mint sprigs. As a variation, grate a carrot into the mixture too, or add some finely chopped celery.

SPINACH SLAW
Vegan
Serves 4

A delicious combination of flavours. Be sure the spinach is really fresh and crisp. If it looks a little droopy, wash it, put it in a bowl of cold water for about half an hour, then drain and put in the fridge in a polythene bag to crisp up. Don't forget to remove the tough main ribs from the leaves.

WHAT YOU NEED
large handful of seedless raisins, soaked
juice of 1 orange and 1 lemon
large bunch of young spinach leaves
75g (3oz) white cabbage
3 apples (preferably sweet red ones)

HERE'S HOW
Soak the raisins in the fresh orange and lemon juice for about an hour. Shred the spinach leaves, grate the cabbage and dice the apples, and put them all into a bowl. Stir in the soaked raisins and juice. Use an oil dressing with a little honey in it.

RAINBOW SLAW
Vegan
Serves 4

This is a nice salad to serve at parties because it is so eye-catching. Choose half a dozen different vegetables of contrasting colour and shred or grate them, then arrange them in curving rows on a large platter to form a rainbow pattern. Clean your processor grater between the different vegetables or you will get the colours staining each other. Try some of the following in quantities of 75g (3oz) or so.

- ❑ red cabbage
- ❑ white cabbage
- ❑ green cabbage
- ❑ carrots
- ❑ beetroot
- ❑ turnips
- ❑ parsnips
- ❑ swedes
- ❑ shredded beet greens or spinach

Put a 'pot of gold' of salad dressing at one end of the rainbow.

THREE-SEED TOPPING
Vegan

Equal amounts of pumpkin, sesame and sunflower seeds mixed together provide an almost perfect combination of protein, essential fatty acids and other nutrients. Mix them, toast them, keep them and use them often.

WHAT YOU NEED
225–450g (8–16oz) sesame, pumpkin and/or sunflower seeds
3 tbsp organic bouillon powder or 1–2 organic vegetable bouillon
  cubes, carefully flaked
1 garlic clove, very finely chopped
1 tbsp onion flakes (optional)

HERE'S HOW
Heat a large, heavy, dry pan on the stove and lightly toast the seeds until they turn a beautiful brown. Be careful not to overcook them. You can also toast them in the oven for 15 minutes at 150°C/300°F/Gas Mark 2. Be sure to stir them frequently. Then add the other ingredients while the seeds are still warm and blend well. Sprinkle them liberally over warm vegetables or fresh salads.

OTHER WAYS TO GO
Seed Power: When you've finished toasting the seeds, grind them in a food processor or coffee grinder until fine, then add the other ingredients and blend well. This is good to add to soups, dressings, muesli – almost anything – for a crunchy, powdery finish.
Wild Ones: To create intriguing, exotic flavours, use only 100g (4oz) of sesame seeds together with 50g (2oz) of any of the following seeds: fennel, celery, poppy, caraway, dill or cumin.

DRESS IT UP

The fresh vegetables, herbs and other delicacies that you put into a salad are only half the story. The other half is the dressing. A good dressing can make a tasty dish of even the simplest salad. So splendid are some of the Powerhouse dressings recipes that they even delight vegetable-haters. Most of the recipes that follow can be used as dips or dressings, depending upon how thick you make them. These dressings will dress a salad for four people, depending on personal taste. Use as little or as much as you like.

Salad Dressings

Let's look first at some recipes for rich, creamy dressings.

MASTER MAYONNAISE
Vegetarian

Mayonnaise is not as difficult to make as people think, particularly since the advent of high-speed blenders and food processors. It does, however, take a little bit of patience and practice. If you don't succeed with your first emulsion, wash and dry your blender or food processor carefully, then use the 'unemulsified emulsion' to drop back, drop by drop, into a new supply of egg yolks as though it were just oil. In effect, go through the process all over again. Naturally, you will have to add a bit more seasoning as you'll end up with some more mayonnaise. If at first you don't succeed, try again. As always, buy your eggs from a good supplier and always insist an organic or, at the very least, free-range.

This mayonnaise is made with extra-virgin olive oil. You can do all sorts of wonderful things to it, like add garlic, herbs or mustards. Commercial mayonnaise – the kind you buy in jars in the supermarket – is something you want to avoid as much as you can. These products are full of transfatty acids and made from the cheapest, nastiest forms of hydrogenated junk fats. Mayonnaise you make yourself will keep for four to five days in the coolest part of the refrigerator. Here's my basic recipe plus some suggestions on how to vary it.

WHAT YOU NEED

2 yolks from large eggs

275ml (10fl oz) extra-virgin olive oil or half olive oil and half flaxseed
     oil

2 tbsp cider vinegar

½ tsp dry mustard

Celtic or Maldon sea salt to taste

freshly ground black pepper to taste

2 tbsp lemon juice

HERE'S HOW

Put the egg yolks in a blender or food processor. Begin to blend on
a low setting. Very, very gradually add the oil – literally drop by drop
as the blender is running. Soon you will see an emulsion beginning
to form. When this starts to happen, the mixture will be thicker with
the consistency of a light face cream. Continue slowly to add oil to the
mixture in a thin stream, all the while keeping the blender low, until
you have added half the oil. Now add the vinegar, mustard, salt and
pepper and the lemon juice, all the while continuing to blend. Finally,
slowly add the remaining olive oil. Taste and adjust seasoning. This
recipe makes about 300ml (10fl oz).

OTHER WAYS TO GO

Orange Zest: Take 225ml (8fl oz) of home-made mayonnaise, but leave
out the mustard, and add 2 tsp grated orange zest as well as 1 tbsp
fresh orange juice and 2 tbsp finely chopped fresh mint leaves.

Curried Mayonnaise: Take 100ml (4fl oz) of home-made mayonnaise
and add 1 tsp mild to medium curry powder as well as 1 tsp finely
grated fresh ginger.

TOFU MAYONNAISE LITE
Vegan

Instead of being made with eggs, this mayonnaise is made with tofu.
You can use it for salads and dips as well as sauces to go on lightly
steamed or wok-fried vegetables. It's easy to make and light as air to
eat. Like conventional mayonnaise, you can vary this recipe by adding
garlic, Cajun seasoning, mustard or fresh herbs to give a totally different
look and flavour.

WHAT YOU NEED
455g (1lb) soft tofu, drained
50g (2oz) granular lecithin
3 tbsp lemon juice
small pinch of stevia, Manuka honey or maple syrup to taste
1 tsp vegetarian broth powder
50ml (2floz) flaxseed oil or extra-virgin olive oil
1 tsp fine lemon zest
Celtic or Maldon sea salt to taste
freshly ground black pepper to taste

HERE'S HOW
Put the tofu into a blender and add the lecithin granules, lemon juice, stevia, Manuka honey or maple syrup to taste and broth powder as well as half of the oil. Blend well until thoroughly mixed. Now slowly, drop by drop, add the remaining oil and blend again for 2–4 minutes until the mixture grows thick and creamy. Finally, stir in the lemon zest and season to taste. This mixture will keep in the refrigerator for 5–6 days.

CASHEW MAYONNAISE
Vegan

A delicious alternative mayonnaise, which goes beautifully with crudités and also as a garnish for lightly steamed vegetables.

WHAT YOU NEED
125g (4½oz) cashews
225ml (8fl oz) spring water
2 garlic cloves, finely chopped
juice of 1 lemon
1 tsp vegetable bouillon powder or sea salt or soy sauce
spring onions, finely chopped, to taste

HERE'S HOW
Blend the ingredients together well in a food processor or blender, chill and serve. This recipe will keep for 4–5 days covered in the refrigerator.

TAHINI MAYONNAISE
Vegan

Once you know the basic ingredients and method for this egg-free mayonnaise, there are lots of delicious variations you can try. This mayonnaise is delicious as a dip for crudités or served over steamed vegetables.

WHAT YOU NEED
juice of 2 lemons or 100ml (4fl oz) cider vinegar
½ tsp vegetable bouillon powder or soy sauce
4 tbsp tahini
100ml (4fl oz) water
1 garlic clove, chopped
50ml (2fl oz) olive oil

HERE'S HOW
Mix all the ingredients except the olive oil in a blender or food processor until thoroughly blended. Add the olive oil very slowly, as much as you need to thicken. Store in a glass jar in the refrigerator and it will keep for 4–5 days.

OTHER WAYS TO GO
Honey and Lemon Mayonnaise: Add caraway or dill seeds perhaps, 1 tbsp cider vinegar, some finely grated lemon rind, a little honey and some finely grated onion if desired. Sprinkle a few sesame or poppy seeds into the dressing just before you serve it.
Mexican Pepper Mayonnaise: Add 2 tbsp finely chopped red and/or green pepper, 1 tbsp finely minced onion, a pinch of cayenne pepper, a little mustard and ½ tsp vegetable bouillon powder. Combine all the ingredients in the blender or put them in a screw-top jar and shake well to mix.

CREAMY LEMON DRESSING
Vegan

WHAT YOU NEED
juice of 2 lemons
2 tbsp chopped cashews
½ tsp vegetable bouillon powder
100ml (4fl oz) extra-virgin olive oil

HERE'S HOW

Combine the ingredients, except the oil, together in a blender or food processor and blend thoroughly. Then add the oil slowly, drop by drop.

Classic Dressings

LIGHT VINAIGRETTE
Vegan

This dressing is especially good for leafy salads such as lettuce and spinach. With the right seasonings such as tasty mustard and specific herbs, it can be very flavourful and not at all the 'plain oil and vinegar dressing' most people know.

WHAT YOU NEED

2 tbsp apple cider vinegar
4 tbsp sesame oil or flaxseed oil
½ tsp Meaux mustard
½ tsp tarragon
½ tsp chervil
½ tsp vegetable bouillon powder or sea salt

HERE'S HOW

Mix the vinegar, oil, mustard, herbs and bouillon powder or salt together and blend well by pouring into a screw-top jar and shaking thoroughly.

FRENCH LIGHT
Vegan

WHAT YOU NEED

175ml (6fl oz) tomato juice
50ml (2fl oz) lemon juice
1 tsp wholegrain mustard or mustard powder
a little vegetable bouillon powder or tamari
1 garlic clove, crushed or a dried tarragon leaf
black pepper to taste

HERE'S HOW

Combine all the ingredients in a blender or pour into a screw-top jar and shake well to mix.

OTHER WAYS TO GO

Rich and Hot: Add to the basic dressing:

1 tbsp soy sauce

1 finely chopped spring onion

a dash of cayenne

Balsamic: Add to the basic dressing 1 tbsp of balsamic vinegar.

Herb: My favourite combination of herbs for dressings is 3 tbsp each of fresh marjoram, basil, thyme and dill or lovage, finely chopped. (Use 2 tsp of each if dried.)

Citrus: Use in the basic dressing:

175g (6oz) seasoned tofu

juice of ½ a lemon

juice of 1 orange

1 tbsp cider vinegar

Add to it:

pinch of nutmeg

1 tsp chervil

1 tsp Manuka honey

Celtic or Maldon sea salt to taste

freshly ground black pepper to taste

zest of a lemon, finely shredded

zest of an orange, finely shredded

Blend all ingredients except the citrus zests until smooth. Then add the zests and mix by hand.

SPICE IT UP

Vegan

A pleasant, light dressing that seems to complement any salad.

WHAT YOU NEED

juice of 2 lemons

2 ripe tomatoes

1 garlic clove

12 chives, chopped finely

1 tsp powdered kelp (optional)

75ml (3fl oz) extra-virgin olive oil or flaxseed oil

1 tsp cayenne

1 tbsp tamari

1 tbsp Dijon mustard

1 tsp vegetable bouillon powder

HERE'S HOW
Blend the ingredients together in a food processor or blender until thoroughly mixed. This dressing may be refrigerated and kept for up to four days.

ITALIAN DRESSING
Vegan

Another classic dressing. It goes well with my favourite greens, such as lamb's lettuce, rocket, American land cress and curly cress, served on their own and sprinkled with parsley.

WHAT YOU NEED
600ml (20 fl oz) extra-virgin olive oil or half olive oil and half flaxseed oil
2 tbsp paprika
2 tbsp finely chopped fresh basil
2 tsp vegetable bouillon powder
½ tsp dried oregano
pinch of cayenne
pinch of kelp (optional)
30g (1oz) chopped fennel
½ tsp finely chopped red pepper

HERE'S HOW
Put the ingredients into a screw-top jar and shake vigorously until well mixed. You may thin this dressing with water if it seems too thick. It will keep well for up to 10 days in the refrigerator.

BASIL AND MORE BASIL DRESSING
Vegan

Since basil is my favourite herb, I'm occasionally accused of overdoing it. So far as I'm concerned there is nothing more uplifting than a basil dressing on a magnificent salad of green leaves. My favourites are rocket – especially wild rocket – and lamb's lettuce, or *mâche* as the French call it.

WHAT YOU NEED
100ml (4fl oz) extra-virgin olive oil
3 tbsp fresh lemon juice
25–50g (1–2oz) fresh basil, chopped
1 tsp vegetable bouillon powder
freshly ground black pepper to taste

HERE'S HOW
Mix all the ingredients in a food processor until smooth, adjusting the flavour as necessary. Use immediately or store in a container in the refrigerator for up to two days.

GREEN DREAM
Vegetarian

This dressing is ideal on finely sliced tomatoes.

WHAT YOU NEED
2 cucumbers
3 spring onions, chopped finely
juice of 1 lemon
1 tsp horseradish
½ tsp vegetable bouillon powder or dash of soy sauce
Celtic or Maldon sea salt to taste
225ml (8fl oz) natural yoghurt or home-made mayonnaise

HERE'S HOW
In a food processor, blend together all the ingredients except the mayonnaise or yoghurt. Fold into the mayonnaise or yoghurt and chill. This dressing will not keep for more than a day.

AVOCADO DELIGHT
Vegan

This is a superb dip or dressing, and very rich indeed. Excellent on a sprout salad or as a dip for crudités.

WHAT YOU NEED
1 avocado, peeled and stoned
juice of 1 lemon
juice of ½ an orange
1 small onion, chopped finely
1 garlic clove, chopped finely
handful of fresh herbs – mint, parsley or basil
freshly ground black pepper to taste

HERE'S HOW
Blend all the ingredients in a food processor or blender and serve. This dressing will not keep for more than a day in a refrigerator.

PARSLEY CREAM
Vegetarian

This is a low-fat salad dressing based on yoghurt. It's particularly good served on salads or sprouts, cucumbers and tomatoes. It also makes a nice addition to a slaw.

WHAT YOU NEED
225ml (8fl oz) natural, low-fat yoghurt
juice of 1 lemon
½ tsp dill
1 small onion, chopped
2 tsp chopped parsley
½ tsp vegetable bouillon powder or soy sauce

HERE'S HOW
Blend the ingredients well together by hand or in a blender. Will keep for 4–5 days in a refrigerator.

GLORIOUS GREEN HERBS
Vegetarian

This dressing is an absolute cinch to make if you have fresh herbs in the garden. You may be amazed to find how many different herb varieties you can use to make it.

WHAT YOU NEED
2 tbsp extra-virgin olive oil or flaxseed oil
2 tbsp lemon juice
175ml (6fl oz) fresh natural yoghurt
8 tbsp fresh herbs from the garden (whatever you have available: lovage, mint, apple mint, lemon mint, chives, spring onions, etc.)

HERE'S HOW
Place all the ingredients in a blender or food processor and blend thoroughly until the dressing turns green. This dressing will keep for 4–5 days in the refrigerator.

WILD CARROT
Vegan

This dressing works well either on a salad or on steamed vegetables.

WHAT YOU NEED
3 large carrots, washed and cut into small pieces
10 chives, chopped finely
1 tsp vegetable bouillon powder
150g (5oz) blanched almonds (preferably soaked overnight in 225–450ml (8–16fl oz) spring or filtered water)
2 tsp chopped parsley

HERE'S HOW
Put all the ingredients into a food processor or blender and blend with as much water as you need to make the dressing the consistency you want. It's best to leave it thick if you want to use it as a dip, or make it thinner as a dressing to pour over salads.

SUNNY TOMATO SPECIAL
Vegan

A surprising combination of the tangy flavour of tomatoes with the richness of fresh sunflower seeds.

WHAT YOU NEED
6 fresh tomatoes

225g (8oz) sunflower seeds
1 tsp vegetable bouillon powder or soy sauce
1 garlic clove, finely chopped
juice of 2 lemons
1 tbsp fresh, finely chopped parsley or fresh basil (if you can't get the
    fresh herbs you may use much smaller quantities of the dried ones)

HERE'S HOW
Put the ingredients together in a blender or food processor and blend
thoroughly. If you want a thicker consistency, add more sunflower seeds
(but remember the dressing will thicken as it stands); if you want a
thinner consistency, add a little water. Chill thoroughly before use. This
dressing will keep for two days in the refrigerator.

Extra-light Dressings
Light, low-fat dressings are especially flavoursome when skilfully
blended for texture and spiked with garlic or fresh herbs. Don't be
afraid to experiment with them. You can make some of them out of
surprising leftovers – a cup of cooked brown rice from the night before
or 100g (4oz) of lentils or sprouted chickpeas can make a great base
for a creamy dressing. Most call for simple ingredients and supermarket
spices such as garlic salt, onion powder or Cajun seasoning. Be sure
to season each to taste and to add an extra ingredient or two whenever you feel it needs it. Always make low-fat dressing to taste. The
more inventive you become, the better they get.

SPROUT SALAD DRESSING
Vegan

WHAT YOU NEED
100g (4oz) tofu or three medium-ripe tomatoes
25g (1oz) fresh garden herbs
1 tbsp sesame seeds
2 tbsp lemon juice
Celtic or Maldon sea salt to taste
coarse-ground black pepper to taste
1 tbsp shallots, finely chopped
1 tbsp celery, finely chopped

HERE'S HOW
Place all the ingredients except the shallots and celery in a blender and mix well. Then remove from the blender and mix in the chopped shallots and celery by hand. This can be used as a dip or a dressing.

SWEET GINGER
Vegan

Another dip dressing, this one has a fine hot flavour perfect for a green salad.

WHAT YOU NEED
225g (8oz) tofu
juice of 1 lemon
zest of 1 lemon, finely shredded
stevia, Manuka honey or maple syrup to taste
1 tsp freshly grated ginger root
1 garlic clove, crushed
1 tbsp red wine
1 tsp vegetable bouillon powder

HERE'S HOW
Blend all the ingredients well in the food processor. Alter the quantity of red wine to adjust the thickness.

MOVABLE FEASTS AND SNACKS

I love food to go. I like to make every meal a picnic – an adventure. Try to keep from falling into habits with food, either by eating the same thing over and over or by eating in the same place with the same plates. If the sun is shining on the landing, then take a tablecloth and eat there. Eat in bed. Sit on your children's beds and have lunch with them when they are ill. Eat as often as you can in the open air. When you travel or head off to work, take a simple but beautifully packed meal with you: a salad topped with free-range chicken breast or fish, a box of buckwheat soba (*see page 272*) – my favourite – or a container of crudités with luscious dipping sauces.

Crudités

There is no more delicious way to reap the benefits of energy-enhancing vegetables than munching on a platter of crudités: crunchy raw vegetables sliced or slivered, garnished with lemon slices, sprigs of watercress or fresh basil and served with rich and wonderful dipping sauces. Whether you tuck them into a lunch box or serve them on a wooden platter in the garden or in bed, these finger foods make ideal on-the-go eating. Most crudités fall short of their potential because people get stuck in a rut when preparing them. For crudités to work you need real variety – not only in the sauces you serve with them but also in the raw materials themselves. Use a mandolin to make chunky chips of carrots, turnips, courgettes and celery. Serve them with knife-sliced hunks of green and red peppers. Don't forget the bigger foods too. Whole leaves of chicory and pak choi torn from the plant, washed and crisped up are great dipped into tapenades or into a mixture of chopped hard-boiled eggs, lean mayonnaise and Cajun seasoning. You can use raw asparagus in salads by cutting it into 1.5-cm/half-inch pieces, and also as crudités with dips, but the thinner asparagus is better for this. Crudités don't have to be all-raw either. An artichoke steamed and chilled makes a wonderful dunking partner as do blanched florets of broccoli or cauliflower. You can create a good selection of crudités from almost anything you happen to have in the fridge. Some of my favourites are young spring onions, button mushrooms, mangetout which have been topped and tailed, cherry tomatoes, radishes, cucumber in big chunks, kohlrabi and small beetroots. Even slices of apple or pineapple make a nice addition. I like to wash my vegetables and cut, tear or slice them, giving as much variety as possible to the combinations, then dip them in iced water and put them in the refrigerator for half an hour before draining and serving. Lemon juice squeezed atop the drained and dried vegetables keeps them fresh. Always offer a great variety of dipping sauces. Some of my favourites are Curried Avocado Dip, Fresh Pesto, Raw Hummus, Fish Dip and Aioli (*see Dip It*).

Whole Vegetables
Button mushrooms with their stalks on, whole baby carrots, the sweet centre shoots from a head of celery, young green beans, topped and tailed, cauliflower florets, radishes, young spring onions – all of these make delicious crudités. All you do is trim and rinse them and dry on a paper towel.

Sticks and Matchsticks
These are very tempting. Carrots, turnips, courgettes, cucumbers, celery and pineapples are naturals for making sticks. To make matchsticks, just keep chopping lengthwise until you get sticks as thin as matches. Green or red peppers also make good matchsticks. To keep sticks fresh, put them in a bowl of cold water with a squeeze of lemon juice in the refrigerator, but don't keep them in the water for longer than half an hour.

Wedges
Orange and tangerine segments make natural wedges for a platter of crudités. So do tomatoes, chicory, Webs Wonder lettuce, apples and pears if you cut them right.

Slices
Some vegetables are particularly good sliced diagonally. This makes larger pieces for better dunking. Try diagonal slices of cucumber, carrot and white radish. Very thin slices of small beetroots, Jerusalem artichokes, kohlrabi and turnips are also nice. Large apples sliced crosswise can be used as bread for open sandwiches. Sweet peppers cut crosswise make attractive rings. Try cutting serviette rings of pepper and placing them around bundles of carrot or celery sticks.

SOBA
Vegan
Serves 2

The Japanese are masters of convenience foods. Some of the lunch-to-go recipes you find on the streets of Osaka or Tokyo are the best in the world. The difference between their foods and ours is that so many of their processed foods – like kudzu, organic tamari and miso – are naturally processed through fermentation and preparations that have traditionally been carried out for centuries. As a result, much of their packaged food is actually good for you.

Buckwheat soba is such a food. It is made from the edible fruit seed of the buckwheat plant, which comes originally from the Orient and is a relative of rhubarb – not at all a grain as many people assume. It is a hearty food, high in protein and potassium as well as B-complex vitamins, calcium, iron and fibre. You can buy buckwheat soba in any Japanese grocers and most good health-food stores. It comes in two forms: soba, which is 100 per cent buckwheat and contains no wheat flour, and the more common soba noodles, made from a combination of both. I strongly prefer the former. Cook the buckwheat noodles, then serve hot or cold. They travel well and are yummy to eat as a lunch or snack any time.

WHAT YOU NEED
2 carrots, finely slivered (optional)
200g (7oz) soba noodles
2 garlic cloves, finely chopped
5-cm (2-inch) piece fresh ginger, finely slivered
2 tbsp finely chopped spring onions
125ml (4fl oz) mirin, white wine or water
a few drops of sesame oil
3 tsp tamari
1 small red pepper, finely chopped

HERE'S HOW
Bring a saucepan filled with water to a rolling boil. Put in the carrots and the soba noodles and follow the manufacturer's instructions to cook. When finished, remove from the heat and rinse under cold water in a colander. Meanwhile, sauté the garlic, ginger and spring onions in the mirin, wine or water in a heavy pan for 5–7 minutes so that some of the liquid evaporates. Now add the sesame oil, tamari and red pepper,

mix and remove from the heat. Pour the sautéed mixture over the cooled soba and serve.

Seaweed Dipping Sauce

Because I so love dipping sauces, I make this seaweed-based one to go with my soba noodles when I choose to serve them hot. It is easy to make, so delicious and good for hair and nails, not to mention overall metabolism thanks to seaweed's mineral content. I make a seaweed stock by soaking several pieces of kombu – kelp leaves – in 375ml (13fl oz) of spring water overnight. Then I simmer this stock for a very few minutes adding 4 tablespoons of tamari, 4 tablespoons of mirin, 1 tablespoon of Manuka honey and a pinch of salt. I add some chopped spring onions and sesame seeds at the last minute, and dip.

Hors D'oeuvres and Snacks

Fun to make and eat, hors d'oeuvres and appetisers should be both beautiful and delicious, either with a meal or on their own. Here are a few decorative ideas, which can raise any lunch box, picnic, starter, or main dish for that matter, several notches up in the eye-appeal scale.

PETE'S CRACKER SUBSTITUTE

These two recipes are from my friend Peter Sim who by chance tried scooping out pâté with Japanese radish – *daikon*. This recipe works well with turnip, swede or large carrots. Turnips are round rather than cylindrical like daikon. You get more even-sized vegetable 'crackers' with daikon. Obviously, anything you would spread on a cracker could be spread on the daikon. Serve with Bachelor's Curried Caviar or see *Dip It* for great dips and spreads.

BACHELOR'S CURRIED CAVIAR
Meat free
Serves 4

WHAT YOU NEED
1 tin sardines
1–2 tsp lemon juice
1 tsp curry powder

HERE'S HOW

Mash the sardines with a fork, adding lemon juice and curry powder. Spread on daikon 'crackers'. Adding minced onion and/or garlic is quite acceptable, especially if using more than one tin of sardines. I'd recommend using minced spring onion and some of the green foliage.

If using sardines canned in water, some drops of olive and/or flax oil should be added to the mashed sardines. I use only sardines that are canned in olive oil or water.

DEVILLED EGGS
Vegetarian
Serves 8

I grew up on devilled eggs. It was one of those American dishes always served at barbecues and get-togethers in the country. I associate it with beautiful summer afternoons and young girls in gingham dresses. Devilled eggs are not only great garnishes for salad dishes and good hors d'oeuvres, they are also an excellent snack food to carry with you during the day.

WHAT YOU NEED
6 large organic or free-range eggs, hard-boiled
12 black olives, chopped
2 tbsp minced red onion
3 tbsp mayonnaise (preferably home-made)
1½ tsp Dijon mustard
Celtic or Maldon sea salt to taste
freshly ground black pepper to taste
80g (3oz) finely chopped celery
a few sliced olives, to garnish
Mexican chilli powder, to garnish

HERE'S HOW
Slice the hard-boiled eggs in half lengthwise. Take out the yolks, put them in a bowl and smash them. Stir in all the other ingredients except the garnish, then spoon back into the egg whites and garnish with the olive slices. Lightly douse with Mexican chilli powder and serve.

Vegetable Flowers

TOMATO LILIES
Vegan

There are two ways of making these; the first is better for smaller tomatoes, and the second for larger, slightly firm ones. For small tomatoes, place them stem end down on a cutting board, and cut almost all the way through them with four crossing cuts so that you end up with eight petals. Gently prise these petals open. For larger tomatoes you make small zigzag cuts around their equators, cutting right through to the centre with each cut. Your knife needs to be very sharp to do this. The smaller the angle between your zigzags, the more petals you will have and the more attractive your lilies will look. When you have cut all the way around, separate the two halves.

CARROT OR COURGETTE ROSETTES
Vegan

Wash your carrots or courgettes, then with a very sharp knife, cut about six regularly spaced grooves along their length and remove the long slivers of flesh. Slice them crosswise into little flowers.

RADISH ROSES
Vegan

Again, there are two ways to tackle them. If your radishes are long, simply cut a criss-cross pattern of four cuts in the bottom end (the end opposite the stalk), cutting about half-way down each radish. Then place the radishes in a glass of cold water in the fridge for the petals to open up. If you have larger, chubbier radishes, you can cut zigzags around the middle as for tomato lilies, then separate the halves.

Stuffed Stuff

GREEN CRÊPES
Vegan
Serves as many as needed

These are stuffed lettuce leaves, but the leaves need to be large and flexible so that they roll without splitting. For the stuffing I use finely chopped vegetables in a creamy dressing.

WHAT YOU NEED
Avocado, tomato, red and green peppers, spring onions, finely grated carrot or beetroot, cucumber, large lettuce leaves.

HERE'S HOW
Finely chop or grate the vegetables and mix them together with the dressing of your choice – a thick, creamy mayonnaise is very good. Put spoonfuls of the mixture on to the lettuce leaves, roll them and spear with a cocktail stick to hold them in place.

STUFFED TOMATOES WITH FRESH BASIL
Vegan
Serves 4

The best tomatoes are home-grown, picked when they are red and ripe and full of flavour.

WHAT YOU NEED
4 large tomatoes
2 spring onions
8 leaves fresh basil
225–450ml (8–16fl oz) tahini mayonnaise
1–2 tbsp French mustard
½ clove garlic, pressed

HERE'S HOW
Slice the tops off the tomatoes and keep them. Scoop out the seeds and pulp and chop with the onions and fresh basil. Mix with the tahini mayonnaise, mustard and garlic. Spoon the mixture back into the tomato shells. Cut the lids in half and stick them into the top of the filling to make butterfly wings. Serve each tomato on a lettuce leaf.

TOFU CHEESE-STUFFED PEPPERS
Vegan
Serves 3

This recipe looks most attractive with red peppers but you can use green. Green peppers turn red as they ripen and become sweeter in taste. The idea is to stuff them with a firm cheese and herb mixture so that they can be sliced crosswise and served as red or green-edged medallions. You can also serve them in halves as a main course, because they are quite filling.

WHAT YOU NEED
2 red peppers
chives, fresh parsley, lovage or marjoram
450g (16oz) Tofu Cheese (*see recipe below*)
1 tbsp vegetable bouillon powder

HERE'S HOW
Remove the stalks and seeds from the peppers by cutting around the stalks with a sharp knife. Be sure to scoop out all the seeds and the white pith as well. Finely chop the chives and other herbs, mix with the tofu cheese, not forgetting to add the bouillon powder. Fill the peppers with the mixture and pack down firmly. Wrap each pepper in clingfilm and chill for about an hour, by which time they should be firm enough to slice crosswise into medallions. Serve on a bed of curly endive garnished with sprigs of parsley.

If you want to make stuffed pepper halves, simply slice the peppers in half lengthwise to begin with, remove the seeds and pith and fill with the cheese mixture. Serve sprinkled with a little paprika and on a lettuce leaf.

TOFU CHEESE
Vegan

This recipe is from my friend Joelle Gregorius. She says: 'I don't really enjoy tofu, as it has no taste, so when my mother-in-law passed this recipe on to me, I found I could not only use it as a spread on vegetables (like aubergine) but also as a salad dressing by diluting it with lemon juice. So enjoy.'

WHAT YOU NEED
500g (18 oz) tofu
1 tbsp extra-virgin olive oil or flaxseed oil (optional)
1 tbsp apple cider vinegar
2 tbsp lemon juice
2 tbsp yeast powder (optional)
½ a small onion, grated
1 tbsp chives, finely cut
2 tbsp dill, finely chopped
½ tsp gomasis (roasted sesame with salt)

HERE'S HOW
Mix half of the tofu and all the other ingredients in a bowl with a mixer until it reaches the consistency of cream. With a fork, crumble the other half of the tofu into the mixture and fold in. Season to taste. This recipe needs to be kept refrigerated.

STUFFED FAIRY BUTTON MUSHROOMS
Vegetarian
Serves 4

Button mushrooms are the immature predecessors of the large, flat-topped, brown mushrooms. Ideally, they should be white, unbruised and perfect, straight from the mushroom farm.

WHAT YOU NEED
8–12 large button mushrooms
30g (1oz) ground almonds
3 tbsp yoghurt
squeeze of lemon juice
stevia, Manuka honey or maple syrup to taste
1 tbsp dill seeds, roasted and crushed
fresh parsley and mint
40g (1½oz) finely grated hard cheese
vegetable bouillon powder

HERE'S HOW
Remove the stalks of the mushrooms, trim and keep. Grind the almonds as finely as possible and mix with the yoghurt, lemon juice and honey. Add the ground dill seeds, the bouillon powder and a little chopped

parsley and mint. Chop the mushroom stalks finely and mix in. Spoon this mixture into the mushroom cups and sprinkle with finely grated hard cheese. Serve in twos or threes on little dishes garnished with mint sprigs.

Avocado Ideas

Avocados make attractive and delicious starters. There is so much more you can do with them than the familiar avocado vinaigrette. Many people do not realise that avocados are a fruit, although they contain very little fructose, and that they go particularly well with other fruits. The Brazilians eat them with cream and sugar. Even the shells have their uses – I often fill them with salad as starters.

CRUNCHY APPLE AVOCADOS
Vegetarian
Serves 4

WHAT YOU NEED
2 ripe avocados
juice of ½ a lemon
1 handful pecans or walnuts
2 eating apples (preferably red)
1 stick celery
1 handful raisins
3 tbsp plain egg mayonnaise
cinnamon

HERE'S HOW
Cut the avocados in half and scoop out the flesh. Keep the shells. Mash the flesh with lemon juice to prevent it going brown. Roughly chop the nuts. Chop the apples and celery finely. Mix apples, celery, walnuts, raisins and avocado together, and add the mayonnaise and a pinch of cinnamon. Fill the avocado shells with the mixture and garnish with a walnut and an apple slice.

SPICY NUTS
Vegan
Serves 5

These are great to carry as a snack. You can make them ahead, cool them and store in a tightly closed jar.

WHAT YOU NEED
2 tbsp coconut oil
250g (9oz) almonds
¼ to ½ tsp Cajun seasoning
¼ tsp vegetable bouillon powder

HERE'S HOW
Place the coconut oil in the bottom of a heavy frying pan – big enough to allow the nuts to sit side by side so they get evenly toasted. Heat the oil until it shows a hint of smoke, toss in the nuts, turning them frequently so they don't burn. Cool on the kitchen worktop on top of paper towels. Meanwhile, mix together Cajun seasoning and bouillon powder. While the nuts are still warm, place them together with this mixture in a paper bag or jar and shake vigorously to coat.

DIP IT

Dips are versatile. They are easy to make and add colour, softness and vibrant tastes to dishes. A beautifully presented dip is a scrumptious accompaniment to a plate of crudités. Dips can be spooned into the centre of dish salads, or if made thick enough, served as delicious pâtés.

CURRIED AVOCADO DIP
Vegan

This dip is great for crudités. I serve it together with a platter of fresh phytonutrient-filled vegetables such as endive, bulb fennel, crunchy lettuce, celery, slices of red, green and yellow pepper and anything else I happen to have around.

WHAT YOU NEED
2 large ripe avocados, peeled and cubed
3 garlic cloves, chopped
3 tbsp lemon juice
1 tsp vegetarian bouillon powder
⅛ tsp Cajun seasoning
Celtic or Maldon sea salt to taste
freshly ground black pepper to taste
1 tsp mild to medium curry powder
1 tbsp lemon zest

HERE'S HOW
Add chunks of avocado plus garlic, lemon juice, bouillon powder and other seasoning to the food processor – everything except the lemon zest. Blend until creamy then add lemon zest and serve. This recipe makes about 225ml (8fl oz).

Aïolis

I was introduced to aïoli years ago when I lived in Paris. As far as I am concerned, the taste is overwhelmingly wonderful. I use the very best olive oil I can find when making this rich sauce because I like it strong and true in the Mediterranean way. You can serve this sauce with many things other than fish soup too, such as hard-boiled eggs, crudités, steamed baby potatoes, fish and sliced cucumbers. You can also use it on cold meat, in sandwiches or on freshly baked and steamed fish and on vegetables such as steamed broccoli, mushrooms, beans or spinach. All sorts of delicious things can be added to aïoli, such as toasted slivered almonds or an anchovy or two, as well as fresh herbs like basil, lovage or fennel tops. I like the simple lemon aïoli best with fish soup.

TRADITIONAL AÏOLI
Vegetarian

WHAT YOU NEED
1 large egg
1 large egg yolk
juice of 2 ripe lemons
Celtic or Maldon sea salt to taste
freshly ground black pepper to taste
dash of tamari or 2 pinches of Cajun seasoning
300ml (10fl oz) extra-virgin olive oil
2 garlic cloves, finely chopped or crushed (less if you are not in love
   with garlic)
1 tsp Dijon mustard
1–2 tbsp chopped fresh basil, parsley, fennel tops or lovage (optional)
1–2 tbsp toasted almond slivers or a couple of anchovies (optional)

HERE'S HOW
Add the egg, egg yolk and lemon juice together with the salt, pepper and tamari or Cajun seasoning to a food processor and blend at high speed. Slowly add the olive oil – drop by drop for if you do it faster it will not emulsify. Once you have added about a third of the olive oil in this way, the sauce will have thickened and you can add the rest in a slow, steady stream. Now turn off the food processor and, either in its own container or after decanting the mixture to a bowl, add the garlic, mustard, any herbs or extras such as almonds, and blend by hand until smooth. Put in a small crock and serve with your other dishes, or place a spoonful over hot dishes and watch it melt.

AÏOLI LITE
Vegetarian

If you want to steer clear of oil – traditional aïoli is almost nothing but oil – why not try mock aïoli? It too gets on well in fish soups and on any kind of vegetable.

WHAT YOU NEED
450ml (16fl oz) soya milk
1½ tbsp arrowroot powder
8 tbsp soya milk powder
1 large egg yolk
juice of 1 large or 2 small lemons
1–2 tbsp extra-virgin olive oil
½ garlic clove, very finely chopped
1 tsp Dijon mustard
1–2 tbsp chopped fresh basil, dill, fennel tops or lovage (optional)
1–2 tbsp toasted almond slivers or a couple of anchovies (optional)
freshly ground black pepper to taste

HERE'S HOW
Place half the soya milk together with the arrowroot powder in a saucepan. Cook and stir to thicken, then allow to cool. Into the food processor put the cooled soya milk, the soya milk powder and the egg yolk. Blend well. Slowly add just enough olive oil to thicken. Add the lemon juice. Remove the ingredients from the food processor and by hand mix together the other ingredients. You can also add some other flavours to make it very special such as basil, dill, chopped roasted seeds or nuts and even chopped fennel tops. Season with black pepper and lemon juice.

SESAME MISO DIPPING SAUCE
Vegan

WHAT YOU NEED
125ml (4fl oz) rice wine
3 tbsp Manuka honey
1 tbsp miso
2 tbsp sesame seeds, ground in a coffee grinder or food processor
1 garlic clove, crushed

HERE'S HOW
Combine all the ingredients. This can be served immediately and is ideal for vegetables.

HONEY AND PINEAPPLE DIPPING SAUCE
Vegan

WHAT YOU NEED
200g (7oz) fresh pineapple
2 garlic cloves, crushed
1–2 tbsp honey
1 tsp allspice
1 tsp freshly ground nutmeg
1 tsp ground cinnamon
¼ tsp ground cloves
Celtic or Maldon sea salt to taste

HERE'S HOW
Mix together all the ingredients and let stand for 15 minutes. Then use as a marinade before cooking or as a dipping sauce afterwards. It is great for salmon, meat and chicken.

LEMON AND RICE WINE DIPPING SAUCE
Vegan

WHAT YOU NEED
125ml (4fl oz) lemon juice
2 garlic cloves, crushed
2 tbsp tamari
6 tbsp rice wine
Celtic or Maldon sea salt to taste

HERE'S HOW
Mix together all the ingredients and refrigerate until needed. This dipping sauce is good on seafood of all kinds.

RAW PESTO
Vegetarian

Probably my favourite dip of all time is Italian pesto. I grew up eating it over pastas and for a time missed it terribly when I wasn't eating pasta. Then I realised that the same sauce goes brilliantly on fish, green beans, spaghetti squash – even a salad of buffalo mozzarella and thinly sliced tomatoes. I make this sauce in a blender, store it in the fridge and use it up within two days. I am notorious for buying huge bunches of fresh basil and making masses. When I want to freeze pesto, I make it without the cheese and then add the cheese when I defrost it. It keeps very well this way.

WHAT YOU NEED
50g (2oz) fresh basil leaves
3 tbsp pine kernels
4 tbsp extra-virgin olive oil
a little lemon juice
25g (1oz) fresh Parmesan cheese, finely grated
1–2 garlic cloves

HERE'S HOW
Pop all of the ingredients except the garlic and the Parmesan cheese into a food processor and blend to break them up (but not so much that you turn it into a purée). Keep stopping and scraping things down from the sides of the food processor and blend again. If you need extra moisture, add a teaspoon or more of fresh lemon juice. Once the sauce takes on a creamy texture (yet hopefully still maintains the pieces of basil so you can see them), add the Parmesan cheese and the garlic and quickly blend again, then chill.

Serve as a dip or spread on buckwheat crackers. You can also put it over cooked vegetables and omelettes. Store the sauce in the refrigerator for two days or serve as soon as it is cool. You can also dilute it whenever you wish by adding a little more lemon juice.

FISH DIP OR PÂTÉ
Meat free

I discovered this recipe one night when I happened to cook too much fish for my son Aaron and myself, and I didn't know what to do with it. So I put it into a blender and began adding various ingredients. I ended up producing a fish pâté or dip so delicious that the whole thing disappeared before I had a chance to store it overnight for the next day's lunch. You can make it with just about any kind of light-tasting fish you can find. I even use smoked salmon but if you do, make sure you buy a form of smoked salmon that doesn't have sugar in it.

WHAT YOU NEED
450g (1lb) cooked white fish or smoked salmon
50g (2oz) mayonnaise (preferably home-made)
handful of chopped fresh parsley, coriander or basil
1–2 tsp vegetable bouillon powder to taste
2–5 tsp filtered or spring water (play this by ear, watch the
    consistency)
a dash or two of Worcestershire sauce
2 tbsp extra-virgin olive oil or half olive oil and half flaxseed oil
2–4 fresh garlic cloves, crushed

HERE'S HOW
Place all the ingredients in a blender and blend until smooth. If you need a little more water, add it now, remembering that once you have chilled the pâté it will firm up. Use more water if you are using it as a dip, and less if you are using it as a pâté. Turn off the blender and adjust the flavouring. Be creative about this. Put in anything else that might be flavourful, such as part of a chopped onion – perhaps this is best blended in by hand afterwards to keep the onions from going liquid, for their crunchiness is a wonderful part of the texture of the pâté itself. Remove from the blender and pour into ramekin dishes. Cover and chill. This will keep in the fridge for 4–5 days.

RAW HUMMUS
Vegan

WHAT YOU NEED
400g (14oz) sprouted chickpeas (sprouted for 2–3 days)
1 garlic clove, chopped finely
3 tbsp tahini
juice of 3 lemons
water to thin

1 tsp vegetable bouillon powder or 2 tsp soy sauce
3 tsp chopped chives or spring onions

HERE'S HOW
Put the ingredients (except chives or spring onions) into a food processor or blender and blend thoroughly. Then mix in the chopped chives or spring onions and chill. This dressing will keep for 2–3 days in the refrigerator.

RACY RED CHEESE
Vegan

This delicious dip or dressing can be served with crudités, over a salad or added to freshly steamed or wok-fried vegetables. It's a beautiful pink colour and has a refreshing zippy taste.

WHAT YOU NEED
150g (5oz) cashews or pine nuts
225ml (8fl oz) filtered or spring water
1 tsp vegetable bouillon powder or sea salt
½ tsp caraway seeds
juice of 2 lemons
50g (2oz) pimentos
4 chopped chives or spring onions

HERE'S HOW
Mix all the ingredients (except the chives or spring onions) in a blender or food processor until smooth. Blend in the chives or spring onions by hand and serve. This dip may be kept in the refrigerator for 4–5 days.

COOL CUCUMBER DIP
Vegetarian

WHAT YOU NEED
1 small cucumber
175ml (6fl oz) yoghurt
squeeze of lemon or dash of vinegar
1 tbsp minced onion

stevia, Manuka honey or maple syrup to taste
1 clove garlic (optional)
fresh mint
Celtic or Maldon sea salt to taste
freshly ground black pepper

HERE'S HOW
Peel and grate the cucumber and drain off any excess juice (you can use it as a drink). Mix with the yoghurt, lemon juice or vinegar, onion, sweetener and garlic, if using. Finely chop a few mint leaves and add. Season and serve in a dish with sprigs of fresh mint.

THOUSAND ISLAND DIP
Vegetarian

WHAT YOU NEED
¼ red pepper
2 hard-boiled eggs
4 green olives (or 1 fresh gherkin)
slice of beetroot
225ml (8fl oz) mayonnaise
1 tbsp Meaux mustard
fresh parsley

HERE'S HOW
Cut the red pepper into tiny pieces, discarding the seeds. Finely chop or grate the eggs. Stone the olives and chop finely. Cut the beetroot slice into tiny squares. Combine the mayonnaise and mustard and add the 'islands' (red pepper, egg, olives and beetroot). Serve with fresh parsley sprigs.

TAPENADE
Meat free
Makes about 450g (16oz)

I love good olives. One of the nicest ways to eat them is to combine them with capers, garlic and fresh herbs to make a tapenade – a paste you can use as a dip, over vegetables or pasta or simply spread on toast at tea. This is one of the easiest spreads to make – it only takes about 5 minutes. It is best served chilled.

WHAT YOU NEED

1 tin good-quality pitted black olives
1 small jar capers, washed and dried
2 tbsp fresh lime juice
4 anchovy fillets, chopped
1 tsp fresh oregano, finely chopped
2–3 tbsp extra-virgin olive oil
1 tbsp fresh basil, chopped
1–2 garlic cloves, peeled and finely chopped

HERE'S HOW

Put all the ingredients except the olive oil, herbs and garlic into a blender or food processor and blend until creamy. Now gently and slowly add the olive oil, drop by drop. Should the mixture become too thick, add a little more olive oil until you get the right consistency. Pour into a bowl or jar, add the herbs and garlic and mix with a fork. Cover and chill. This will keep for 2–3 days in the refrigerator.

SPARKLING RAW SOUPS

Soups make an excellent first or even second course. A blender, food processor or juicer is invaluable for soup making. It saves time but also allows you to achieve a smooth consistency and a thorough blending of flavours.

Raw soups have a vegetable juice base. Even people who wouldn't dream of drinking a glass of carrot juice can be seduced by the subtle flavours of Carrot Chowder. Whereas many cooked soups have a washed-out appearance, raw soups sparkle with brilliant colours to entice you. Fruit and vegetable soups can be tasty, nutrient-packed additions to a main meal. If you prefer your soups warm, heat them gently to 32°C/90°F and serve. This way you do not destroy the valuable enzymes.

Vegetable Soups

RAW ASPARAGUS SOUP
Vegan
Serves 2–4

A very special uncooked but heated protein soup, this is a delicate marriage of the unusual taste and aroma of the asparagus with the rich, sensuous quality of the cashews.

WHAT YOU NEED
100g (4oz) cashew nuts
700ml (25fl oz) spring water
1 bunch raw, fresh asparagus (tips only)
3 sticks celery
2 tsp vegetable bouillon powder
2 tbsp fresh lovage, chopped finely (optional)
2 tbsp minced parsley, to garnish

HERE'S HOW
Place the cashew nuts in a food processor with 225ml (8fl oz) of hot water and blend thoroughly until they have been reduced to a cream. Add the other ingredients, saving the parsley for garnish. Heat thoroughly but do not boil. Serve with a sprinkling of parsley.

CHILLED CUCUMBER SOUP
Vegetarian
Serves 2–4

You can't beat this delightful soup on a hot summer day.

WHAT YOU NEED
1 large cucumber
450ml (16fl oz) natural yoghurt, chilled
ice (optional)
2 tsp vegetable bouillon powder
4 tbsp finely chopped mint
¼ tsp crushed poppy seeds (optional)

HERE'S HOW
Chop the cucumber and blend in a blender or food processor with the chilled yoghurt. You may add a few cubes of ice to make it colder if you wish. After blending for two minutes, add the vegetable bouillon powder and continue to blend with ice. Finally, add the chopped mint and blend again very briefly. Pour into bowls and serve immediately with a little chopped mint or crushed poppy seeds sprinkled on top.

GAZPACHO
Vegan
Serves 2–4

Another delicious cold summer soup which you can make as spicy as you like.

WHAT YOU NEED
6 ripe tomatoes, chopped
½ cucumber, chopped
juice of 1 lemon
2 tsp vegetable bouillon powder
1 tsp kelp (optional)
1 garlic clove, finely chopped
½ red pepper, finely chopped
½ green pepper, finely chopped
4 spring onions, finely chopped

3 tbsp parsley, finely chopped
Mexican chilli to taste

HERE'S HOW

Keeping aside a small portion of the tomatoes and cucumber, put the rest of the tomatoes and cucumber, the lemon juice, the bouillon powder, kelp (if desired) and garlic in a food processor or blender and liquidise. Add the peppers, spring onions and parsley and mix well, season to taste with the chilli and serve with the tomatoes and cucumber you have kept aside.

CARROT CHOWDER
Vegetarian
Serves 4

WHAT YOU NEED
100g (4oz) nuts (almonds, hazels or pecans)
225ml (8fl oz) goat's milk yoghurt
2 egg yolks
small garlic clove
juice of ½ a lemon
1 tbsp extra-virgin olive oil
2 tsp vegetable bouillon powder
700ml (25fl oz) carrot juice (you will need about 12 large carrots for this)
ice cubes
½ green pepper
2 spring onions
chopped parsley

HERE'S HOW

Grind the nuts finely and blend them with the yoghurt, egg yolks, pressed garlic, lemon juice, olive oil and bouillon powder. Juice the carrots into a jar with ice cubes in it then slowly add the juice and ice to the yoghurt mixture, stirring well. Serve sprinkled with a mixture of finely chopped green pepper, spring onion and parsley.

FRESH GREEN SOUP
Vegan
Serves 2–4

WHAT YOU NEED
2 avocados, peeled and stoned
700ml (25fl oz) apple juice
juice of ½ a lemon
parsley
2 tsp tamari
1 tsp vegetable bouillon powder
ground ginger
1 courgette
1 stick of celery
handful of mung sprouts
sliced mushrooms or flaked almonds

HERE'S HOW
Combine the avocados, apple juice, lemon juice, parsley, tamari, vegetable bouillon and a pinch of ginger in the blender. Grate the courgette and finely dice the celery and mix them with the sprouts. Now pour on the avocado sauce. Serve sprinkled with sliced mushrooms or flakes of almond.

Fruit Soups

BLACK CHERRY SOUP
Vegan
Serves 2–4

WHAT YOU NEED
450g (16oz) sweet black cherries
juice of 3 oranges
2 tbsp Manuka honey
450ml (16fl oz) water
fresh mint sprigs
grated coconut

HERE'S HOW
Stone the cherries and blend with the orange juice, Manuka honey and water. Serve chilled, decorated with mint sprigs and some grated coconut.

STRAWBERRY SURPRISE SOUP
Vegetarian
Serves 2–4

WHAT YOU NEED
75g (3oz) cashew nuts
550ml (20fl oz) soya milk
½ tsp nutmeg
½ tsp ginger
1 tbsp vegetable bouillon powder
2 small punnets of strawberries
fresh mint

HERE'S HOW
Place the nuts, milk, nutmeg, ginger and bouillon powder in the blender and mix until smooth. Blend the strawberries to a cream (keeping aside a few for decoration). Add the strawberry mixture to the milk mixture and stir in well. Serve in individual bowls garnished with fresh chopped mint pieces and slices of strawberry.

FISH IS BEST

Delicious and easy to prepare, fish is my favourite form of protein. A diet that revolves around fish as a primary source of protein and fat helps protect against many degenerative diseases from gallstones and colitis to arthritis, diabetes, heart disease and cancer. Part of the reason why fish is so wonderful is that it is very high in polyunsaturated omega-3 fatty acids. The best sources of omega-3 are cold-water fish such as anchovies, sardines, swordfish, bass, mackerel and wild salmon.

Quick and Easy Fish

SALMON DELIGHT
Meat free
Serves 2

Salmon is such a delightful dish with a unique and delicate flavour. My friend Belinda Hodson, who gave me this recipe, was pondering one day what marinades she could invent for two superb salmon fillets. She stumbled across the idea of using lemon as a base. I really love this dish because it is easy to prepare and very tasty. The marinade enhances the natural flavours of the fish, and the spring onion really gives it a special zest.

WHAT YOU NEED
2 large spring onions
juice of 4 medium-sized lemons
freshly ground black pepper to taste
Celtic or Maldon sea salt to taste
2 fillets of salmon
1 dsp coconut oil
zest of 1 lemon, 2 lemon wedges and parsley for garnish

HERE'S HOW
Finely chop the spring onions and place in a mixing bowl. Add the lemon juice, pepper and salt, and blend. Place the salmon fillets into the marinade (pink side down) and leave for 45 minutes. Turn the fillets over and leave for a further 15 minutes. Heat the coconut oil in

a frying pan. Sauté the fillets until tender then garnish with lemon zest, wedges and parsley. Serve immediately or eat cold. It is great with salad as a lunch to go.

SAUTÉED SEA BASS WITH GARLIC
Meat free
Serves 2

Sea bass is my favourite fish. Its delicate flavour and texture invite equally delicate seasoning and handling. This recipe works well with any fish – sole, halibut, cod, salmon, tuna, fresh herring and mackerel – and is quick and easy to prepare.

WHAT YOU NEED
1 tbsp coconut oil
450g (1lb) bass fillets or other fish
4 garlic cloves, chopped
¼ red onion, finely diced
2 tbsp fresh coriander or broad-leafed parsley, finely chopped
juice of 1 large lemon

HERE'S HOW
Melt the coconut oil on a teppenyaki grill or in a heavy frying pan. Add the fish and sauté for 5 minutes, turning over only once. Remove the fish from the pan and pour in all the other ingredients, allowing them to heat through for about a minute and a half. Pour these other ingredients over the fish and serve immediately.

SUCCULENT SASHIMI
Meat free
Servings depend entirely on appetite

You can't get faster or easier than succulent slices of raw fish. Nor can you get higher-quality protein foods anywhere. Delightful, summer or winter served with a cup of Oolong, Sencha or green Assam tea, is a plateful of bright-coloured sashimi. It is not only beautiful to look at but, when it comes to fish, there is no better way of eating it than raw, assuming the source of the fish is a good one – absolutely fresh and caught in unpolluted waters. Alternatively, there is a growing number of excellent organic food emporia that are extremely careful about the fish they sell.

Flash Freezing

To make absolutely sure that the dish is parasite-free – although I do believe this compromises the flavour – you can always flash-freeze it for between 24 and 48 hours or freeze it in an ordinary freezer for a week then thaw, slice and serve immediately. In 1990, the Food and Drug Administration in the United States recommended that any fish served raw be blast-frozen to –35°C for 15 hours, or frozen by ordinary methods to –23°C for seven days before thawing and eating. If I'm going to freeze it (which I rarely do), I like to cut my fish into portions of about 150g (5oz) each, so that when I'm ready to prepare the sashimi, slicing is a simple task. When eating sashimi as a main course you need about 100–150g (4–5oz) of fish per person. If eating it as a starter or a small meal, you need about half that amount.

I make my sashimi out of two or three kinds of fish at one time. Among the fish I particularly like are wild salmon, tuna – especially the huge, red tuna, squid (I use the body rather than the tentacles), large white fish such as sea bass or grouper, terakihi, sole, scallops, and even crayfish or lobster (which makes some of the most delicious sashimi in the world).

NUT-CRUSTED TUNA
Meat free
Serves 2

This is a great way of cooking fish steaks, whether they be salmon, swordfish, tuna or any other kind of large fish. You can use almonds, pecans, walnuts or macadamia nuts – whatever you prefer.

WHAT YOU NEED
120g (4oz) chopped nuts (the best way to do this is in a coffee grinder)
Celtic or Maldon sea salt to taste
freshly ground black pepper to taste
2 tbsp melted coconut oil
2 tbsp melted butter
150g (5oz) boneless fish steaks
2 tsp fresh chopped parsley

HERE'S HOW

Preheat your oven to 200°C/400°F/Gas Mark 6. Grease a baking sheet. Mix the chopped nuts together with the seasoning and put on a plate. Melt the coconut oil and butter in a pan. Remove from the heat. Dip the fish in the oil and butter mixture and then into the nut mixture, pressing down to make sure the nuts hold. Place the nutted fish steaks on the baking sheet and pop into the oven for 6–10 minutes until cooked through. Sprinkle with chopped parsley and serve.

LA BOURRIDE PACIFICA
Meat free
Serves 6

I like this one-bowl meal so much that I could quite literally live on it. It is so easy to make and completely adaptable to whatever fish you can find. Because I adore the fish you can get in the southern hemisphere – especially for their wide variety and unbeatable freshness – this recipe calls for a number of fish available in the South Pacific.

Go to your fishmonger or your supermarket and ask for all the parts of fresh fish they usually throw away – the skeletons, the heads, the fins. Throw it all into a pot and make your fish stock. This you can keep in the refrigerator for 2–3 days or in the freezer for 2–3 months. You will use this not only for La Bourride Pacifica but for a number of other dishes. If you are feeling really lazy, go and buy fish sauce which you will find in any Oriental shop or speciality section of a good supermarket, and mix it with water to make your fish stock. But making your own fish stock is so much more delicious – and fun too.

FISH STOCK
Makes 3 litres.

WHAT YOU NEED
Select a few things from the following list to a total weight of 2kg (4½lb):

- ❑ fish heads
- ❑ fish bones (oily fish bones are not so good, so go for others if you have a choice)
- ❑ fish fins and tails
- ❑ bits and pieces from crabs, prawns, lobsters or crayfish

- ❏ 2 onions, roughly cut
- ❏ 2 stalks of celery, roughly cut
- ❏ 1 fat leek, roughly sliced
- ❏ 2 fat carrots, roughly sliced
- ❏ small handful of fresh parsley
- ❏ 1 head of garlic in its skin, broken up
- ❏ 1 fresh bay leaf
- ❏ 2 sprigs of thyme
- ❏ 1 tsp Cajun seasoning
- ❏ juice of 1 lemon
- ❏ 1 tsp grated fresh ginger

HERE'S HOW

Choose a pot large enough to hold 3 litres (5 pints) of water plus everything else. Toss everything into the pot. Bring to a rapid boil and let simmer for 20 minutes. While it is simmering, keep skimming off the froth. Remove from the heat and pass through a fine sieve to make sure any tiny bones are removed. Use immediately or store for later.

LA BOURRIDE PACIFICA

WHAT YOU NEED

100g (4oz) julienned carrots
100g (4oz) leek circles
100g (4oz) fennel
100g (4oz) chopped broccoli
100g (4oz) spring onions, sliced
1 tbsp extra-virgin olive oil
Celtic or Maldon sea salt to taste
freshly ground black pepper to taste
1½ litres (2½ pints) fish stock
1½kg (3½lb) five to eight varieties of fish and shellfish. Try to mix the two so you end up with large pieces of fish, some clams or mussels and some small pieces of fish or even tiny whole fish. Look for variety in colour too. Here are some of my favourites, but go for whatever is cheap and easy to come by: snapper, cod, grouper, turbot, bass, terakihi, salmon, eel, halibut, mussels, clams, prawns, shrimp.

HERE'S HOW

To the fish stock add the olive oil, all the vegetables and seasoning. Cook for 20 minutes. Toss in your fish and cook for another 5–8 minutes. Serve immediately with aïoli.

LOBSTER OR CRAYFISH WITH DIPPING SAUCES
Meat free
Serves 4

Not only are lobster and crayfish some of the most beautiful foods in Nature, they are also some of the most nutritious – especially when it comes to supporting immune functions and reproductive health. Rich in iodine for the thyroid gland and the sex glands, these crustaceans are excellent sources of zinc in a form that your body fairly laps up, of selenium – an essential antioxidant – and of the omega-3 fatty acids, which are strongly linked with heart-protective and anti-inflammatory properties. Serve with Green Goddess, Blood of Angels or Midnight Sun sauces (*see Salsas and Sauces*).

WHAT YOU NEED

4 lobsters or crayfish, 400–500g (14–18oz) apiece

HERE'S HOW

Once you have chosen your crayfish or lobsters, take them home and put them under a wet towel so they go to sleep. When you are ready to cook them, take a very sharp knife and pith them by sticking the knife through the centre of the neck. It only takes an instant to do. This severs the spinal cord so that when you put them into boiling water they do not suffer. Fill a big pot with enough water to cover and then some. Bring to a rolling boil. Now drop the crayfish or lobsters into the water and cover.

Cook for 3–6 minutes, depending on their size. Take them from the pot and put on a board. Now, with a good sharp knife placed just behind the eyes, split them down the top end and then turn around and split the other end so that you are cutting along the entire length. Remove the dark vein that runs down the tail, the stomach sac, which is inside the head, and the gills. Crack open the claws with the base of a large knife. Serve flesh side up with an aïoli or dipping sauce (*see Dip It*).

MUSSELS STRAIGHT UP
Meat free
Serves 6

Mussels are my favourite shellfish. The best in the world are New Zealand's green-lipped mussels from the sea. They are not only highly nutritious, they are also some of the biggest. This recipe works perfectly well with any good clean mussels. Whatever mussels you buy, make sure they come from unpolluted waters and are alive. If you think they are likely to be sandy then soak them overnight in a bucket of water to which you have added a couple of tablespoons of cornflour. The mussels will feed on the cornflour and in return expel any sand they have collected.

WHAT YOU NEED
2g (4½lb) green-lipped mussels
6 tbsp olive oil
1 large onion, finely chopped
3 garlic cloves, slivered
225ml (8fl oz) dry white wine
a finger fresh ginger, finely shredded
handful of arami seaweed – soak for 1–2 hours and then drain (optional)
zest of 1 lemon, finely shredded
Celtic or Maldon sea salt to taste
freshly ground black pepper to taste
small bunch of fresh basil, chopped
small bunch of fresh broad-leafed parsley, chopped
2 red peppers, chopped in medium pieces (you can also use chilli peppers if you want it hotter, but I find too much heat obscures the delicious flavour of the mussels themselves)
2 green chillies, finely chopped

HERE'S HOW
Scrub the outer shells of the mussels with a stiff brush in cold water and pull out the beards that stick to the sides. Throw away any mussels with broken shells and any that remain open when you are handling them. They are not only not for human consumption, I would not even let my cats have them. Now, in a large pot heat the olive oil and gently fry the onion and garlic for five minutes, stirring regularly. Add the wine, ginger, arami (if using), zest of lemon and salt and pepper and bring to the boil. Toss in the mussels and cover tightly, steaming them

for no more than 2–3 minutes – just long enough for the shells to pop open. Discard any that have remained shut after cooking. Now add the fresh chopped basil, parsley, peppers and green chillies, tucking it into the open shells with your fingers to garnish the mussels. The contrast between the vibrant colours of these garnishes and the rich, sea-earth shades of the mussels is one of the great pleasures of making this dish. Serve immediately in the sauce. And don't forget to drink the sauce. It is not only delicious, it is rich in minerals too – great for hair and nails, not to mention hormones. Sometimes – especially on summer afternoons – I drain off the sauce and serve the mussels themselves garnished in glass dishes with the sauce on the side – much as the Japanese serve miso soup in a little covered wooden bowl.

PEPPERED SKATE WINGS
Meat free
Serves 4

Skate wings are one of the least expensive yet most delicious and unusually-textured of all seafoods. Because this particular fish has a reputation for supporting the body on a hormonal level, it is eaten in many parts of the world as an aphrodisiac. The bones of the skate (a ray in fact) – which are not bones at all, but cartilage – are easy to manage and help create the beauty of the dish. Traditionally, skate is cooked in an oven and served with a nut-brown butter. I prefer to cook mine on a teppanyaki grill, simply because it is quick and easy, and I love the way that the grill creates a beautiful pattern in the shape of the wing itself as it's cooking.

WHAT YOU NEED
400–500g (14–18oz) skate wings (cut into pieces if you wish)
½ tsp red peppercorns, cracked with a mortar and pestle
50g (2oz) butter
1 medium-hot red pepper, finely chopped
1 medium-hot green pepper, finely chopped
4 garlic cloves, slivered
Celtic or Maldon sea salt and coarsely ground red peppercorns to taste
50g (2oz) capers
1 fresh lemon, cut into quarters

HERE'S HOW

Prepare the skate wings by covering them with a layer of cracked red peppercorns. Heat a teppanyaki grill or heavy frying pan and melt the butter, continuing to heat it until it takes on a dark, golden-brown colour. Pour it off immediately into a dish and add the peppers and garlic to the darkened liquid. Now place the skate wing on the teppanyaki grill or frying pan with the thickest part facing the grill. Cover with a piece of aluminium foil and cook for five minutes. Turn the skate wing and cook on the other side until brown and the wing curls. This whole process usually takes about 10–12 minutes, depending upon the thickness of the wing. Remove to a serving dish, season to taste, strew with capers, butter and lemon wedges and serve immediately with a mixture of brown rice and wild rice, and a fresh green salad.

SNAPPER IN BANANA LEAVES
Meat free
Serves 4

This recipe calls for banana leaves – just because they are so beautiful with the red snapper and because this is how I learned to cook fish in the South Pacific. But greaseproof paper will do just as well if you can't come by the banana leaves. I use aluminium foil only as a last resort. When you cook anything acidic such as a protein food or a fruit like tomato in aluminium, it leaches some of the metal into the food, and aluminium is something we are all better off without. Don't feel that you have to use red snapper. Try other types of fish, such as red mullet, John Dory or what looks freshest when you are shopping.

When buying ginger, look for a firm ginger root. In truth, ginger is not really a root at all. It is part of the stem of this tropical plant, which happens to grow beneath the ground. Make sure the ginger you buy has no mould on it. When you bring it home, keep it wrapped in a paper bag in the refrigerator. This way it will stay fresh for several weeks. You can also freeze ginger very easily. Another way you can keep it fresh is to seal it in a tightly closed jar in the refrigerator.

WHAT YOU NEED

2 snappers (approximately 500g/18oz) cleaned, scaled and dorsal fins removed
banana leaves, greaseproof paper or aluminium foil

1 tbsp extra-virgin olive oil
limes

FOR THE PASTE
3 green chillies, deseeded and chopped
1 stalk of lemon grass, chopped
6 garlic cloves, peeled and finely chopped
1 onion, peeled and chopped
6-cm (2½-in) piece of fresh ginger, chopped
25g (1oz) bunch of coriander (root and all), chopped
15g (½oz) fresh mint, chopped
zest of 1 lime, finely shredded
1 tsp ground roasted cumin
1 tsp fennel seeds, dry toasted
½ tsp freshly ground black pepper
2 tbsp Manuka honey
juice of 2 limes
60g (2½oz) unsweetened creamed coconut, grated

HERE'S HOW
Place all the paste ingredients in a food processor and purée. If the paste seems too thick, add a little warm water to get the right consistency so that it is moist and sticks together well. Wash and dry the fish and make a few diagonal slits through the skin on each side. Rub half the paste all over the fish, inside and out. Wrap in banana leaves, greaseproof paper or aluminium foil to enclose the fish completely and secure with string. It is essential to create a really tight package so the juices don't escape while the fish is cooking. Refrigerate until ready to cook.

Heat the grill or oven to 200°C/400°F/Gas Mark 6. Rub the parcels all over with oil and grill or bake for about 8–10 minutes. The outside leaves will char, but the fish inside will cook gently. Mix the remaining paste with 2–3 tablespoons of warm water if it is too stiff and serve with the fish and wedges of lime.

OTHER WAYS TO GO
Fast and Easy: Fill a greaseproof paper parcel with fish, clams, prawns and scallops. Add some lemon juice, Oriental fish sauce, garlic and Cajun seasoning and bake in a hot oven for 5–8 minutes. Serve immediately.
Salt Crust: This is a particularly good way of cooking salmon. Spread 500g (18 oz) of rock salt on a dish, lay the fish on this, then cover it

with another 500g (18oz) of salt and bake at 200°C/400°F/Gas Mark 6 for about 20 minutes.

Simple Seasoning: Fish can be seasoned with something as simple as oregano, olive oil and the juice and zest of half a lemon, and pan-fried or grilled for a fast, simple meal.

CRUNCHY GREEN PRAWNS
Meat free
Serves 4

When it comes to prawns, green means raw. These are the best. You can buy them fresh or frozen in every form – shelled, unshelled, whole or heads removed. If you are lucky enough to find fresh ones, make sure they really are fresh since, like other shellfish, prawns go off fast. Plan to eat them the day you buy them. I love to eat them whole, partly because they are so beautiful and partly because I like the crunchy texture of the shells. I always eat the shells – usually not the heads unless they are very small.

Sadly, most prawns we buy these days are farmed – milder in flavour than their wild cousins. Great spices and herbs can make up for this – lemon, lime, garlic and chillies used either in the cooking of the shellfish itself or in the sauces you serve with it. Crunchy Green Prawns can be cooked under a grill or on a barbecue. You can even flash-fry them on a teppenyaki grill or in a heavy frying pan if you like. They are delicious hot, but you can also make them for a picnic and serve them cold.

WHAT YOU NEED
750g (1½lb) king prawns, uncooked (you may peel and de-vein them
    if you wish)
2 limes, cut in wedges

FOR THE MARINADE
3–4 tbsp olive oil
1 tbsp spring onions, finely chopped
50g (2oz) fresh ginger, finely shredded
small handful of fresh coriander, chopped
juice and finely shredded zest of 2 small limes (if you can't get limes
    then use 1 lemon)
2 tbsp sake or dry sherry

5 garlic cloves, finely chopped
½ tsp mustard seeds, broken up with a mortar and pestle
coarse-ground black pepper to taste

HERE'S HOW
Wash the prawns carefully in cold water and dry with a tea towel. To make the marinade, place the oil, spring onions, ginger, half the coriander, lime juice, black pepper and sake into a food processor or blender. Purée to a paste. Pour into a bowl, add the garlic, the lime or lemon zest and the remaining chopped coriander and mustard seeds then mix into the paste by hand. Place the prawns in the bowl and, using your hands, turn them over and over until they are covered with the paste. Transfer to a flat glass dish and cover. Set it in a cool place – the fridge itself if it happens to be the middle of summer – for at least three hours.

Cook on a teppenyaki grill, a barbecue or under a grill until crunchy. It takes only a couple of minutes a side to fry these and very little more under a hot grill or on a barbecue – all you want is for them to turn opaque. Serve with lime wedges and don't throw away any of the marinade – cooked or uncooked – that still remains. It is delicious to spread over the crunchy prawns. However you cook them, eat them with your fingers – shell and all. All sensuous food tastes better this way, but prawns especially. I serve them with a combination of brown rice and wild rice – about half and half – and a bright-green salad with wild rocket and whatever fresh herbs, from basil to lovage, that I can harvest from the garden or find at the market.

MEAT MATTERS

All meals need power foods – top-quality proteins like our ancestors got. Proteins from the architectural structure of the body's living matrix – the bones, tendons, ligaments, skin and tissues. The word protein quite literally means 'primary substance'.

It is an appropriate name. Every tissue in your body from your brain to your little fingernail is built of and repaired with protein. Amino acids, the building blocks of protein, are central factors in most of the processes of the body – like making antibodies against infection, and creating hormones and overall strength.

The following dishes act as a perfect complement to the crunchy, light, biophoton-rich raw fare you eat with them. You can cook your meat pretty much any way you like. Grill your fish and meat teppenyaki style, bake them in greaseproof paper or banana leaves, slow-roast chicken, game or turkey, and serve them with surprising redcurrant and pear fruit freeze. What follows are just a few of my favourite recipes.

Teppenyaki

Teppenyaki is a way of cooking protein foods as well as vegetables that couldn't be healthier, and is also incredibly delicious. Developed in the last 30 years in Japan, teppenyaki sears into foods their intrinsic flavour and protects the integrity of their nutritional value. Foods like meat, fish, shellfish, chicken and game as well as vegetables like pak choi, bamboo shoots, sprouts and carrots are quickly grilled on a flat heated sheet. The ultimate in fast-food preparation, it takes 1–2 minutes to cook squid, 5 minutes for scallops, 10 minutes for boneless chicken and 15 minutes for pork.

Ideally, you need a teppenyaki grill. Good ones are just beginning to come on the market. The best consist of stainless-steel electric flat plates. They plug into the wall and can be used on the kitchen work surface or directly on the table itself. Prepare the raw ingredients, such as spare ribs, prawns, tofu or finely sliced steak plus the vegetables to go with them, by chopping them and placing on a dish. Then you cook the food as you need it, making sure never to overcook anything (this is easy to do when cooking teppenyaki since it cooks so quickly). Either eat the food as is or serve with simple sauces, pestos or salsa. You can even skewer fish and vegetables and cook things this way.

If you don't have a teppenyaki grill, you can begin to experience the delights of this way of cooking using a heavy crêpe pan or even a large frying pan – electric or otherwise. But somehow these substitutes are never as good as the real thing. Once you get into teppenyaki food preparation, I predict you will want to buy an Oriental grill to make the whole process more graceful and simple. Many of the sauces in *Dip It* – from Basil Pesto to the dipping sauces – are ideal companions for teppenyaki-grilled foods.

What to Use for Teppenyaki-grilled Food

Beef: sirloin, rump, ribeye, fillet
Chicken: breast fillet, thigh fillet
Lamb: fillet, cutlets, sliced leg or shoulder
Fish: fillets
Shellfish: prawns in shells or shelled, mussels in shells, clams in shells, shelled scallops

A TEPPENYAKI FEAST
Serves 4

The single most important nutritional feature of meat is its cellular structure, which is very similar to our own. This means that the nutrients absorbed from meat are very quickly and easily transformed into our tissue and blood. Consequently, small amounts of meat can be enormously beneficial to people who are deficient in strength and energy. This recipe can be adapted for vegetarians who eat fish and even vegans who like to use tofu as a protein source.

WHAT YOU NEED
sesame oil (if not using a non-stick grill)
500g (18oz) pork, lamb, chicken breasts and beef sirloin, cut into 6–12-mm (¼–½-in) strips **or**
500g (18oz) prawns, scallops, squid, fish or tofu
1 tbsp sesame oil
garlic cloves, sliced
500g (18oz) raw fresh vegetables, e.g. pak choi, carrots, onions, spring onions, shallots, courgettes, sliced or shredded
a finger of ginger, finely shredded
chillies, chopped (optional)

tamari to season (optional)
Celtic or Maldon sea salt to taste
freshly ground black pepper
1–2 dipping sauces (optional)

HERE'S HOW

Heat the grill or pan to hot so that a few drops of water flicked on the grill jump off. Add sesame oil (if you have a non-stick grill you don't even need the oil). You can cook garlic slivers before placing other foods on the grill to add flavour. Place the food on the grill and cook for the appropriate time. Beef: 3 to 4 minutes each side. Pork: 4 minutes each side. Chicken slices: 2 to 3 minutes each side. Lamb: 2 minutes each side. Fish: 4 to 5 minutes each side. Scallops: 1 minute each side. Squid: 30 seconds each side. Prawns: 3 minutes each side. Vegetables: 2 to 3 minutes. Tofu: 3 minutes each side. Garlic, ginger, chillies: 3 to 5 minutes. Remove and serve immediately with dipping sauces.

JAPANESE TERIYAKI MARINADE
Vegan
Makes about 125ml (4fl oz)

I love teriyaki but so often the marinades in which fish, chicken and meat are soaked to get a teriyaki taste are full of sugar and sake. This is my alternative. It's equally delicious and easy to make.

WHAT YOU NEED

100ml (3fl oz) tamari or soy sauce, with no sugar added
2 tbsp soya oil (or olive oil at a pinch)
2 tbsp spring or filtered water
2 tsp wine vinegar
a finger of fresh ginger, finely grated
2 garlic cloves, crushed or chopped
¼ tsp stevia, Manuka honey or maple syrup to taste

HERE'S HOW

Combine all your ingredients in a flat, low pan then marinate your beef, pork, chicken or tofu from 1½ hours to overnight in the fridge if you have time, before teppenyaki grilling, stir-frying or barbecuing. If you are stir-frying, you can pour the remaining sauce into the pan once the meat and vegetables are cooked to season the food further.

HERBED LAMB SHANKS
Serves 4

Lamb shanks are just about the most delicious and the cheapest cut of lamb. Cook them slowly and they fall off the bone, bringing out the most wonderful flavour. I serve mine with simple mashed potatoes or brown rice mixed with wild rice plus some roasted vegetables or a crunchy salad. I like to follow lamb with white wine and rosemary sorbet, which cuts beautifully through the tendency lamb has to be a bit fatty.

WHAT YOU NEED
1 tsp black peppercorns, hand-ground with a mortar and pestle if possible
1 tbsp fresh rosemary, chopped
1 tbsp fresh marjoram, chopped
4 lamb shanks
1 tbsp extra-virgin olive oil
3–6 garlic cloves, finely chopped
3 medium shallots, quartered and finely chopped
1 large carrot, quartered and finely sliced
225ml (8fl oz) dry white wine
6 large leaves of fresh sage plus a sprig more to garnish
Celtic or Maldon sea salt to taste

HERE'S HOW
Mix the freshly ground pepper with the chopped fresh herbs and roll the lamb in this mixture. Heat the bottom of a large casserole with the oil and brown the meat on all sides, then remove. Add the garlic, shallots and carrot and sauté them until soft. Return the lamb shanks to the pot. Add the white wine, sage and seasoning, and allow to simmer very, very slowly for 1½–2 hours until the meat falls off the bone. Skim off any fat. Serve immediately with wild rice or mashed potatoes and coriander salsa.

MEATBALLS
Serves 4

Meatballs are a traditional New Zealand favourite for people of all ages. This tasty recipe is simple to prepare, and the meatballs go well with a number of different sauces. They are also great for picnics and barbecues.

WHAT YOU NEED

1 dsp coconut oil
750g (1½lb) lean mince (beef or lamb)
½ tsp garlic powder
Celtic or Maldon sea salt to taste
freshly ground black pepper to taste
4 garlic cloves, finely chopped
1 egg
1 large onion, diced
1 tbsp fresh parsley, finely chopped
1 tbsp fresh thyme, finely chopped
1 tbsp fresh marjoram, finely chopped
1 tbsp fresh sage, finely chopped

HERE'S HOW

Heat the oil in a frying pan. Mix the remaining ingredients together in a large bowl and roll into balls. Spoon into the frying pan and cook gently for 20–25 minutes. Drain the meatballs on paper towels, then serve with your favourite sauce.

CHICKEN CURRY
Serves 4

This curry is a dream to make, creamy thick, full of spices, with a rich fragrance and flavour. I often prepare it using leftover pieces of chicken, tossing them into a frying pan, mixing in all my sauce ingredients, then serving over a plate of lightly steamed broccoli or cauliflower florets. Another way I do curry – a real lazy way – is to take a chicken cut in pieces, and put it into a large cast-iron pot with a lid. I then toss in all the ingredients (except coconut oil), pop it into the oven with the lid on, and cook for about an hour at 200°C/400°F/Gas Mark 6. I turn the chicken so the sauce covers it and cook for another 15 minutes. This way you end up with curried chicken pieces rather than a true curry, but it is so quick to prepare – in all it takes about five minutes – and once it's done you can use it any time for snacks or main courses. Here is my recipe for a more conventionally made chicken curry.

WHAT YOU NEED
2 tbsp coconut oil
3 tbsp chives
6 garlic cloves, chopped
1 good-sized finger of ginger, finely sliced
2 tsp mild to medium curry powder
pinch or two of cayenne pepper
pinch of turmeric
1 large chicken, skinned, de-boned and cut into bite-sized pieces
1 large can coconut milk
handful of fresh parsley, chopped
2 tbsp chopped spring onions
Celtic or Maldon sea salt to taste
freshly ground black pepper to taste

HERE'S HOW
Melt the coconut oil in a heavy pot. Add the chives, garlic and ginger and lightly brown. Toss in the curry powder and spices. Put in the chicken pieces and coat with the sauce, allowing them to cook lightly for 2–3 minutes. Now cover and turn the heat down until the chicken pieces cook through, stirring every 5 minutes to make sure nothing burns. Finally, pour on the coconut milk, add a little water if you need more juice, bring to a sizzle and cook gently for another 4 minutes. Season with parsley, spring onions, salt and pepper and serve, either on its own, over a bed of grated raw vegetables or with brown rice or kasha (*see following recipe*).

KASHA
Serves 4–6

Kasha has been a favourite for me ever since a Russian lover taught me how to make this traditional dish. It also makes a wonderful breakfast – especially to share in bed on a Sunday morning.

WHAT YOU NEED
250g (9oz) buckwheat
1 litre (1¾ pints) spring water
2 tsp low-salt vegetable bouillon powder
1 garlic clove, crushed
2 tbsp chopped fresh parsley

HERE'S HOW

Place the buckwheat in a heavy-bottomed pan and roast it dry over a medium heat while stirring with a wooden spoon. As it begins to darken, pour hot water over it and add the vegetable bouillon powder, garlic and one teaspoon of the parsley. Cover and simmer very slowly for about 15–20 minutes until all the liquid has been absorbed. Serve sprinkled with the remaining parsley or pour a light gravy over the top.

CHICKEN AND WATER CHESTNUT WRAPS WITH THAI PEANUT AND GINGER SAUCE
Serves 3–6

This is one of those dishes you can make ahead, chill and then pop into a lunch box or take on a picnic. I prefer to use skinless chicken breasts. I find they make wonderful additions to salads as well as good snacks to carry around with me when all that seems to be available is convenience foods. Generally, I make this recipe from breasts of chicken I have already cooked. Once the cooked chicken is available, it takes virtually no time to make the wraps. These wraps I have made with Cos lettuce. However, you can use cabbage or red cabbage – in fact, practically any green vegetable that is leafy and tough enough to hold the stuffing.

WHAT YOU NEED

1 tbsp sesame oil
6 skinless breasts of chicken, cut into 1-cm (½-in) cubes
8 spring onions, finely chopped
150g (5oz) mangetout, de-stringed and sliced diagonally in thin pieces
1 green pepper, diced
1 red pepper, diced
4 kaffir lime leaves, sliced (optional)
5-cm (2-in) finger of fresh ginger, finely shredded
Celtic or Maldon sea salt to taste
freshly ground black pepper to taste
juice of 2 lemons or limes
1 ripe avocado, mashed
200g (7oz) can of water chestnuts, drained and sliced
Thai fish sauce or Thai sweet chilli sauce to taste
8 strong edible green leaves
peanut ginger dressing

FOR THE PEANUT AND GINGER SAUCE

400g (14oz) organic non-hydrogenated peanut butter
2 tbsp tamari
3 tbsp Manuka honey
juice of 2 limes
1 tsp turmeric
1 tsp Tabasco sauce
Thai fish sauce to taste
freshly ground black pepper to taste
2–4 tsp water to blend
1 small finger of fresh ginger
3 garlic cloves, finely chopped

HERE'S HOW

Place the sesame oil in the bottom of a large frying pan or wok and heat. Toss in the chicken and onions first. Once they have begun to brown, put in the mangetout, peppers, lime leaves (if using) and ginger. Cook only as much as necessary to braise the vegetables and herbs and see that the chicken is cooked through. Remove from the heat and, when cool, season. Add the lemon or lime juice and mashed avocado as well as the chopped water chestnuts and fish or sweet chilli sauce. Chill this in the refrigerator for a couple of hours. Next, wrap your green leaves around a small handful of the mixture to make rolls that you can either pick up with your fingers or eat with a knife and fork. Hold with a cocktail stick if necessary. Drizzle with the peanut and ginger sauce and either refrigerate until you need them – as long as the lettuce is a hardy one or it will wilt under the strain – or serve immediately.

To make the sauce, place all the ingredients except the water, ginger and garlic in a food processor or blender and pulse until smooth. Add whatever water is necessary to get a good consistency, but do so only a teaspoon at a time. At the last moment add the finely chopped garlic and ginger and pulse once or twice to blend in, being careful not to liquidise the garlic so it still maintains its chunkiness. Cover and chill in the fridge for half an hour to let the flavours develop and serve chilled.

MARJORAM QUAIL WITH MANUKA HONEY
Serves 4

These little members of the pheasant family are easy to prepare and a delight to eat. I like to cook them for small dinner parties as they take very little preparation yet taste so good. You need a good heavy pot with a lid, some fresh herbs from the garden and not a lot else.

WHAT YOU NEED
4–6 quail, cleaned
Celtic or Maldon sea salt to taste
freshly ground black pepper to taste
plenty of sprigs of fresh marjoram
2 tbsp extra-virgin olive oil
1 tbsp fresh savory, chopped
725g (1½lb) tiny potatoes, scrubbed but not peeled
good handful of raisins
1 glass dry white wine
3 tbsp Manuka honey

HERE'S HOW
Wash and dry the quail and rub them inside and out with salt and pepper. Place a couple of sprigs of marjoram inside each. Heat the olive oil in the bottom of a heavy pan and put the quail in to brown, turning frequently. Remove from heat, add the chopped savory, potatoes, raisins, white wine and Manuka honey as well as more sprigs of marjoram, and bake for half an hour. Garnish with more marjoram and serve. These little birds are delicious served cold later.

VEGETARIAN GOURMET

Once you have tasted the delicate balance of fresh organic vegetables enhanced by the potent flavours of herbs and spices, the doors of creative vegetarian cooking are opened. Although these recipes take a little more time to prepare, the delicious results are well worth the effort.

If you are a vegetarian or a vegan it can be more of a challenge to ensure you get the good-quality protein you need to thrive. But it can be done. Eggs, some cheese, some soya tofu, nuts and seeds – all these can be brought together to make delicious and highly nutritious dishes. You'll even find a number of all-raw protein main dishes here which are great for Sunday lunches outdoors. And don't forget the omelettes topped with Powerhouse Salsa (*see Salsas and Sauces*).

TEPPENYAKI TOFU
Vegan
Serves 2–3

A good vegan form of protein, tofu is something all of us should include regularly in our diet. The problem with tofu or soya bean curd is that it has no flavour of its own, so you need to marinate it well before cooking. I like to cook tofu in strips or chunks, some of which I eat immediately at one meal and some that I store to be used the next day at another, or even eaten cold as a snack. You can add these tofu strips to a stir-fry or a phytonutrient-rich salad.

WHAT YOU NEED
500g (18oz) firm tofu

FOR THE MARINADE
60ml (2fl oz) tamari or soy sauce (without sugar)
1 tbsp extra-virgin olive oil or coconut fat
4 garlic cloves, crushed
a small finger of fresh ginger, finely shredded
1 tbsp lemon juice

½ tsp wasabi or 1 tsp Meaux mustard
pinch of stevia

HERE'S HOW
Slice the tofu into long strips. Separate them and lay them in a shallow baking dish. Mix together the marinade ingredients and pour over the tofu. Allow to marinate for an hour or two (best overnight). Remove the tofu strips and fry on a teppenyaki grill or in a heavy frying pan using coconut fat or extra-virgin olive oil, turning until gently browned on all sides.

NEW AGE PIZZA
Vegetarian
Serves 4

If you are a pizza lover, chances are you are going to miss it more than any other food when you start high-raw, low-grain eating. Here's my version of a pizza sauce which you can spread on teppenyaki tofu strips (cut them wider than usual) or over grilled slices of aubergine. It ain't the same as the gooey dough you will find in pizza, but it's quite delicious in its own right and lots of fun to make.

WHAT YOU NEED
450g (1lb) teppenyaki tofu slices or aubergine, cooked and cooled (best made from ultra-firm tofu)
2 tbsp fresh oregano or ½ tsp dried oregano
Celtic or Maldon sea salt to taste
freshly ground black pepper to taste
handful of fresh basil leaves, chopped
200g (7oz) shredded mozzarella
anchovies, pepperoni and/or olives to garnish
2 tbsp extra-virgin olive oil

FOR THE SAUCE
1 tin of tomatoes
4 garlic cloves, crushed
1 tsp vegetarian bouillon powder
1 tbsp extra-virgin olive oil
Celtic or Maldon sea salt to taste

freshly ground black pepper to taste
pinch of cayenne pepper
1 tbsp fresh oregano, finely chopped or ½ tsp dried oregano

HERE'S HOW
Make the sauce first by heating a pan and adding all of the ingredients, then allowing the sauce to reduce until it becomes thick. This usually takes about five minutes. Now place the slices of pre-cooked tofu or aubergine on a baking sheet, sprinkle with olive oil, oregano and seasoning and spread with the pizza sauce, topping off with basil leaves and fresh oregano as well as the cheese and garnishes. Place under the grill for 3 or 4 minutes until the cheese melts. This sauce will keep for 3–4 days in the fridge if you make extra, and this recipe makes a delicious snack which you can eat the next day.

CORIANDER TOFU
Vegan
Serves 4

The intense flavour of coriander works well to enhance the blandness of tofu. This recipe goes particularly well with steamed vegetables – especially broccoli – and brown rice. Or add this tofu to a salad to make a one-bowl meal rich in protein and plant factors for health.

WHAT YOU NEED
400g (14oz) firm tofu
2 tbsp extra-virgin olive oil or sesame oil
25-cm (10-in) piece of fresh ginger, finely shredded
handful of fresh coriander, finely chopped
1 tbsp tamari
1 tsp Manuka honey
Celtic or Maldon sea salt to taste
freshly ground red or black peppercorns

HERE'S HOW
Cut the tofu crosswise into slices approximately 1cm (½in) thick. Mix together all the other ingredients except the seasoning in a bowl, then dip each tofu slice into the mixture. Heat a heavy frying pan, grill or teppenyaki grill. Spray or brush just enough olive oil on top of the grill or in the pan so the tofu will not stick. Place the tofu on the grill

or in the pan, sprinkle with salt and peppercorns and cook at a high temperature until browned. Turn and brown again. Serve immediately as a 'tofu sandwich' (use the tofu like slices of bread and fill with salad or steamed vegetables) or in a tofu salad, or simply as is with loads of beautifully coloured fresh vegetables. The whole cooking process takes no more than 3–5 minutes.

Croquettes, Patties and Loaves

When people start eating a high-raw diet they often complain that salad and fruit simply don't satisfy them. The dishes in this section are designed to do just that, to supplement the main course of your meal (a large salad) with extra protein and calories in the form of nuts, seeds and sprouts to give you that 'full' feeling. After eating lots of raw foods for a while, you will find that your 'hunger pangs' decrease, that you no longer want to eat a lot of heavy foods such as nuts, and that a large salad for a main meal will be quite enough to leave you feeling satisfied, but not bloated.

SANDSTONE LOAF
Vegan
Serves 2–4

This dish has a beautiful pink/orange colour. It is very easy to prepare with a food processor.

WHAT YOU NEED
6–8 carrots
3–4 sticks of celery
juice of ½ a lemon
2 tbsp vegetable bouillon powder
50g (2oz) almonds or peanuts
2 tbsp tahini
½ an onion, finely chopped
handful of fresh parsley or 1 tbsp dried parsley

HERE'S HOW
Wash the carrots and celery. If the celery is stringy, peel away the tougher fibres. Roughly chop the carrots and celery and put into a food processor. Blend thoroughly, adding the lemon juice and bouillon powder, and transfer to a separate bowl. Now grind the nuts as finely

as possible. Add them to the carrots and celery mixture, then stir in the tahini, onion and parsley. Pack into a bread tin. Garnish with parsley leaves and serve.

FERMENTED SEED LOAF
Vegan
Serves 2–4

This loaf needs to be fermented for 24 hours so make it at least a day before you want it.

WHAT YOU NEED
50g (2oz) almonds
50g (2oz) sesame seeds
2 tbsp tamari
1 garlic clove, chopped
bunch of basil
bunch of parsley
1 tsp caraway seeds
100–225ml (4–8fl oz) cup water
100g (4oz) cauliflower or broccoli florets
2 sticks of celery
4 mushrooms
radish slices, to garnish

HERE'S HOW
Finely chop the nuts and seeds. Add the seasonings – tamari, garlic, basil, parsley and the caraway seeds – and the water. Finely chop or grate the cauliflower or broccoli and dice the celery and mushrooms. Mix all the ingredients together and pack into a bread tin. Cover with a tea towel and leave to ferment for 24 hours in a warm place. Add radish slices just before serving.

PHONEY PHEASANT LOAF
Vegan
Serves 4

The cranberry sauce finishes this recipe off nicely. Cranberries have an affinity for game. The American Indians used to mix their venison with cranberries to preserve it for winter. Nowadays people drink cranberry juice to help fight off infections. You could substitute blackcurrants or redcurrants if you cannot get cranberries.

WHAT YOU NEED
225g (8oz) pumpkin seeds
150g (5oz) cashew nuts
100g (4oz) brazil nuts
4–6 sticks of celery
1–2 spring onions
fresh parsley
1 tsp sage
100g (4oz) cranberries (or blackcurrants or redcurrants)
Manuka honey to taste

HERE'S HOW
Grind the seeds and nuts in a food processor. Add the chopped celery and spring onion and process (for a crunchier loaf, chop them finely and combine without processing). Add the herbs and mix well. Turn into a loaf tin. Make a sauce with the berries by blending them, straining most of the juice off (use it as a drink) and adding Manuka honey to taste. Spread the berries over the top of the loaf and garnish with parsley.

SPRUNG SPROUT CROQUETTES
Vegan
Serves 2–4

A good way of using up sprouts if you find you have grown too many.

WHAT YOU NEED
75g (3oz) cashew nuts
100g (4oz) sunflower seeds
1–2 spring onions, chopped
1 tsp dried oregano
1 tsp vegetable bouillon powder
1–2 tbsp tamari
handful each of mung bean, lentil and fenugreek sprouts
a few radish sprouts

HERE'S HOW

Grind the cashews and sunflower seeds finely, adding the chopped spring onions, oregano, bouillon powder and tamari. Add the sprouts and process for just a few seconds so that they retain their crunchiness. Form the mixture into croquettes or balls, chill and serve.

CHICKPEA CROQUETTES
Vegetarian
Serves 2–3

WHAT YOU NEED
200g (7oz) chickpea sprouts
100g (4oz) sunflower seeds or peanuts
1 egg yolk
1 tbsp tamari
juice of ½ a lemon
¼ tsp cayenne pepper
2–4 carrots
1 shallot
pinch of cumin
handful of poppy or sesame seeds
fresh parsley

HERE'S HOW

Mix together the chickpea sprouts, sunflower seeds or peanuts, egg yolk, tamari, lemon juice and cayenne pepper in the food processor. Finely grate the carrots and shallot and add to the chickpea mixture. Season with a little cumin. Form into croquettes and sprinkle with poppy or sesame seeds. Serve on a bed of lettuce and garnish with fresh parsley.

CARROT YOGHURT PATTIES
Vegetarian
Serves 4

These are an old family favourite and very simple to make.

WHAT YOU NEED
225g (8oz) sunflower seeds or 100g (4oz) mixed nuts

6–8 carrots
2 sticks of celery
3 spring onions
100ml (4fl oz) yoghurt
wheatgerm
juice of 1 lemon
1 tsp vegetable bouillon powder
bunch of fresh basil
freshly ground black pepper to taste

HERE'S HOW
Grind the sunflower seeds or nuts finely or coarsely, depending on how crunchy you want the patties to be. Grate or process the carrots and finely chop the celery and spring onions and add them to the sunflower seeds or nuts. Mix together in another bowl the yoghurt, wheatgerm, lemon juice, bouillon powder, herbs and seasonings. Make a well in the centre of the sunflower and vegetable mixture and pour in the yoghurt and wheatgerm mixture. Mix together, adding more wheatgerm if necessary to get the right consistency. Form the mixture into balls and flatten. Eat plain or garnish with chopped parsley or toasted sesame seeds.

SALSAS AND SAUCES

Delicious salsas, light sauces and relishes have replaced many of the heavy sauces of the past. They are a great way to add zing to anything from cooked or raw vegetables to buckwheat soba or kasha to fish and crudités. You can even eat them on brown rice. Make and use as little or as much as you like. Let's look at the raw sauces first.

POWERHOUSE SALSA
Vegan

I adore salsa. You can eat this salsa hot or cold. I like to spoon it on to omelettes for brunch or breakfast, and to eat it with crudités. This recipe is all raw. It makes the best possible use of the phytonutrients in the herbs and vegetables that go into it. I like to cut my salsa rougher than most so you get a great mixture of textures as well as flavours. Make it in the food processor, as far as I'm concerned, and you turn a salsa into a delicious gazpacho.

WHAT YOU NEED
2 garlic cloves, finely chopped
½ a red onion, finely chopped
handful of fresh coriander, chopped
handful of fresh basil, chopped, or 2 tbsp fresh mint, chopped
handful of broad-leaved parsley, chopped
green or red chilli pepper, seeded and roughly chopped
1 large tomato, roughly chopped
1 large green pepper, roughly chopped
Celtic or Maldon sea salt to taste
freshly ground black pepper to taste
3 tbsp extra-virgin olive oil
3 tbsp lemon or lime juice

HERE'S HOW
Mix everything together in a bowl and chill in the refrigerator. It takes this chilling process to let the ingredients in salsa meld properly. I like

to eat my salsa fresh and would never keep it in the fridge for longer than 48 hours.

BLOOD OF ANGELS SAUCE
Meat free

WHAT YOU NEED
2 small tomatoes
small handful of sun-dried tomatoes
small handful of cashews
1 tsp fresh oregano, finely chopped
dash or 2 of Worcestershire sauce
juice of 1 lemon
1 tsp ginger, finely grated

HERE'S HOW
Place the tomatoes, the sun-dried tomatoes, the cashews, oregano, Worcestershire sauce and lemon juice in a blender and blend until smooth. Now add the grated ginger and stir in by hand. Put in the fridge to chill so the flavours blend.

MIDNIGHT SUN SAUCE
Vegan

WHAT YOU NEED
2 yellow peppers
1 shallot
1 fresh garlic clove
225ml (8fl oz) mayonnaise or soya mayonnaise
1 feather of saffron
½ tsp turmeric
juice of 1 lemon

HERE'S HOW
Blend all the ingredients together in a food processor or blender and serve.

GREEN GODDESS SAUCE
Vegan
Makes a medium-sized bowlful

WHAT YOU NEED
1 ripe avocado
handful of watercress leaves, finely chopped
2 tbsp spring onions
juice of 1 lime
½ tsp vegetable bouillon powder
1 garlic clove

HERE'S HOW
Place all the ingredients in a food processor and pulse on and off to blend, being careful not to blend too much so that you preserve the texture of the vegetables.

COCONUT CURRY SAUCE
Vegan
Serves 4–6

My friends from the Cook Islands taught me this recipe. It's easy to make and will turn meat, fish or chicken into a delicious meal. If I'm feeling really energetic, I serve it over a bed of unsweetened hand-shredded coconut in place of rice.

WHAT YOU NEED
½ an onion, finely chopped
3 garlic cloves, crushed
1 tbsp coconut fat
1 tin unsweetened coconut cream
2 tsp mild, medium or hot curry powder
1 pinch stevia, Manuka honey or maple syrup to taste
pinch of turmeric (optional)

HERE'S HOW
Place the onion and garlic in a pan. (I often use the pan in which I have stirfried the meat, fish or chicken for the curry so that the crispy crunchy bits of protein carry the flavour over into the curry sauce.) Add the coconut fat and brown the garlic and onions, picking up any

leftover residue from protein foods you have cooked. Pour on the coconut cream and add all the other ingredients. Bring to a gentle simmer for a minute or two, then it's ready to serve.

COCONUT CREAM SAUCE
Vegan
Serves 4

I cringe when I think of the traditional sauces that were served in my mother's time. They were so full of flour and complicated to make. I prefer simple sauces you can whip up in a minute, which are bright and clear in flavour, spiked with herbs and spices. You can use this sauce just about anywhere and it works. This recipe uses the spice turmeric, which has wonderful health-giving properties. I frequently add turmeric to vegetables and fish just because I love the brilliant yellow colour.

This sauce is easy to make and works beautifully over steamed cabbage, broccoli, cauliflower, spinach, fish, chicken or lamb – in fact just about anything. You can make it with fresh coconut liquid, in which case you need to mix it with a bit of arrowroot powder in order to thicken it, or you can make it – as I usually do – with canned coconut milk.

WHAT YOU NEED
3 tbsp cold-pressed sesame oil
1 small onion, finely chopped
2 garlic cloves, finely chopped
300ml (10½fl oz) coconut milk
⅛ tsp Cajun seasoning
Celtic or Maldon sea salt to taste
freshly ground red peppercorns to taste
½ tsp ground turmeric
2 tbsp broad-leaved parsley or fresh coriander, finely chopped

HERE'S HOW
Put the sesame oil in a pan and fry the onion and garlic until very light brown. Now add the coconut milk, Cajun seasoning, salt, pepper and turmeric and cook for 2–3 minutes until heated through, then remove from the heat. Add the fresh herbs, reserving a teaspoonful as a garnish, and pour into a bowl or directly over vegetables or fish.

Garnish with the rest of the chopped fresh herbs. If you prefer your sauce thicker, add a little arrowroot or cornflour.

HOLLANDAISE SAUCE
Vegetarian

I adore hollandaise sauce. For years I did not eat it because I, like so many people, was afraid of the fat it contains. This recipe is easy to make and tastes great over eggs, spinach or asparagus. Use it as a dipping sauce for artichokes as well.

WHAT YOU NEED
100g (3½oz) butter
4 egg yolks, beaten
juice of 1 lemon
Celtic or Maldon sea salt to taste
freshly ground black pepper to taste
1 tsp Dijon mustard (optional)
sprinkling of Mexican chilli powder (optional)

HERE'S HOW
Melt one-third of the butter in a *bain-marie*, then remove from the heat. Beat the egg yolks in a bowl, using either a hand-held electric beater or a whisk. Very slowly add the melted butter to the egg yolks, continuing to mix all the time. Pour this mixture into the *bain-marie* and put back over simmering water. Gradually add the rest of the butter, little by little, all the while continuing to whisk. Once the butter is completely melted and integrated with the sauce, remove it from the heat and stir in the lemon juice, salt, pepper and other additions.

SUMMER COOLERS AND WINTER WARMERS

Drinking plenty of water and fresh juices throughout the day is a key strategy for health and beauty. We need to replace the vital body fluids which are constantly lost through perspiration and breathing. A good fluid intake helps flush out your system. A glass of fresh vegetable or fruit juice is also a tonic and energy booster. On an empty stomach the vitamins and minerals are absorbed into your bloodstream in a matter of minutes and leave you feeling clear-headed, refreshed and energised. The drinks in this section range from fruity summer thirst-quenchers to protein-rich breakfast drinks.

Fruit Drinks

Make fruit drinks by juicing any kind of fresh fruit – apples, oranges, grapes, pineapples – in a centrifuge or citrus press, or blending them with a little water in the blender. Often it is worth buying a crate of oranges or apples from a wholesaler specifically for juicing. Fresh juice is the only thing worth drinking.

GARDEN PUNCH
Serves 4

This is my favourite summer drink. The recipe comes from a family friend who has a most beautiful garden full of flowers, fruit, vegetables and honey bees. Drinking her version of the drink on a hot summer's day surrounded by her wonderful flowers is pure paradise.

WHAT YOU NEED
fresh mint
fresh lemon balm
450ml (16fl oz) water
handful of raspberries or blackcurrants (mainly for their colour effect)
2 oranges
1 lemon

450–700ml (16–25fl oz) apple juice
225ml (8fl oz) pineapple or orange juice
50g (2oz) fresh or dried elderflowers (de-stalked)
Manuka honey
ice

HERE'S HOW

Blend the fresh mint and lemon balm with the water and berries until the leaves are finely chopped. Add the grated rinds of the oranges and lemon and leave the mixture to soak in the blender for about 15 minutes. Strain into a jug and discard the leaves, berry pulp and rinds. Pour in the other juices (apple and pineapple or orange). Juice the lemon and slice the orange and add them to the jug, then add the elderflower heads (these can be strained off later, but a few poured into the glasses with the drink are particularly attractive). Sweeten with a little Manuka honey and chill. Serve in tall glasses with ice and fresh mint. As a variation, try replacing the apple juice with grape juice.

SPICED APPLE JUICE
Serves 4

A very simple way of doing something special with plain juice.

WHAT YOU NEED

1 lemon and/or orange
1–1¼ litres (2–2½ pints) apple juice (or organic cider)
2 tbsp Manuka honey
6 cloves
4 cinnamon sticks
2 cardamom pods
pinch of nutmeg and allspice
ground cinnamon

HERE'S HOW

Cut the lemon and orange into thin slices and place in a jug. Pour the apple juice over them and add the honey and spices (but not the cinnamon sticks). Cover and leave to stand for an hour. Strain the juice and serve in glasses with a stick of cinnamon in each.

LEMONADE
Serves 4

Lemons have many known health benefits (not to mention that they were once used to keep clothes moths out of cupboards before moth-balls were invented). Their high hesperidin content helps to strengthen collagen in the skin and blood vessels, and their vitamin C soothes sore throats. Lemon juice is also supposed to be an excellent cure for hiccups.

WHAT YOU NEED
2–4 lemons
1–1¼ litres (2–2½ pints) water
150g (5oz) raisins
1 tbsp Manuka honey
4 lemon slices

HERE'S HOW
Grate the rind off one of the lemons and put the rind into a saucepan with about 450ml (16fl oz) of water and heat to just below boiling. Strain this liquid into a bowl and add the raisins. Leave them to soak until they are plump. Pour the raisins and soak water into the blender and add the juice of all the lemons (including the rindless one). Blend well and add Manuka honey to taste. Serve in tall glasses with crushed ice and a slice of lemon.

Fruit Smoothies

These are made by blending a combination of fruits with a little apple juice, spring water or carbonated water, and adding Manuka honey if desired. You will need about 225g (8oz) of chopped fruit (peeled if necessary) and just under 225ml (8fl oz) of liquid per person. Here are some nice combinations, which are even more scrumptious if you chill the fruit in the freezer for an hour or so first:

❑ Banana and Peach
❑ Banana and Strawberry/Raspberry/Blackberry/Blueberry
❑ Banana and Apple
❑ Pear and Apple
❑ Mango and Orange
❑ Peach and Apricot
❑ Orange with a pinch of ground ginger

GOLDEN SMOOTHIE
Serves 2

WHAT YOU NEED
2 oranges
2 peaches
1 banana
1 tsp vanilla essence
a little Manuka honey if desired
1 tsp nutmeg

HERE'S HOW
Peel the oranges and remove the pips. Process in a blender or food processor with the peaches and banana. Add the vanilla, the Manuka honey (if using) and the nutmeg. Combine well. Pour into two tall glasses with crushed ice and serve.

PINEAPPLE OR ORANGE SHAKE
Serves 1

WHAT YOU NEED
75g (3oz) pineapple or orange
50ml (2fl oz) pineapple or orange juice
squeeze of lemon
2 ice cubes

HERE'S HOW
Peel the fruit, remove the pips, cut into chunks and blend with the juice and a squeeze of lemon until smooth. Add the ice cubes and process until crushed. Serve in a tall glass with a sprig of mint and a twist of orange or slice of pineapple.

PINEAPPLE BLACKBERRY FRAPPÉ
Serves 2

WHAT YOU NEED
300g (10oz) fresh pineapple chunks
50g (2oz) blackberries
juice of ½ a lime (optional)
spring or filtered water (optional)

HERE'S HOW

Place all the ingredients into the blender and liquidise. This can be thinned using a little spring or filtered water and chilled with an ice cube or two.

APPLE RASPBERRY FRAPPÉ
Serves 2

WHAT YOU NEED

2 sweet apples, cored but not peeled, cut into small pieces
½ tsp finely chopped lemon balm or mint
50g (2oz) fresh or frozen raspberries
spring or filtered water (optional)
ice cubes (optional)

HERE'S HOW

Place all the ingredients into the blender and liquidise, adding a little spring or filtered water to thin if you wish and ice cubes if you want a chilled drink.

CREAMY DATE DELIGHT
Serves 2

WHAT YOU NEED

2 very ripe bananas
4 fresh dates
1 tbsp shredded coconut
100–225ml (4–8fl oz) sparkling spring water

HERE'S HOW

Blend the bananas, dates and coconut together thoroughly in the blender or food processor, then add the sparkling water and mix gently. Pour into chilled glasses and serve immediately.

STRAWBERRY CREAM SHAKE
Serves 1

Not a breakfast recipe – this shake is a full fruit meal in itself and makes a lovely light supper for hot summer evenings.

WHAT YOU NEED
75g (3oz) fresh cashews
225ml (8fl oz) spring or filtered water
50g (2oz) strawberries
1 tbsp Manuka honey
75g (3oz) pineapple chunks (optional)

HERE'S HOW
Blend all the ingredients (including the pineapple chunks, if desired) in a food processor or blender and serve in a tall frosted glass. The quantities above make one very large shake.

ORANGE PINEAPPLE COCKTAIL
Serves 4

Pineapple is an excellent aid to digestion because it contains the enzyme bromelain, which encourages the secretion of hydrochloric acid in the stomach and helps to digest proteins. In Hawaii, pineapple is often eaten at the end of a meal as a digestive.

WHAT YOU NEED
1 small pineapple
225–450ml (8–16fl oz) orange juice
several ice cubes
ground ginger
fresh mint
lemon slices

HERE'S HOW
Peel the pineapple, cut it into chunks and process in the blender or food processor with the orange juice. Add the ice cubes, ginger and mint and blend again. Serve immediately in tall or stemmed glasses with a slice of lemon hooked over the rim.

MIXED ENERGY COCKTAIL
Serves 4

WHAT YOU NEED
2 tomatoes

2 carrots
2 sticks celery
1 lemon
fresh parsley
basil and marjoram
several ice cubes
1 tbsp vegetable bouillon powder
enough water to give the desired consistency

HERE'S HOW

Peel the tomatoes. Roughly chop the carrots, celery and tomatoes and put them in the blender. Add the juice of the lemon, herbs, bouillon powder and ice cubes, and blend. Serve in glasses with a sprig of fresh parsley, a slim swizzle stick of cucumber and a dash of Tabasco or Worcestershire sauce if desired.

Nut and Seed Milks

These are simple to make, highly nutritious and easy to digest. They can also replace cow's milk in certain dishes. Nut milks and seed milks can be made separately or together – the principle is the same.

ALMOND MILK
Serves 2

This is an ambrosial introduction to these milks, and it is my favourite. I remove the almond skins as they are rather bitter and contain a high quantity of prussic acid, which should be avoided. Some people blanch the almonds first, but I find it easiest to prepare the milk with unskinned almonds and then strain it through a fine sieve or piece of cheesecloth to remove the pulp. As a general rule, you need one part nuts to three parts water.

WHAT YOU NEED

150g–225g (5–8oz) almonds
1 litre (1¾ pints) water
Manuka honey to taste
dash of cinnamon or nutmeg
vanilla essence (optional)

HERE'S HOW

Combine the almonds and water in your blender and process really well for a minute or so until the mixture is very smooth. Add the Manuka honey, cinnamon or nutmeg and vanilla essence (if using). Strain and serve. As a variation, blend a ripe banana with the almond milk. You can use other nuts instead of almonds. Cashews are particularly good, but you may find you need a little more water. Nuts and sunflower or sesame seeds also make a nice drink.

SWEET SEED MILK
Serves 4

WHAT YOU NEED

200g (7oz) sunflower and sesame seeds (3 parts sunflower to 1 part sesame)
generous litre (1¾ pints) water
10 dried dates or 8 dried figs (minus the hard stalks)
squeeze of lemon (optional)

HERE'S HOW

Grind the seeds very finely in the blender with some of the water. When smooth, add the dates or figs and process again. The figs give a pleasing crunchy texture because of their seeds. Add the remaining water and a squeeze of lemon juice if desired. Serve immediately. Try making this as a breakfast drink, soaking the seeds and dried fruit together in the blender overnight. Next morning, blend all the ingredients together well. The extra soaking makes the seeds and fruit even tastier and more digestible. You can use raisins or apricots instead of the dates.

OTHER WAYS TO GO

Seed and nut milks can be flavoured in many different ways.
Banana Milk: Add 2 ripe bananas to the basic recipe for 4 people. You will need to add a little extra water, especially if you want to drink it through a straw. Blend the bananas with the milk until creamy.
Carob Milk: Add 50g (2oz) of carob powder to the basic recipe for 4 people, plus a teaspoon of vanilla essence and a little extra water. Blend the ingredients together well.

Teas and Tisanes

RASPBERRY, GINSENG AND VANILLA TEA
Serves 2

Ginseng is full of phytosteroids – natural plant chemicals which not only improve our ability to deal with stress, but also act as mild sexual stimulants. A delicious combination of fruits and flavours, this tea is one I serve in tall, clear-glass cups with a few raspberries sitting in the bottom. Vanilla pods contain vanillin – also a mild stimulant. Raspberries are rich in potassium, and are not only beautiful to look at, but soothing to the spirit too. A combination of the three is hard to beat. You can serve this tea either hot or cold. The colour is like a summer sunset and the taste is sensuous beyond belief.

WHAT YOU NEED
100g (4oz) raspberries, either fresh or frozen
½ tsp dried ginseng root, crushed, or a bag of good ginseng tea, or a packet of freeze-dried ginseng granules
2 vanilla pods
275ml (10fl oz) boiling water
100ml (4fl oz) maple syrup or Manuka honey

HERE'S HOW
Wash the fruit. Put the raspberries in a saucepan with enough water to cover the base of the pan to prevent burning. Simmer over a low heat to extract the flavour from the raspberries. Stain the liquid into a cup and put the cup to one side. Put the ginseng and one vanilla pod into a teapot and pour boiling water over them. Steep for 3 minutes then pour through a strainer into the raspberry liquid. Add the maple syrup or Manuka honey. Rinse the vanilla pods and place in tall glasses or cups. Fill each cup with the mixture and serve immediately. You can also chill this and keep it in the refrigerator. I generally add a few more raspberries and a little more ginseng if I chill it, because things tend to lose their flavour when they are iced. If chilled, serve over crushed ice. It's as good for a midsummer picnic as it is for an afternoon of love.

LAVENDER TEA
Serves 1

There is no more beautiful tea to take at bedtime than this dark midnight brew of tiny fresh lavender flowers. It is relaxing, light and gentle. To brew you need a cafetière and a handful of flowers. Place the flowers in the cafetière, pour boiling water over them and let them steep for 5–15 minutes, depending on how strong you want it. The longer it brews, the deeper the violet colour. Press down with the plunger and pour into a glass mug. Serve with a teaspoon of Manuka honey just before bed.

SWEET TREATS

Sweets and puddings can be the crowning enjoyment to a meal, leaving you feeling satisfied and energised. Some fruits contain enzymes which aid digestion and are an ideal and refreshing way to end a meal. Here are some recipes for fruit desserts and sweet treats that are as delicious as they are fulfilling.

Fruit Salads

TROPICAL FRUIT SALAD
Vegan
Serves 2–4

Coconut, papaya, mango, bananas and feijoas (if you can get them – a wonderful tropical fruit that grows almost wild in the southern hemisphere) are one of my favourite fruit salad combinations.

WHAT YOU NEED
1 papaya, peeled, seeded and sliced
2 ripe bananas, sliced lengthwise twice then chopped into small pieces
1 ripe mango, peeled and diced
1 fresh lime, sliced, to garnish

FOR ANGEL SAUCE
225g (8oz) tofu
75ml (3fl oz) maple syrup
1 tsp vanilla
2 tbsp coconut flakes, either from a fresh coconut or unsweetened packaged coconut
2 tsp fresh lime juice
a sprinkling of freshly ground nutmeg

HERE'S HOW
Cut the fruit into different sizes so you get a good variation in size and texture in this salad. Mix together the ingredients for Angel Sauce and blend in a blender until smooth. Sprinkle with nutmeg and serve immediately with a slice of lime on the side of each dish.

SATIN SALAD
Vegan
Serves 2–4

This is made mainly from soft fruits, to create a smooth texture. The most common types of peaches are yellow, but look out for the white variety. They are a pale, creamy colour tinged with pink and have a beautiful, fruit blossom aroma. When choosing peaches, make sure they are not bruised or green. Unlike other fruits, peaches do not ripen after they have been picked; they merely soften and begin to lose their flavour.

WHAT YOU NEED
2 sweet plums or a few cherries
4 peaches or nectarines
1 pear
150g (5oz) seedless green grapes or 150g (5oz) soaked raisins
2 bananas
desiccated coconut (optional)

HERE'S HOW
Slice the plums or halve the cherries, dice the peaches and peel and dice the pear. Put them in a bowl and add the grapes, whole or halved, or the raisins. Slice and add the bananas. As a topping, blend a cupful of the fruit with a little fruit juice or the soak water from some dried fruit. Pour this over the fruit salad. Alternatively, serve plain or sprinkled with a little desiccated coconut.

FRESH CITRUS SALAD
Vegan
Serves 2–4

When buying grapefruit, avoid those that feel light or have puffy skins – they are likely to be dry and pithy inside. Look out for the pink/ruby-red grapefruit – they are sweeter than the yellow ones and twice as delicious.

WHAT YOU NEED
2 oranges
1 grapefruit or 3 satsumas

1 small pineapple
fresh mint, to garnish

HERE'S HOW
Peel the oranges and the grapefruit or satsumas. Slice them into segments, removing each from its envelope of skin. Now slice each segment across to give small bite-sized pieces. Scoop the fruits and their juices into a bowl. Peel the pineapple, dice it and add to the citrus fruit. Serve garnished with a little fresh mint.

ORCHARD SALAD
Vegan
Serves 4

This beautiful salad is a combination of subtle reds and pinks.

WHAT YOU NEED
1 pear
2 large red apples
1 banana
juice of ½ a lemon
225g (8oz) cherries
1 punnet strawberries
mint sprigs, to garnish

HERE'S HOW
Dice the pear, apples and banana and sprinkle with lemon juice. Halve the cherries and remove the stones. Slice the strawberries lengthwise. Mix all the fruits together and decorate with the mint sprigs.

ALL MELON SALAD
Vegan
Serves 4

Of melons it is said, 'Eat alone or leave alone'. Here is a good salad which combines three different types of melon and makes a delicious summer breakfast or starter.

WHAT YOU NEED
1 small watermelon
1 cantaloupe
1 honeydew melon
a little Manuka honey
fresh flowers and mint leaves, to garnish

HERE'S HOW
Cut the watermelon in half lengthwise. Scoop out the pulp and dice all but a cupful – this you can blend or juice to make a drink. Halve the other melons and scoop out balls with a melon scoop, or cut in cubes while still in the skin and scoop out the pieces with a spoon. Mix all the melon balls or cubes together and fill the watermelon 'baskets'. Drizzle with a little Manuka honey and decorate with fresh flowers (marigold, elderflowers, waterlilies) and mint leaves.

Stuffed Fruit Salads

MULLED STUFFED APPLES
Vegan
Serves 4

The best apples to buy are organic ones. Most of the nutritional value of an apple lies in its skin, or just below it, so wash apples well but don't peel them. Softish apples are best for this recipe as their insides have to be scooped out.

WHAT YOU NEED
225ml (8fl oz) grape juice or red wine
1 tsp cinnamon
3 cloves
½ tsp nutmeg
2 crushed white cardamom pods
½ tsp allspice
150g (5oz) blanched almonds
4 large apples
juice of ½ a lemon
75g (3oz) dates or raisins

HERE'S HOW
'Mull' the grape juice or wine by putting it in a bowl with the spices

and leaving for at least an hour. Discard the cloves and cardamom and blend the remaining mixture with the almonds. Slice the tops off the apples and keep them. Remove the cores, saving small pieces to plug the bottoms. Scoop out the apple pulp, leaving a shell about 1cm (½in) thick. Lightly blend the pulp with the juice and almond mixture until smooth, adding a squeeze of lemon juice. If the mixture is not thick enough, add a few more ground almonds. Chop the dates or raisins and fill the apple shells with the dried fruit and almond mixture. Replace the 'lids'. Using the same method, you can make stuffed apples with apple sauce and blackberries. Blend the apple pulp with a little lemon juice, honey and spices, then combine it with the blackberries and spoon into the apple shells.

STUFFED PINEAPPLE
Vegan
Serves 4

WHAT YOU NEED
1 pineapple
1 orange, peeled and sliced
1 mango or papaya, peeled and sliced
100g (4oz) raspberries or strawberries, sliced
2 figs (fresh or soaked dried ones)
coconut milk (optional)
dried coconut, to garnish

HERE'S HOW
Slice the pineapple in half lengthwise and remove the flesh from each half, leaving a 1cm (½in) shell. Dice the flesh and mix it with the sliced orange, mango or papaya and raspberries or strawberries. Finely chop the figs and add. Mix all the ingredients with the coconut milk, if desired. Spoon the mixture into the pineapple shells and sprinkle with dried coconut.

Fruit Purées

These are an alternative to fruit salads and are particularly good for babies or elderly people for whom chewing is a problem. You can combine almost any fruits, but soft tropical fruits and berries are especially delicious. Most of these these recipes will serve 4 people – or 2 to 3 people generously.

SUNSHINE BLEND
Vegan

WHAT YOU NEED
½ a pineapple
1 mango or papaya
2 seedless oranges
1 peach
Manuka honey to taste
2 tbsp dried coconut

HERE'S HOW
Peel and roughly chop the pineapple, mango or papaya and oranges. Halve and stone the peach. Combine all these ingredients in a blender until smooth. Sweeten with a little Manuka honey if you like. Spoon into frosty chilled dessert glasses. Serve with a little coconut. As a variation, use two bananas instead of the mango or papaya.

CHERRY WHIP
Vegetarian

WHAT YOU NEED
225ml (8fl oz) natural yoghurt
100g (4oz) pitted black cherries
2 tsp Manuka honey
double cream (optional)

HERE'S HOW
Blend the yoghurt, cherries and honey and pour into a tall glass. Top with a spoonful of double cream, if desired, and garnish with a pair of cherries hung over the edge of the glass. As a variation, use strawberries or raspberries instead of cherries.

BERRIES PURE AND SIMPLE
Vegan

Fresh blueberries and raspberries smothered in a simple sauce of raspberries blended with maple syrup, eaten from the dish with your fingers.

RASPBERRY CHOCOLATE MOUSSE
Vegetarian
Serves 4

This is a fun dessert that everybody seems to enjoy. You can make it with or without the double cream. If you don't use cream, you can use microfiltered whey protein instead, giving you a mousse that is high in protein.

WHAT YOU NEED
120ml (4fl oz) filtered or spring water
2 tsp unflavoured vegetarian gelatine
120g (4oz) unsweetened baker's chocolate, grated or finely chopped
stevia or Manuka honey to taste
240ml (8½fl oz) double cream
1 tsp pure vanilla extract or pure vanilla oil
100g (4oz) fresh raspberries

HERE'S HOW
Heat the water to boiling and add the gelatine, stirring until dissolved. Toss in the shredded chocolate and the stevia or Manuka honey. Mix well then remove from the heat and set aside. Beat the cream in a chilled mixing bowl until almost thick (or use a couple of scoops of microfiltered whey mixed with enough water to give a cream-like consistency). Add the vanilla and beat again to mix. Fold in the chocolate mixture and pour into four serving dishes. Garnish with fresh raspberries and chill for half an hour before serving.

EXOTIC GINGERED FRUIT
Vegan

Some exotic fruits are best eaten separately to appreciate their subtle flavours. Try mangoes, lychees, papayas, persimmons, kiwi fruits, and so on, sliced and sprinkled with a little lemon juice, powdered ginger and Manuka honey.

STALKED STRAWBERRIES
Vegetarian

One of my all-time favourites. First I wash large strawberries with long stems still attached, and place them in a bowl. Then I fill another bowl with thick yoghurt or soured cream, and another bowl with raw sugar and place them on the table. Everyone can dip their own strawberries into the yoghurt and then into the sugar. Delicious.

STRAWBERRIES AND CASHEW CREAM
Vegan
Serves 4

Make your own 'non-dairy' cream from cashew nuts and pour it over a bowl of ripe fresh strawberries (or any other fruit).

WHAT YOU NEED
150g (5oz) cashew nuts
100ml (4fl oz) of water
1–2 tbsp Manuka honey
nutmeg
strawberries or other fruit

HERE'S HOW
Blend the nuts and liquid as finely as possible in the blender or food processor. Add a little Manuka honey and nutmeg and use as a topping for any fruit.

BROWN RICE PUDDING
Vegan
Serves 4

This has to be one of the oldest and most comforting foods in the Western world. Eating rice pudding can put you into a soporific state. You can prepare it way ahead and keep it in the fridge for late-night raids. Coconut gives this old favourite a new twist.

WHAT YOU NEED
75g (3oz) brown rice

1 litre (1¾ pints) coconut cream
75ml (3fl oz) Manuka honey
stevia or maple syrup to taste
pinch of salt
pinch of fresh grated nutmeg
3 tbsp grated almonds
slivered almonds, roasted, to serve (optional)

HERE'S HOW
Preheat your oven to 130°C/250°F/Gas Mark ½. Stir all the ingredients together in a casserole dish and bake, covered, for three hours, stirring a couple of times during the first two hours. Either serve immediately garnished with crystallised rose petals or slivered almonds, or refrigerate for future raids.

EASY-GOING PIECRUST
Vegan

This piecrust made from fresh almonds and flaxseeds is healthfully rich in omega-3 and omega-6 fatty acids. I use it for just about everything, from a frozen raspberry pie to a cheesecake. I like to grind up my flaxseeds in a coffee grinder, and I do the same with the almonds. I find that coffee grinders reduce everything to a beautiful powder that you can easily manipulate into whatever you want.

WHAT YOU NEED
60g (2oz) flaxseeds, ground to a fine powder
1 tsp fresh lemon juice
2–4 tbsp iced water
stevia, Manuka honey or maple syrup to taste
pinch of salt
180g (6oz) almonds, ground to a fine powder
1½ tbsp coconut oil, melted

HERE'S HOW
Soak the flaxseeds in lemon juice and a couple of teaspoons of iced water for about 20 minutes. Mix together with a fork and put aside. In another bowl, mix the stevia, Manuka honey or maple syrup with the salt, almonds and the melted coconut oil. Now combine the seed and nut mixtures and knead gently like pastry until they are mixed

thoroughly. Pour into a 22cm (9in) flan dish and, using your fingers, press the mixture into the dish all along the bottom and sides. Prick with a fork and bake at 170°C/325°F/Gas Mark 3 for a quarter of an hour. Let cool and you are ready to fill.

Fillings

The simplest fillings are sliced or chopped fruits such as plums, peaches or apples, sprinkled with a little orange or lemon juice, drizzled with Manuka honey and dusted with cinnamon or powdered allspice. But experiment with your own ideas. You will need about 1–1½ pieces of fruit for each person.

Mince Pie Filling: 150g (5oz) of raisins and 150g (5oz) of dates, soaked for several hours, 3 apples, Manuka honey, cinnamon and nutmeg to taste. Grate or process the apples finely and process the dates. Stir in the raisins and other ingredients and spoon into the crust. (This filling is delicious eaten on its own, topped with yoghurt.)

Apple and Blackberry Filling: Grate the apples and mix with blackberries, lemon juice and Manuka honey. This makes a traditional and delicious filling.

LEMON CREAM PIE
Vegetarian
Serves 8

I love to use this creamy and yummy filling. You can make similar recipes using pumpkin, strawberries or rhubarb, or even chocolate cream pies and strawberry cream pies – all it takes is a little imagination.

WHAT YOU NEED
120ml (4fl oz) fresh lemon juice
125g (4½ oz) unflavoured vegetarian gelatine
A little stevia, Manuka honey or maple syrup to taste
450g (1lb) cottage cheese
200g (7oz) soured cream
200ml (7fl oz) thick cream, whipped
1 tsp finely shredded lemon zest
120ml (4fl oz) fresh strawberries, raspberries, blueberries or blackberries, crushed

HERE'S HOW

Heat half of the lemon juice gently in a saucepan, sprinkling the gelatine into it and stirring over a low heat until dissolved. Mix the stevia, honey or maple syrup together with the cottage cheese, blending in the soured cream and the remainder of the lemon juice, and blend well. Cool in the refrigerator until the mixture thickens but does not set completely. Fold in the whipped cream. Fill the piecrust with the mixture, chill for several hours and serve sprinkled with lemon zest with the crushed berries as a topping.

Cakes

Raw cakes are every bit as tempting as baked cakes for birthdays and special occasions. The first two recipes contain oats.

SPICY FRUIT CAKE
Vegan
Serves 6

WHAT YOU NEED

50g (2oz) mixed nuts and seeds (walnuts and sunflower seeds, for example)
3 tbsp dried coconut
dried fruit – 30g (1oz) raisins, 4 peaches (or 6 apricots), 4 pear halves, 4 figs, 4 dates, pitted
1 banana
¼ tsp each of cinnamon, nutmeg and allspice
vanilla essence
1 orange
1 lemon
100g (4oz) rolled oats

HERE'S HOW

Put the seeds, nuts, coconut and dried fruit in the food processor and grind coarsely. Turn into a bowl. Blend the banana with the spices and a few drops of vanilla essence and add ½ tsp orange rind and ½ tsp lemon rind, finely grated. Juice the orange and lemon and keep separate. Mix the banana and the dried fruit/nut mixture together in a bowl and add the oats. Stir well and add some juice to give a firm binding consistency. Spoon the mixture into a cake tin with a removable base, or simply shape into a loaf and wrap in greaseproof paper. Refrigerate for a couple of hours. Serve the cake in thin slices – it's rich.

CAROB AND APPLE CAKE
Vegan
Serves 4

WHAT YOU NEED
225g (8oz) sunflower seeds or a 2:1 mixture of sunflower and sesame seeds
100g (4oz) carob powder (or a good organic cocoa)
30g (1oz) dried coconut
75g (3oz) dates
3 apples (red ones are nice)
½ tsp vanilla essence
1 tsp allspice
apple slices or strawberries, to garnish

HERE'S HOW
Grind the seeds very finely and mix with the carob powder, coconut and finely chopped dates. Core, then finely grate or process the apples. Add them to the carob mixture, put in the vanilla essence and allspice, and stir well. Form the mixture into a loaf or log shape and refrigerate for a couple of hours. Serve sliced, garnished with the apples and strawberries.

Sweet Dreams
These munchy snacks can replace those mid-morning chocolate bars or biscuits. They are particularly good for children (babies too), and can quickly take the place of 'sweets'. They are also helpful as an energy booster and sustainer between meals. Each recipe makes a good number for a family of four.

EASTER EGGS – BASIC RECIPE
Vegan

WHAT YOU NEED
30g (1oz) sesame seeds
175g (6oz) sunflower seeds
150g (5oz) nuts (a mixture such as pecans and hazels or almonds and brazils)
175g (6oz) mixed dried fruit (apricots, peaches, pineapple and bananas, or pears with raisins, figs and dates)

3 tbsp dried coconut
1 tbsp Manuka honey
juice of ½ an orange or 1 tbsp apple or grape juice
carob powder or sesame seeds to coat the eggs

HERE'S HOW

Finely grind the sesame seeds in the food processor. Add the sunflower seeds and nuts and grind well. Roughly chop the dried fruit and process with the seeds and nuts. Add the coconut, Manuka honey and a little fruit juice and process once more. You should end up with a slightly sticky wodge. Powder a board with carob powder or sesame seeds and form the mixture into little balls or sausages, rolling it in the powder or seeds. Chill and keep in the fridge.

SWEET TREATS
Vegan

These attractive little sweets can be wrapped in coloured paper and given in boxes as gifts for Easter and Christmas and all other celebrations.

WHAT YOU NEED

150g (5oz) almond and hazelnut mixture
175g (6oz) mixed dried fruit (such as date and apricot, peach and raisin, sultana and pear)
1 tbsp Manuka honey
juice of 1 orange or 50ml (2fl oz) apple juice
dash of orange liqueur (optional)
coconut flakes
sesame seeds

HERE'S HOW

Put the nuts and the dried fruit in the food processor and chop thoroughly. Add the honey and enough fruit juice to make the mixture bind, plus a dash of orange liqueur if desired. Remove from the processor and roll into spheres the size of large marbles. Sprinkle a plate with the coconut flakes (toasted if desired) and sesame seeds and roll the balls in either one or both. Chill in the fridge and serve on a platter decorated with fresh fruit.

PROTEIN FUDGE TREATS
Vegan

These nice sweets are perfect for kids' lunch boxes. They look quite a lot like the sweets that all the other kids munch and are delicious.

WHAT YOU NEED
50g (2oz) unsweetened dried coconut
50g (2oz) walnuts or almonds, finely ground (use a coffee grinder if possible)
1 heaped tsp coconut fat or almond butter
50g (2oz) unsweetened organic cocoa powder
stevia or Manuka honey to taste
1 small quantity iced water
another 25g (1oz) unsweetened coconut for rolling

HERE'S HOW
Mix everything but the water and 25g (1oz) of dried coconut in a big bowl. Using your fingers, work it all together well, adding the water drop by drop until you get a malleable dough, then form into balls. Roll in the extra coconut until completely coated. Refrigerate until chilled thoroughly (best overnight). These will keep in the fridge for three or four days.

CAROB FUDGE
Vegan

Once chilled, these wonderful fudge balls have the texture of ordinary fudge, and their carob flavour makes them ideal chocolate substitutes.

WHAT YOU NEED
100g (4oz) sesame seeds
30g (1oz) dried coconut
50g (2oz) carob powder (or a good organic cocoa)
1 dsp Manuka honey
½ tsp vanilla essence

HERE'S HOW
Grind the seeds very finely in the food processor. Add the other ingredients and process again. Form the mixture into little balls and chill.

SUNFLOWER SNACKS
Vegan

WHAT YOU NEED
100g (4oz) sunflower seeds
50g (2oz) carob powder
¼ tsp cinnamon
a little apple juice

HERE'S HOW
Finely grind the sunflower seeds and mix with the carob and cinnamon. Add a few drops of the apple juice, just enough to make the mixture bind. Form into a roll about 2.5cm (1in) thick, chill and then slice. Alternatively, break off little bits, press into coin-size wafers and chill.

SESAME STICKS
Vegan

It's not easy to find yummy sweet treats that don't contain wheat. Almost all the biscuits, cookies and bars you can buy are full of wheat flour. Sesame sticks fit the bill perfectly. These delicious sweets are great with afternoon tea. They are high in calcium and phosphorus as well as important essential fatty acids. Easy to make, they can either be little cookies or long sticks. Personally, I like the sticks best. Make sure you leave them in the oven long enough to get the surface golden-brown, so that they go ultra-crunchy when they cool.

WHAT YOU NEED
350g (12oz) raw, unbleached sesame seeds
50–75g (2–3oz) cups finely shredded coconut
50g (2oz) chopped almonds
4 tbsp almond butter or cashew butter (you can use peanut butter if you can't find the other two, but it's nowhere near as good)
100ml (4fl oz) Manuka honey
½ tsp salt
zest of 1 lemon, finely shredded
100g (4oz) golden granulated sugar or date sugar

HERE'S HOW
Mix all the ingredients together and then, if you choose to make the

sticks, smooth them out to a thickness of 1 cm (½in) on a greased baking tray. Bake for 20–30 minutes at 150°C/300°F/Gas Mark 2, then cut into fingers. The other way of making them is to drop them from a spoon to form small cookies, and baking them that way. Do be careful because the cookies will tend to stick together once cold.

APPLE SPICE BALLS
Vegan

These do not keep as well as some of the other treats because of the fresh apple. Nevertheless, they taste wonderful.

WHAT YOU NEED
175g (6oz) of mixed sesame, sunflower and pumpkin seeds
3–4 apples
¼ tsp nutmeg
½ tsp freshly ground cloves
1 tsp cinnamon
75g (3oz) raisins
30g (1oz) coconut
dried coconut

HERE'S HOW
Finely grind the seeds and place in a bowl. Core the apples and process to a sauce, adding the spices. Stir the raisins, coconut and apple sauce into the ground seeds, form the mixture into balls and sprinkle with some coconut. Chill and serve.

INDIAN BALLS
Vegan

These have an unusual and spicy taste.

WHAT YOU NEED
150g (5oz) dried figs (clip off the rough stem)
6 dried dates
50g (2oz) dried coconut
1 tbsp Manuka honey
1 tbsp grated orange peel
1 tsp powdered cardamom

HERE'S HOW

Grind the dried fruit finely and add the coconut, honey and orange peel. Crush several cardamom pods, remove the seeds and crush to a powder. Add to the rest of the ingredients and combine well. Form into tiny balls and refrigerate.

Ices

When food is frozen, as in the preparation of sorbets and freezes, the enzymes in it are temporarily inactivated but not destroyed. When you eat it and it warms up inside you, the enzymes become active again and behave just as beneficially as those in all raw foods. These raw sorbets and freezes are more delicate in flavour than the kind you buy. Each recipe serves from two to four people, depending on how sweet their teeth are!

FRUIT FREEZES

I make these simply by blending my favourite fruits with a little fruit juice or water (if needed) and freezing. To prevent large crystals forming and to make the mixture lighter and easier to spoon, stir every half hour or so during the freezing process. Here are a few combinations you might like to try.

Blackberry and Peach: Blend 225g (8oz) of blackberries with 4 finely grated peaches and a little Manuka honey, then freeze.

Redcurrant and Pear: Blend 225g (8oz) of redcurrants with 3 finely grated pears.

Berry and Banana: Blend 225g (8oz) of blueberries, raspberries or strawberries with 3 mashed bananas.

STRAWBERRY ICE
Vegan

For this recipe you will need a good blender or food processor with a 1.7-litre (3-pint) capacity.

WHAT YOU NEED

700g (1½lb) strawberries, frozen
lemon juice
4 tbsp Manuka honey

HERE'S HOW

Tip the frozen strawberries into a food processor or blender with the juice of the lemon and the honey. Process until smooth and bright scarlet. Pour into chilled dishes and pop in the freezer for 5–10 minutes to chill. Alternatively, you can pour the unfrozen mixture into the bowl of an ice-cream machine and continue, following the manufacturer's instructions.

CAROB AND HONEY ICE CREAM
Vegetarian

This is one of my family's favourite recipes. I find the combination of carob and honey unbeatable.

WHAT YOU NEED

½ litre (1 pint) milk (I use goat's milk but you can use cow's or even skimmed milk if you like)

2 egg yolks

3 tbsp granular lecithin (optional but very nice since it gives a creamier texture)

100g (4oz) unheated carob powder

100ml (4fl oz) Manuka honey

1 tsp pure vanilla essence

HERE'S HOW

Freeze the milk in a shallow plastic container. When frozen, remove from the freezer and let sit for about ½ an hour until just soft enough to slice into pieces. Put the egg yolks into the food processor, add about 225ml (8fl oz) of the frozen milk, the lecithin (if using), the carob powder, honey and vanilla, and blend thoroughly using the blade attachment. Add the rest of the frozen milk and continue to blend until it is just mixed (don't over-blend or you will make the ice cream too liquid). Should it become too liquid, simply return it to the freezer for a few minutes then stir before serving. Serve immediately.

ROCKY ROAD BANANAS
Vegan

This is a great recipe if you have too many ripe bananas on your hands. Once frozen, the bananas will keep for weeks – unless they are eaten immediately, as in my house.

WHAT YOU NEED
4 ripe bananas
Manuka honey
50–100g (2–4oz) coarsely ground brazil nuts

HERE'S HOW
Simply peel the bananas and push a skewer or ice lolly stick through each one. Roll in honey and then in the chopped nuts. Put on a freezer-proof plate and freeze until hard. Eat straight from the stick. If you prefer, you can first slice the bananas crosswise, coat in honey and sprinkle with nuts, then freeze to make bite-sized treats. As a variation, try mixing a few tablespoons of carob powder into the honey to make chocolate-coated bananas and then roll them in coconut, dates or nuts . . . or all three.

FURTHER READING

Allan, Christian B., Lutz, Wolfgang, *Life Without Bread. How a Low-Carbohydrate Diet Can Save Your Life*, Los Angeles, Keats Publishing, 2000

Andes, Karen, *A Woman's Book of Strength*, New York, Perigee Books, 1995

Antczak Drs S. & G., *Cosmetics Unmasked*, London, Thorsons, 2001

Audette R., *Neanderthal*, Dallas, Paleolithic Press, 1996

Balch, James F., *The Super Antioxidants*, New York, M. Evans & Co. Inc., 1998

Bank, David MD, & Sobel E., *Beautiful Skin*, MA, Adams Media Corporation, 2000

Batmanghelidj Dr, *Your Body's Many Cries for Water*, Vienna, Global Health Solutions, Inc., 1992

Beachel, Thomas & Westcott, Wayne, *Strength Training Past 50*, Leeds, Human Kenetics, 1998

Becker, R.O., *Electromagnetism and Life*, Albany, NY, State University of New York Press, 1982

Becker, Robert O., & Selden, Gary, *Body Electric: Electromagnetism and the Foundation of Life*, New York, William Morrow & Co., 1987

Bennett, Peter MD, Barrie, Stephen MD, Faye, Sara *7-Day Detox Miracle*, Roseville, CA, Prima Publishing, 2001

Benson, Herbert, *Beyond the Relaxation Response*, New York, Times Books, 1984

Berkson, Burton MD, Challem, Jack, Smith, Melissa Diane, *Syndrome X. The Complete Nutritional Program to Prevent and Reverse Insulin Resistance*, Canada, John Wiley & Sons, 2000

Bertalanffy, L. von. *Problems of Life: An Evaluation of Modern Biological Thought*, New York, Harper Torchbook, 1980

Bircher, Ralph, '*A Turning Point in Nutritional Science*', Lee Foundation for Nutritional Research, Milwaukee, Wisconsin reprint, n.d.

Bircher-Benner, M.O., *Food Science for All*, London, C.W. Daniel, 1928

Bircher-Benner, Max, *The Meaning of Therapeutic Order*, Unpublished translation by Hilda Martin

Bircher-Benner, Max, *The Prevention of Incurable Disease*, Unpublished translation by Hilda Martin

Bircher-Benner Nutrition Plan for Raw Food and Juices, translated by Timothy McManus, New York, Jove/HBJ Books, 1977

Blauer, Stephen, *The Juicing Book*, New York, Avery Publishing Group Inc., 1989

Brand-Miller, Jennie, et al. *The Glucose Revolution*, New York, Marlowe, 1999

Brekhman, I.I. *Man and Biologically Active Substances*, Oxford, Pergamon Press, 1980

Burkitt, Denis, *Refined Carbohydrate Foods and Disease*, New York, Academic Press, 1975

Calbom, Cherie and Keane, Maureen, *Juicing For Life*, New York, Avery Publishing Group, 1992

Carson, Rachel, *Silent Spring*, London, Penguin, 1962

Charmine, Susan E., *The Complete Raw Juice Therapy*, Wellingborough, Thorsons Publishers Limited, 1977

Cichoke, Anthony J., *Enzymes & Enzyme Therapy*, New Canaan, Connecticut, Keats Publishing Inc., 1994

Colburn T., Dumanoski D. & Myers J.P., *Our Stolen Future: Are we Threatening our Fertility, Intelligence and Survival? A Scientific Detective Story*, New York, Plume, 1996

Colgan, Michael with Colgan, Lesley, *The Flavonoid Revolution, Grape Seed Extract and Other Flavonoids Against Disease*, Vancouver, Apple Publishing Company, 1997

Colgan, Michael, *Hormonal Health: Nutritional & Hormonal Strategies for Emotional Well-Being & Intellectual Longevity*, Vancouver, Apple Publishing Company, 1996

Cordain L. PhD, *The Paleo Diet*, New York, John Wiley & Sons Inc., 2002

Crile, George, *The Bipolar Theory of Living Processes*, New York, Macmillan, 1926

Crile, George, *The Phenomenon of Life*, New York, W.W. Norton, 1936

Dadd, Debra Lynn, *Non-Toxic, Natural and Earthwise*, New York, Jeremy P. Tarcher Inc., 1990

Dadd, Debra Lynn, *The Non-Toxic Home and Office*, New York, Jeremy P. Tarcher Inc., 1990

Erickson K., *Drop Dead Gorgeous*, Chicago, Contemporary Books, 2002

Evans W. & Rosenberg I.H., *Biomarkers*, New York, Simon & Schuster, 1991

Fagan D. & Lavelle M., *Toxic Deception*, Secaucus, NJ, LPC, 1999

Fairley J. & Stacey S., *Feel Fabulous Forever – The Anti-Ageing Health and Beauty Bible*, Australia, Penguin Books Australia Ltd., 1999

Fallon, Sally, Enig, Mary PhD, Connolly, Pat, *Nourishing Traditions*, Indiana, New Trends Publishing, 1999

Fisher, J.A. MD, *The Plague Makers: How we are Creating Catastrophic*

New Epidemics – And What we Must Do to Avert Them, New York, Simon & Schuster, 1994

Frankel, P. & Madsen, F., *Stop Homocysteine Through the Methylation Process*, Thousand Oaks, California, TRC Publications, 1998

Green, Lawrence MD, *The Dermatologist's Guide to Looking Younger*, CA, Crossing Press, 1999

Hampton A., *What's in Your Cosmetics?*, Tucson, Odonian Press, 1995

Hayflick L., *How and Why We Age*, New York, Ballantine Books, 1994

Heinerman, John, *Heinerman's Encyclopedia of Healing Juices*, West Nyack, New York, Parker Publishing Co., 1994

Hoffer, Abram & Walker, Morton, *Orthomolecular Nutrition*, New Canaan, Conn., Keats Publishing, 1978

Horne R., *Cancer Proof Your Body*, Australia, Angus & Robertson, 1996

Howell, Edward, *Enzyme Nutrition*, Wayne, New Jersey, Avery Publishing Group Inc., 1985

Kenton, Leslie, *Age Power*, London, Vermilion, 2002

Kenton, Leslie, *The New Ageless Ageing*, London, Vermilion, 1995

Kenton, Leslie, *The New Joy of Beauty*, London, Vermilion, 1995

Kenton, L. & S. *The New Raw Energy*, London, Vermilion, 1995

Kenton, Leslie, *Passage to Power*, London, Vermilion, 1998

Kenton, Leslie, *The X Factor Diet*, London, Vermilion, 2002

Kordich, Jay, *The Juiceman's Power of Juicing*, New York, Warner Books, 1993

Krimsky, Sheldon & Goldman, Lynn, *Hormonal Chaos: The Scientific and*

Social Origins of the Environmental Endocrine Hypothesis, Baltimore, The John Hopkins University Press, 2000

Lee J.R. MD, *Natural Progesterone: The Multiple Roles of a Remarkable Hormone*, California, BLL Publ., 1993

Lee J.R. MD & Hopkins, Virginia, *What Your Doctor May Not Tell You About Menopause: The Breakthrough Book on Natural Progesterone*, New York, Warner Books Inc., 1997

Lee J.R. MD & Hopkins, Virginia, *What Your Doctor May Not Tell You About Pre-menopause: Balance Your Hormones and Your Life from Thirty to Fifty*, New York, Warner Books Inc., 1999

Lee, William, *Getting the Best out of Your Juicer*, New Canaan, New York, Keats Publishing Inc., 1992

Lees, Mark, et al., *Skincare – How to Save Your Skin*, NY, Delmar, 2002

Lees M., *Skin Care – Beyond the Basics*, NY, Milady, 2001

Lewis W., *The Lowdown on Facelifts and Other Wrinkle Remedies*, London, Quadrille Publishing Ltd., 2001

Liberman, Jacob O.D. PhD, *Light: Medicine of the Future*, Bear & Company, 1991

Lininger, Schuyler W., et al. (editors), *The Natural Pharmacy*, Rockland CA, Prima Publishing, 1999

Loftus, J.M. MD, *The Smart Woman's Guide to Plastic Surgery*, Illinois, Contemporary Books, 2000

Lowe, Prof. N. & Sellar, P., *Skin Secrets*, London, Collins & Brown Ltd., 1999

Lust, John, *Drink Your Troubles Away*, New York, Benedict Lust Publications, 1967

Meyerowitz, S., *Juice Fasting and Detoxification*, Summertown, TN, Book Publishing Co., 1999

Meyerowitz S., *Sproutman's Kitchen Garden Cookbook*, Mass., Sproutman Publications, 1999

Meyerowitz S., *Sprouts the Miracle Food*, Mass., Sproutman Publications, 1999

Murray, Michael, *The Complete Book of Juicing*, Prima Health, 1992

Murray, Michael T., *Dr. Murray's Total Body Tune-Up*, New York, Bantam Books, 2000

Murray, Michael MD, *Encyclopedia of Nutritional Supplements*, Rocklin CA., Prima Publishing, 1996

Perricone N. MD, *The Perricone Prescription*, New York, Harper Collins, 2002

Perricone N. MD, *The Wrinkle Cure*, New York, Warner Books, 2001

Price, W., *Nutrition and Physical Degeneration* (6th ed.), New Canaan, Connecticut, Keats Publishing Inc., 1997

Roberts, Arthur J. MD, O'Brien, Mary E. MD & Subak-Sharpe, Genell MS (editors), *Nutraceuticals: The Complete Encyclopedia of Supplements, Herbs, Vitamins and Healing Foods*, New York, Penguin Putnam, 2001

Schmidt, Michael A., *Smart Fats. How Dietary Fats and Oils Affect Mental, Physical and Emotional Intelligence*, Berkeley, California, Frog Ltd, 1997

Seigel, Bernie S. MD, *Peace, Love & Healing*, New York, Harper & Row, 1989

Stauber J.L. & Rampton S., *Toxic Sludge is Good For You*, Monroe Maine, Common Courage Press, 1995

Steingraber, Sandra Dr, *Living Downstream: An Ecologist Looks at Cancer and the Environment*

The Science and Politics of Endocrine Disrupters, The John Hopkins University Press, November 18, 1999

Toxic Toy Story, Greenpeace USA. Available at www.greenpeaceusa.org

Vance, Judi, *Beauty to Die For*, New York toExcel, 2000

Walker, N.W., *Fresh Vegetable and Fruit Juices*, 1970

Weil, Andrew MD, *Spontaneous Healing: How to Discover and Enhance Your Body's Natural Ability to Maintain and Heal Itself*, New York, Ballantine Books, 2000

What's Wrong with the Body Shop? London Greenpeace, 21 March

Wheater, Caroline, *Juicing For Health*, London, Thorsons, 1993

REFERENCES

Move into Power

Allan, Christian B. & Lutz, Wolfgang, *Life Without Bread: How a Low Carbohydrate Diet Can Save Your Life*, Los Angeles, Keats Publishing, 2000

Atkins, Robert, *Dr Atkins' Diet Revolution*, New York, David McKay, 1972 (reissued 1989)

Avoiding Heart Attacks, Department of Health and Social Services, London, HMSO, 1981

Bircher, R., 'A Turning Point in Nutritional Science', reprint from *Lee Foundation for Nutritional Research*, No. 80, Milwaukee, Wisconsin

Bircher, R. (ed.), *Way to Positive Health*, Erlenbach-Zurich, Bircher Benner Verlag, 1967

Challem, Jack et al., *Syndrome X – The Complete Nutritional Program to Prevent and Reverse Insulin Resistance*, New York, John Wiley & Sons, 2000

Cleave, T.L., *The Saccharine Disease*, New Canaan, Connecticut, Keats Publishing, 1978

Colgan, M., *Your Personal Vitamin Profile*, Quill, New York, 1982

Compendium of Health Statistics (4th ed.), London, Office of Health Economics, 1981

Eades, Michael & Eades, Mary Dan, *Protein Power*, New York, Bantam Books, 1997

Eaton, S.B. et al., 'An evolutionary perspective enhances understanding of human nutritional requirements', in the *Journal of Nutrition*, 1996, 126

Eaton, S.B., Eaton, S.B. III & Konner, M.J., 'Paleolithic nutrition revisited: A twelve-year retrospective on its nature and implications', in the *European Journal of Clinical Nutrition*, 1997

Eaton S.B., Shostak, M. & Konner, M., *The Paleolithic Prescription*, New York, Harper & Row, 1988

Ehret, Arnold, *Mucusless Diet Healing System*, Cody, Wyoming, Ehret Literature Publishing Co., 1953

First Health and Nutrition Examination Survey, United States 1971–1972, DHEW publication, No. 76, Rockville, Maryland, 1976

Foster, D.W., The Banting Lecture 1984: From glycogen to ketones – and back', In *Diabetes*, 1984, 33

Gerson, Max, *A Cancer Therapy: Results of 50 Cases*, Del Mar, California, Totality Books, 1977

Healthy People: The Surgeon General's Report on Health Promotion and Disease Prevention, DHEW publication, Nos. 79–55071 and 79–55071A, Washington DC, 1979

Heinrich, Richard L., *Starch Madness: Paleolithic Nutrition for Today*, Nevada City, California: Blue Dolphin Publishing, 1999

Heroditus, *The Histories (III/2)* translated by Aubrey de Selincourt, London, Penguin Classics, 1954

Kollath, W., 'Der Vollwert der Nahrung und seine Bedeutung für Wachstum und Zellersatz', *Experimentelle Grundlagen*, Stuttgart, 1950

LeBlanc, J., 'Hormonal and metabolic responses to meals of various composition', in *Obesity: Dietary Factors and Control*, ed. Romsos et al., Tokyo, Japan Scientific Societies Press, 1991

Levy, R.I., *Address to the National Institute of Health*, 27 Nov. 1979

Lieb, C.W., 'The effects of an exclusive, long-continued meat diet', in *Journal of the American Medical Association*, 1926, 87 (1)

Lieb, C.W., 'The effects on human beings of a twelve month exclusive meat diet', in *Journal of the American Medical Association*, 929 (3)

Mackarness, R., *Eat Fat and Grow Slim*, New York, Doubleday, 1959

Morgenthaler, J. & Simms, M., *The Smart Guide to the Low-Carb Anti-Aging Diet*, Petaluma, California, Smart Publications, 2000

National Cancer Institute Monograph 57, National Cancer Institute Publication No. 81–2330, Bethesda, Maryland, June 1981

Nolfi, Kristine, *My Experiences with Living Foods*, Humlegaarden, Humlebaek, Denmark (undated)

O'Dea, K., 'Glucose and insulin responses to carbohydrate ingestion: acute and long term consequences', in *Obesity, Dietary Factors and Control*, ed. Rosmos et al., Tokyo, Japan Scientific Societies Press, 1991

Ornstein, Robert & Sobel, David, *Healthy Pleasures: Discover the Proven Medical Benefits of Pleasure and Live a Longer, Healthier Life*, Cambridge, Massachusetts, Perseus Books, 1989

Pelletier, Kenneth R., *Holistic Medicine – From Stress to Optimal Health*, New York, Delacorte Press/Seymour Lawrence, 1979

Pottenger, F.M. Jr., 'The Effect of Heat Processed Foods', in *American Journal of Orthodontistry and Oral Surgery*, Vol. 32, No. 8, 1946

Pottenger, F.M. Jr. & Simonsen, D.G., 'Heat Labile Factors Necessary for the Proper Growth and Development of Cats', in *Journal of Laboratory and Clinical Medicine*, Vol. 25, 1939

Pottenger, F.M. Jr., *Pottenger's Cats*, La Mesa, California, Price-Pottenger Nutrition Foundation, 1983

Price, Weston A., *Nutrition and Physical Degeneration*, La Mesa, California, Price-Pottenger Nutritional Foundation, 1970

Savarin, A.B., *Physiologie du gout*, Munich, Bruckmann Querschnitte, 1962

Schwartz, H., *Never Satisfied: The Cultural History of Diets, Fantasies and Fat*, New York, The Free Press, 1985

Straus, Charlotte Gerson, *A lecture presented before the Second Annual Cancer Convention of the Cancer Control Society*, Los Angeles, California, 1974

Steffanson, V., *Cancer, Disease of Civilization*, New York, Hill and Wang, 1960

Steffanson, V., *The Fat of the Land*, New York, Macmillan Publishing, 1956

Swislocki, A.L.M., et al., 'Insulin resistance, glucose intolerance and hyperinsulinemia in patients with hypertension', in *American Journal of Hypertension*, May 1989, 2

Torjeson, P.A., et al., 'Lifestyle changes may reverse development of insulin resistance syndrome', in *Diabetes*, 1997, 20

Walker, Norman W., *Natural Weight Control*, Phoenix, Arizona, O'Sullivan Woodside and Co., 1981

Williams, R.J. & Kalita, Dwight K. (eds), *A Physician's Handbook on Orthomolecular Medicine*, New Canaan, Connecticut, Keats Publishing Co., 1977

Yudkin, J., *Sweet and Dangerous*, New York, Van Rees Press, 1972

Escape from the Twilight Zone

Angel, J.L., Health as a crucial factor in the changes from hunting to developed farming in the Eastern Mediterranean, in *Paleopathology at the Origins of Agriculture*, eds. M.N. Cohen & G.J. Armelagos, New York, Academic Press, 1984

Avoiding Heart Attacks, op. cit.

Bircher, R., 'A Turning Point in Nutritional Science' op. cit.

Bircher, R., (ed.), *Way to Positive Health*, op. cit.

Bower, B., 'The two million year old meat and marrow diet resurfaces', in *Science News*, 3 January 1987

Carpenter, K.J., 'Protein requirements of adults from an evolutionary perspective', in the *American Journal of Clinical Nutrition*, 1992, 55

Cassidy, C.M., 'Nutrition and health in agriculturalists and hunter-gatherers: A case study of two prehistoric populations', in *Nutritional Anthropology, Contemporary Approaches to Diet and Culture*, eds., N.M. Jerome, R.F. Kandel & G.H. Felto, Pleasantville, New York, Redgrave Publishing Co., 1980

Cohen, M.N., *Health and the Rise of Civilization*, New Haven, Yale University Press, 1989

Colgan, M. op. cit.

Compendium of Health Statistics (4ᵗʰ ed.) op. cit.

Eaton, S.B., Eaton, S.B. III & Konner, M.J. op. cit.

Eaton, S.B. et al. op. cit.

Eaton, S.B., Shostak, M., & Konner, M. op. cit.

Eaton, S.B. & Konner, M.J. 'Paleolithic Nutrition: A consideration of its nature and current implications', in the *New England Journal of Medicine*, 1985

Eaton, S.B. et al., 'Stone agers in the fast lane: Chronic degenerative diseases in evolutionary perspective', in the *American Journal of Medicine*, 1988, 84

Eaton, S.B., 'Humans, lipids and evolution', in *Lipids*, 1992, 27

Ehret, Arnold, *Mucusless Diet Healing System*, Cody, Wyoming, Ehret Literature Publishing Co., 1953

First Health and Nutrition Examination Survey – op. cit.

Gerson, Max op. cit.

Gordon, K.D., 'Evolutionary perspectives on human diet', in *Nutritional Anthropology*, ed. F.E. Johnston, New York, Alan R. Liss, 1987

Healthy People: The Surgeon General's Report on Health Promotion and Disease Prevention, op. cit.

Kollath, W. op. cit.

Levy, R.I. op. cit.

National Cancer Institute Monograph 57 op. cit.

Nolfi, Kristine op. cit.

Pelletier, Kenneth R., New York op. cit.

Pottenger, F.M. Jr. 'The Effect of Heat Processed Foods' op. cit.

Pottenger, F.M. Jr., *Pottenger's Cats* op. cit.

Pottenger, F.M. Jr. & Simonsen, D.G. op. cit.

Price, Weston A. op. cit.

Straus, Charlotte Gerson op. cit.

Walker, Norman W. op. cit.

Williams, R.J. & Kalita, Dwight K. (eds.), op. cit.

Endless Payoffs

Armstrong, Bruce, *American Journal of Clinical Nutrition*, December 1979

Bailey, Covert, *Fit or Fat*, London, Pelham Books, 1980

Beinhorn, G., *Food for Fitness*, Mountain View, California, World Publications, 1975

Bircher-Benner, M.O., *Food Science For All*, London, C.W. Daniel, 1928

Bircher, R., '*A Turning Point in Nutritional Science*' op. cit.

Bircher, R., '*The Question of Protein*', photocopied report from author

Bircher, R., (ed.), *Way to Positive Health* op. cit.

Bircher, Ruth, *Eating Your Way to Health*, London, Faber and Faber, 1961

Chittenden, Russell H., *Physiological Economy in Nutrition*, London, Heinemann, 1905

Chittenden, Russell, *The Nutrition of Men*, New York, Stokes, 1907

Douglass, John, 'Nutrition, Nonthermally-Prepared Foods and Nature's Message to Man', in *Journal of the International Academy of Preventative Medicine*, Vol. VII, No. 2, July 1982, also private communication with author

Eimer, K., '*Klinik Schwenkenhacher*', Zeitschrift für Ernahrung, July 1933

Formica, Palma, Article in *Current Therapeutic Research*, March 1962

Fridovich, I., 'Superoxide Dismutase: a dramatic new enzyme discovery that protects against radiation and prevents disease', in *Bestways*, August 1980

Goulart, F.S., *Eating to Win*, New York, Stine and Day, 1980

Issels, Josef, '*Nutritional Protection Against Cancer*', Tjidskrift fur Halsa, Stockholm, Nos. 1, 2 & 3, 1972

Karstrom, Henning, *Ratt Kost*, Gavle, Skandinavska Bokforlaget, 1982

Katenkamp and Stiller, Histochemistry of Amyloid, E.H. *Voeding*, 30/5, 1969

Katenkamp and Stiller, 'Das Amyloid', in *Hippokrates*, Vol. 41, no. 1, 1970

Kruijswijk H., Oomn, H.A. & Hipsley, E.H. *Voeding*, 30/5, 1969

McCay, Clive M., 'Effects of restricted feeding on aging, etc.' in *American Journal of Public Health*, Vol. 37, May 1947

McCay, Clive M., *Notes on the History of Nutrition Research*, Bern, Hans Huber, 1973

McCully, Kilmer S., *American Journal of Clinical Nutrition*, Vol. 28, May 1975 and *American Journal of Pathology*, Vol. 59 and Vol. 61, 1970

Meneely, George, R., *Nutrition Review*, 1976

Mirkin, Gabe, *The Sportsmedicine Book*, Boston, Little, Brown & Co., 1978

Nutrition Today, Vol. 3, No. 2, June 1968

Ostrand, Per-Olaf & Rodahl, Kaare, *Textbook of Work Physiology*, New York, McGraw-Hill, 1970

Pfeiffer, C., *Mental and Elemental Nutrients*, New Canaan, Connecticut, Keats Publishing Co., 1975

Pfeiffer, C. & Banks, J., *Total Nutrition*, New York, Simon and Schuster, 1980

Physician and Sportsmedicine Magazine, January 1976

Roberts, S.E., *Exhaustion: Causes and Treatment*, Emmaus, Pennsylvania, Rodale Books Inc., 1967

Rosenfield, Albert, *Pro-longevity*, New York, Avon, 1976

Szekely, E.B., 'The Essene Science of Life', in *International Biogenic Society*, Cartago, CostaRica, 1978

Thomas, W.A. et al., *American Journal of Cardiology*, January 1960 and *American Journal Association*, new release, 21 June 1965

Trowel, Hugh, *The Lancet*, 22 July 1978

Walford, Roy L., *Maximum Life Span*, London, W.W. Norton & Co., 1983

Winick, M., 'Slow the Problems of Aging and Quash its Problems With Diet', in *Modern Medicine*, 15 February 1978

Raw Power Slim

Almond S. & Logan, R.F.I., 'Carotenemia', in *British Medical Journal*, Vol. 2, pp. 239–41, 1942

Bernstein, D.S. & Wachman, A., 'Diet and Osteoporosis', in *The Lancet*, Vol. 7549, p.958, 1968

Clemetson, C.A.B., 'Bioflavinoids as Antioxidants for Ascorbic Acid', in *Symposium sui Bioflavinoidi*, Stresa, 23–25 April 1966

Clemetson, C.A.B. et al., 'Estrogens in Food: The Almond Mystery', in *International Journal of Gynaecology and Obstetrics*, Vol. 15, pp. 515–21, 1978

Clemetson, C.A.B. & Anderson, L., 'Plant polyphenols as antioxidants for ascorbic acid', in *Annals of the New York Academy of Sciences*, Vol. 136, Art. 14, 00.339–78 (date unknown)

Curry, S.B., 'Aspects morpho-histochimiques et biochimiques du tissu adipeau dans la dermohypodermose cellulitique', paper given at Cème Journées de Médicine Esthétique, Monte Carlo, 14–15 May 1978

Dukan, Pierre, *La Cellulite en Question*, Paris La Table Ronde Eds.

First Health and Nutrition Examination Survey, United States, 1971–1972, DHEW publication, 76–1219–1 Rockville, Maryland, 1976

Kemmann, E. et al., 'Amenorrhea associated with carotenemia', in *Journal of the American Medical Association*, Vol. 249, No. 7, pp. 9206–929, 18 February 1983

Pfeiffer, Carl C., op. cit.

Schroeder, H.A., *American Journal of Clinical Nutrition*, Vol. 24, p.562, 1971

Taska, Richard Jr., *Life in the Twentieth Century*, Woodstock Valley, Connecticut, Omangod Press, 1981

Wild Woman

The work of the following researchers is referred to in J. Raloff's 'The Gender Benders': Michael Fry, Devra Lee-Davis, Louis J. Guillette, Neils Skakkebaek, Ana Soto, John P. Sumptor and Mary S. Wolf. Raloff's 'Eco-Cancers' refers to the work of David E. Blask, Steven M. Hill and Robert Liburdy. R. Weiss's 'Estrogen in the Environment' refers to the work of David Crews and Herman Aldercreutz.

Almond, S. and Logan, R.F.L. op. cit.

Bavalve R. et al., 'Vegetables inhibit in vivo the mutagenicity of nitrate combined with nitrosable compounds', in *Mutation Research*, 1983, Vol. 120, 145

Bernstein, D.S. & Wachman, A. op. cit.

Clemetson, C.A.B., 'Bioflavinoids as Antioxidants for Ascorbic Acid' op. cit.

Clemetson, C.A.B. et al., 'Estrogens in Food: The Almond Mystery' op. cit.

Clemetson, C.A.B. & Anderson, L. op. cit.

Curry, S.B. op. cit.

Dickinson, L.E. et al., 'Estrogen profiles of oriental and caucasian women in Hawaii', in *New England Journal of Medicine*, 1974, 921, 1211–1213

Dukan, Pierre, op. cit.

First Health and Nutrition Examination Survey, op. cit.

Kemmann, E. et al., 'Amenorrhea associated with carotenemia', in *Journal of the American Medical Association*, Vol. 249, No. 7, pp. 9206–929, 18 February 1983

McDougall, J., 'Balancing the estrogen issue', in *Vegetarian Times*, August 1986, 44

Mercola, Josef., 'Vegetables Prevent Wrinkles', in *Journal of American College of Nutrition*, 2001

Nakashima, H., et al., 'Inhibitory effect of glycosides like saponin from soybean on the infectivity of HIV in vitro', in *AIDS*, 1989, 3, 655–658

Pfeiffer, C. op. cit.

Raloff, J., 'The Gender Benders', Part Two, 'That Feminine Touch', in *Science News*, January 8 1994 & February 22 1994

Schroeder, H.A. op. cit.

Steinman, David, *Diet for a Poisoned Planet*, New York, Ballantine Books, 1990

Taska, Richard Jr. op. cit.

Wilcox, G., et al., 'Estrogenic effects of plant foods in postmenopausal women', in *British Medical Journal*, 1990 (6757) 905–906

Williams, D., 'The forgotten hormone', in *Alternatives for the Health Conscious Individual*, 1991, Vol. 4 (6) 41–46

Wolf, G., 'Is Dietary Beta-Carotene an Anti-Cancer Agent?', in *Nutritional Reviews*, 1982

Cooking May Damage Your Health

Aly, Karl-Otto., '*Cancer defeated by the body's own defenses*', Tjidskrift fur Halso, 9 September 1965

Anderson, James W., *Diabetes*, London, Martin Dunitz, 1981

Bircher, R. (ed.) *Way to Positive Health* op. cit.

Bircher-Benner, M., *The Prevention of Incurable Disease*, Cambridge, James Clarke & Co., 1981

Brekhman, I.I., *Man and Biologically Alive Substances*, Oxford, Pergamon Press, 1980

Cheraskin, E., Ringsdorf, W.M. & Clark, J., *Diet and Disease*, Emmaus, PA, Rodale Press, 1968

Douglass, J.M., 'Raw Diet and Insulin Requirement', in *Annals of Internal Medicine*, Vol. 82, 1975

Douglass, J.M. & Douglass, S.N., 'Sugar, Cereals and Sharks', in *New England Journal of Medicine*, Vol. 295, 1976

Douglass, John op. cit.

Douglass, J.M. & Rasgon, I., 'Diet and Diabetes', in *The Lancet*, December 1976

Gerson, M. op. cit.

Goldin, Barry et al., 'Effect of Diet and Lactobacillis acidophilus Supplements on Human Fecal Bacterial Enzymes', in *Journal of Natural Cancer Institute*, Vol. 64, 1980

Hare, D.C., 'A Therapeutic Trial of a Raw Vegetable Diet in Chronic Rheumatoid Conditions', in *Proceedings of the Royal Society of Medicine*, Vol. XXX, 1936

Kelley, W.D., *One Answer to Cancer*, The Kelley Research Foundation, 1971

Kuhl, Johannes, *Checkmate for Cancer*, Braunlage, Germany, Viadrina Verlag A. Trowitzh

Liechti-von Brasch, D., '*70 Jahre Erfahrungsgut der Bircher Benner Ordnungstherapie*', Erfahrungsheilkunde, Band XIX, Heft 6,7,8, 1970

Livingston, Virginia & Wheeler, Owen, *Food Alive*, The Livingston Wheeler Medical Clinic, San Diego, 1977

Manner, Harold, *Natural Health Federation Conference*, Chicago, September 1977

Neiper, Hans, Lecture given at the Royal Society of Medicine, London, May 1980

Peto, R., Doll, R. et al., 'Can dietary beta-carotene materially reduce human cancer rates?' in *Nature*, Vol. 290, March 1981

Shamburger, R.J. & Willis, C.E.J., *National Cancer Institute*, Vol. 48, No. 5, 1972

Tropp, K., 'Die Pflanzenfermente der Rohkotst und ihre Bedeutung fur den Verdauungskanal des Menschen', in *Der Wenderpunkt*, May 1948

Raw Beginnings

Bicknell, F. & Prescott, F., *The Vitamins in Medicine*, Lee Foundation for Nutritional Research, Milwaukee, Wisconsin, 1953

Bircher, R., 'A Turning Point in Nutritional Science' op. cit.

Culverwell, M., 'Cooking Methods Linked With Cancer', in *University of California Clip Sheet*, 29 December 1981

Douglass, J.M., 'Is "How Vitamin C Works" Medicine's Best Discovery?' in *Nutrition Today*, March/April 1980 (also personal communication with author)

Evans, R.J. & Butts, H.A., 'Inactivation of Amino Acids by Autoclaving', in *Science*, Vol. 109, 1949

Gerber, Donald, *Medical World News*, 13 February 1970

Glatzel, H., *Verhaltensphysiologie der Ernarung*, Berlin, 1973

Greiser, Norburt, 'Zur Biocemie der Vorspeise', in *Deutsches Medizineisches Journal*, 1964

Hein, R.E. & Hutchings, I.J., *Nutrients in Processed Foods*, ed. American Medical Association on Foods and Nutrition, Acton, Massachusetts, Publishing Sciences Group, 1974

Kollath, W. op. cit.

Kollath, Werner., *Die Ordnung Unserer Nahrung*, Stuttgart, Hippocrates-Verlag, 1955

Kouchakoff, Paul, 'The Influence of Food Cooking on the Blood Formula of Man', Proceedings of First International Congress of Microbiology, Paris, 1930

Kuratsune, Masanore, 'Experiment of Low Nutrition with Raw Vegetables', in *Kyushu Memoirs of Medical Science*, Vol. 2, June 1951

Pottenger, F.M. Jr., *Pottenger's Cats* op. cit.

Priestley, R.J. (ed.), *Effects of heating on Foodstuffs*, London, Applied Science Publishers, 1979

Schroeder, H.A. op. cit.

Senti, F.R., *Nutrients in Processed Foods*, ed. *American Medical Association Council on Foods and Nutrition*, Acton, Massachusetts, Publishing Sciences Group (date unknown)

Walsh, Michael J., Article in *Modern Nutrition*, March 1968

Yamaguchi, T. et al., Article in *Journal of Vitaminology*, Vol. 5, 1959

Living Matrix Healing

Abrams, G.D. & Bishop, J.E., 'Normal Flora and Leukocyte Mobilization', in *Archives of Pathology*, Vol. 70, February 1965

Airola, P., *There is a cure for Arthritis*, New Jersey, Pearson Education, 1991

Alvarez, Walter C., 'Enzyme defects can induce cell ageing', in *Geriatrics*, August 1970

Berridge, M.J., Rapp, P.E., Treherne, J.E., 'Cellular oscillators', in *J. Exp. Bio.* 81, Cambridge University Press, Cambridge, 1979

Berry, M.N., Gregory, R.B., Grivell, A.R., Henley, D.C., Phillips, J.W., Wallace, P.G. & Welch, G.R., 'Linear Relationships Between Mitochondrial Forces and Cytoplasmic Flows Argues for the Organized Energy-coupled Nature of Cellular Metabolism', in *FEB* 224, 1987

Bircher, Ralph, *Gesünder durch weniger Eiwess, Geheimarchiv der Ernährungslehre, Höchstleistungskost für Sport, Berg, Eis, Wüste und Dschungel, Sturmfeste Gesundheit and HUNSA Das Volk, das keine Krankheit kannte.* All published in the series 'Edition Wenderpunkt', Bicher-Benner Verlag, 1980/1

Bircher-Benner, M., '*The Meaning of Therapeutic Order*', unpublished translation by Hilda Martin

Brekhman, I.I. & Dardymov, I.V., 'New Substances of Plant Origin which increase Non-specific Resistance', in *Annual Review of Pharmacology*, Vol. 9, 1969

Breithaupt, H. 'Biological Rhythms and Communications', in *Electromagnetic Bio-Information* 2nd Ed. (F.A. Popp, U. Warnke, H.L. Konig and W. Peschka, eds.), Munich, Urban Schwarzenberg, 1979

Cheney, G., 'Anti-peptic ulcer dietary factor', in *American Dietary Association*, Vol. 26, September 1950

Cheney, G., 'Prevention of histamine induced peptic ulcers by diet', in *Stanford Medical Bulletin*, Vol. 6, 1948

Cheney, G., 'The nature of the anti-peptic ulcer dietary factor', in *Stanford Medical Bulletin*, Vol. 8, 1950

Davydov, A.S., 'Energy and Electron Transport in Biological Systems', in *Bioelectrodynamics and Biocommunication* (M.W. Ho, F.A. Popp and U. Warnke, eds.), Singapore, World Scientific, 1994

Dineen, P., 'Effect of alteration in intestinal flora on host resistance in systemic bacterial infection', in *Infectious Diseases*, 109, November/ December 1961

Harold, F.M., *The Vital Force: A Study of Bioenergetics*, New York, W.H. Freeman, 1987

Hill, M.J. et al., 'Bacteria and Etiology of Cancer of the Large Bowel', in *The Lancet*, Vol. 1, 1970

Ho, M.W. & Popp, F.A., 'Biological Organization, Coherence and Light Emission from Living Organisms', in *Thinking About Biology*, (W.D. Stein and F. Varela, eds), New York, Addison-Wesley, 1994

Hume, E.D., *Bechamp or Pasteur?: A Lost Chapter in the History of Biology*, London, The C.W. Daniel Co., 1932, R.A. Montana, Kessinger Publishing Co., print on demand, 1996

Karstrom, Henning, *Protectio Vitae*, February 1972

Karstrom, Henning, *Ratt Kost*, Gavle, Skandinavska Bokforlaget, 1982

Lai, Chiu-Nan, 'Anti-mutagenic activities of common vegetables and their chlorophyll content', in *Mutation Research*, Vol. 77, 1980

Lai, Chiu-Nan, 'The active factor in wheat sprout extract inhibiting the metabolic activation of carcinogens in vitro', in *Nutrition and Cancer*, Vol. 1 (date unknown)

MacDonald, S.M., *Detoxification and Healing*, New York, McGraw Hill, 1998

Offenkrantz, W.G., 'Water Soluble Chlorophyll in the Treatment of Peptic Ulcers of Long Duration', in *Review of Gastroenterology*, Vol. 17, 1950

Oschman, J.L., *Energy Medicine – The Scientific Basis of Bioenergy Therapies*, New Hampshire, USA, Churchill Livingstone, 2000

Oschman, J.L., 'Structure and Properties of Ground Substances', in *American Zoologist* 24 (1984)

Pahlow, Mannfried, *Living Medicine*, Wellingborough, Thorsons, 1980

Pearson, D. & Shaw, S., *Life Extension*, New York, Warner Books, 1982

Peterson, Vicki, *Eating Your Way to Health*, London, Allen Lane, 1981

Pizzorno J.P. & Murray, M., *Encyclopedia of Natural Medicine*, London, Century Hudson, 1990

Reddy, Bandaru, 'Effects of High Risk and Low Risk Diet for Colon Carcinogenises of Fecal Microflora and Steroids in Man', in *Journal of Nutrition*, July–December 1975

Rose, Geoffrey, 'Colon cancer and blood cholesterol', in *The Lancet*, 9 February 1974

Schmidt, Siegmund, '*Cancer and Leukemia*', reprint article from Dr Schmidt, 4502 Bad Rothenfelds, T.W., Bez, Osnabruck, Germany

Talbot, John, 'Role of dietary fibre in diverticular disease and colon cancer', in *Federation Proceedings*, Vol. 40, July 1981

Thornton, J.R., 'High Colonic pH Promotes Colerectal Cancer', in *The Lancet*, 16 May 1981

Tsong, T.Y. & Gross, C.J., 'The Language of Cells – Molecular Processing of Electric Signals by Cell Membranes', in *Bioelectrodynamics and Biocommunication* (M.W. Ho, F.A. Popp and U. Warnke, eds.), Singapore, World Scientific, 1994

Virtanen, A.I., *Angewandte Chemie*, Vol. 70, 1958

Virtanen, A.I., 'Die Enzyme in Lebendigen Zellen', in *Suomen Kemisstilehti*, B.XV, 1942

Virtanen, A.I., *Suomen Kemisstilehti*, No. 4, 1964

Virtanen, A.I., 'Report on primary plant substances and decomposition reactions in crushed plants', in *Biochemical Institute*, Helsinki, 1964

Energy Raw and Free

Alfin-Slater, R.B. & Aftergood, I., 'Lipids' in *Modern Nutrition in Health and Disease*, 6th ed., R.S. Goodheart and M.E. Shils, eds., Philadelphia, Lea and Febiger, 1980

Becker, R.O., *Cross Currents: The Promise of Electromedicine, the Perils of Electropollution*, Los Angeles, Jeremy P. Tarcher Inc., 1990

Becker, R.O., 'Electromagnetic forces and life processes', in *Technological Review*, December 1972

Berridge, M.J., Rapp P.E. & Treherne J.E. (eds.), 'Cellular Oscillators', in *J. Exp Biol.* 81, Cambridge University Press, 1979

Berry M.N., Gregory R.B., Grivell A.R., Henley D.C., Phillips J.W., Wallace P.G. & Welch, G.R. op. cit.

Bircher, R., 'A Turning Point in Nutritional Science', op. cit.

Bircher, R. (ed.), *Way to Positive Health* op. cit.

Bircher-Benner, M., *The Essential Nature and Organization of Food Energy and the Application of the Second Principle of Thermo-Dynamics to Food Value and its Active Force*, London, John Bale Sons & Curnow, 1939

Bircher-Benner M., '*The Meaning of Therapeutic Order*' op. cit.

Bircher-Benner, M., *The Prevention of Incurable Disease* op. cit.

Bohm, David, *Wholeness and the Implicate Order*, London, Routledge & Kegan Paul, 1980

Bray, H.G. & White, K., *Kinetics and Thermodynamics in Biochemistry*, London, Churchill, 1957

Breithaupt, H., Rhythms op. cit.

Brekhman, I.I. op. cit.

Bruce, E., *Living Foods for Radiant Health*, London, Thorsons, 2002

Burr, Harold Saxton, *Blueprint for Immortality: The Electric Patterns of Life*, London, Neville Spearman, 1952

Chen, Junshi, *Diet, Lifestyle and Mortality in China: A Study of the Characteristics of 65 Chinese Counties*, CA, Cornell University Press, 1993

Coats, C., *Living Energies: Viktor Schauberger's Brilliant Work with Natural Energy Explained*, Bath, Gateway Books, 1996

Crile, George, *The Bipolar Theory of Living Processes*, New York, Macmillan, 1926

Crile, George, *The Phenomena of Life: A Radio-Electrical Interpretation*, New York, W.W. Norton, 1936

Dakin, H.S., *High Voltage Photography*, 2nd ed., 3101 Washington St, San Francisco, California, 1975

Davydov, A.S., 'Energy and electron Transport in Biological Systems', in *Bioelectrodynamics and Biocommunication* (M.W. Ho, F.A. Popp & U. Warnke, eds.), Singapore, World Scientific, 1994

Eppinger, Hans, '*Die Permeabilitatspathologie als Lehre vom Krank-heits-beginn*', Vienna, 1949

Eppinger, Hans, 'Transmineralisation und vegetarische Kost', in *Ergebnisse der Inneren Medizin und Kinderheilkuinde*, Vol. 51, 1936

Eppinger, Hans, 'Uber Rohkostbehandlung', *Wiener Klinische Wochenschrift*, No. 26, 1938

Fallon, Sally, *Nourishing Traditions*, Indiana, New Trends Publishing, 1999

Galvani, Luigi, 'Commentary on the Effect of Electricity on Muscular Motion – a Translation of Luigi Galvani's De Virbis Electricitatis', in *Motu Musculari Commentarius*, Cambridge, Massachusetts, E Light, 1953

Gerson, Max op. cit.

Gittleman, Ann Louise, MS, *Beyond Pritikin*, New York, Bantam Books, 1980

Harold, F.M. op. cit.

Hauschka, Rudolph, *The Nature of Substance*, London, Vincent Stuart, 1966

Holzman, Neil A. et al., *Modern Nutrition in Health and Disease*, 6th ed., Goodheart and Shils, eds., Philadelphia, Lea and Febiger, 1994

Hume, E.D. op. cit.

Irons, V.E., *There is a Difference*, pamphlet published by V. Irons, Natick, Massachusetts on Pfeiffer's work, undated

Kang. J. Ho, et al., 'Archeological Pathology', 1971 Mann, G.V. et al., in *American Journal of Epidemiology*, 1972

Karstrom, Henning, *Ratt Kost*, op. cit.

Kuhn, Thomas, *The Structure of Scientific Revolutions*, University of Chicago Press, 1962

Lakhovsky, G., *L'Origine de la Vie*, Paris, Editions Nilsson, 1925

Lund, E.J., *Bioelectric Fields and Growth*, University of Texas Press

MacDonald, S.M. op. cit.

Moore, Thomas J., *Lifespan: What Really Affects Human Longevity*, New York, Simon and Schuster, 1990

Moss, T., *The Probability of the Impossible*, Los Angeles, J.P. Tarcher, 1974

Oschman, J.L., *Energy Medicine – The Scientific Basis of Bioenergy Therapies*, New Hampshire, USA, Churchill Livingstone, 2000

Page, Melvin, DDS, *Degeneration, Regeneration*, San Diego, CA, Price-Pottenger Nutrition Foundation, 1949

Pardee, A.B. and Ingraham, L.L., 'Free energy and entropy in metabolism', in *Metabolic Pathways*, Vol. 1, ed. D.M. Greenberg, (date unknown)

Pfeiffer, E., *Formatic Forces in Crytstallization*, London, Rudolph Steiner Publications

Price, Weston, op. cit.

Rattemeyer, M. & Popp, F.A. 'Evidence of Photo Emission from DNA in Living Systems', in *Naturwissenschaftn*, 68, 1981

Schrodinger, Erwin, *What is Life?* and *Mind and Matter?*, Cambridge University Press, 1980

Seeger, P.G., *Archive experimentelle Zellforschung*, Vols. 20 and 21, 1938

Simoneton, A., *Radiations des aliments oindes humaines, et sante*, Paris, Le Courrier du Livre, 1971

Szent-Gyorgyi, Albert, et al., 'How vitamin C really works . . . or does it?' in *Nutrition Today*, September/October 1979

Thompkins, P. & Bird, C., *The Secret Life of Plants*, London, Allen Lane, 1974

Warburg, Otto, Article in *Naturwissenschaften*, Vol. 21, 1954

Willett, W.C. et al., *AM J Clin Nutr*, June 1995; Perez-Llamas, F., et al., *J Hum Nutr Diet*, Dec 1996; Alberti-Fidanza, A., et al., *Eur J Clin Nutr*, Feb 1994

Williams, R., 'A Renaissance of Nutritional Science is Imminent', in *Perspectives in Biology and Medicine*, Vol. 17, 1973

Zukav, G. *The Dancing Wu Li Masters*, New York, William Morrow, 1979

Energy Breaks The Rules

Becker, R.O., 'Electromagnetic forces and life processes' op. cit.

Bircher, R., 'A Turning Point in Nutritional Science' op. cit.

Bircher, *Way to Positive Health* op. cit.

Bircher-Benner, M., *The Essential Nature and Organization of Food Energy and the Application of the Second Principle of Thermo-Dynamics to Food Value and its Active Force* op. cit.

Bircher-Benner, M., *The Prevention of Incurable Disease* op. cit.

Bohm, David op. cit.

Bray, H.G. & White, K. op. cit.

Brekhman, I.I. op. cit.

Burr, Harold Saxton op. cit.

Crile, George, *The Bipolar Theory of Living Processes* op. cit.

Crile, George, *The Phenomena of Life: A Radio-Electrical Interpretation* op. cit.

Dakin, H.S., *High Voltage Photography* op. cit.

Eppinger, Hans, 'Die Permeabilitatspathologie als Lehre vom Krank-heits-beginn' op. cit.

Eppinger, Hans, 'Transmineralisation und vegetarische Kost' op. cit.

Eppinger, Hans, 'Uber Rohkostbehandlung' op. cit.

Galvani, Luigi op. cit.

Gerson, Max op. cit.

Hauschka, Rudolph op. cit.

Irons, V.E. op. cit.

Karstrom, Henning, *Ratt Kost* op. cit.

Kuhn, Thomas op. cit.

Lakhovsky, G. op. cit.

Lund, E.J. op. cit.

Moss, T. op. cit.

Pardee, A.B. & Ingraham, L.L. op. cit.

Pfeiffer, E. op. cit.

Schrodinger, Erwin op. cit.

Seeger, P.G. op. cit.

Simoneton, A. op. cit.

Szent-Gyorgyi, Albert, et al. op. cit.

Thompkins, P. & Bird, C. op. cit.

Warburg, Otto op. cit.

Williams, R. op. cit.

Zukav, G. op. cit.

Plant Powers

Becker, R.O., *Cross Currents: The Promise of Electromedicine, the Perils of Electropollution* op. cit.

Becker, R.O., 'Electromagnetic forces and life processes' op. cit.

Bircher, R., 'A Turning Point in Nutritional Science' op. cit.

Bircher, R., *Way to Positive Health* op. cit.

Bircher-Benner, M., *The Essential Nature and Organization of Food Energy and the Application of the Second Principle of Thermo-Dynamics to Food Value and its Active Force* op. cit.

Bircher-Benner, M., *The Prevention of Incurable Disease* op. cit.

Blauer, Stephen, *Rejuvenation*, Boston, Hippocrates Health Institute, 1980

Bohm, David op. cit.

Bray, H.G. & White, K. op. cit.

Brekhman, I.I. op. cit.

Burr, Harold Saxton op. cit.

Crile, George, *The Bipolar Theory of Living Processes* op. cit.

Crile, George *The Phenomena of Life: A Radio-Electrical Interpretation* op. cit.

Dakin, H.S., *High Voltage Photography*, op. cit.

Eastwood, M.A. & Mitchell W.D., 'The place of vegetable fibre in the diet', in *British Journal of Hospital Medicine*, January 1974

Eppinger, Hans, '*Die Permeabilitatspathologie als Lehre vom Krank-heitsbeginn*' op. cit.

Eppinger, Hans, 'Transmineralisation und vegetarische Kost' op. cit.

Eppinger, Hans, '*Uber Rohkostbehandlung*' op. cit.

Ershoff, B.H., 'Antitoxic effects of plant fibre', in *American Journal of Clinical Nutrition*, Vol. 27, December 1974

Gabor, M., 'The anti-inflammatory action of flavonoids', in *Akademial Kiado*, Budapest, 1972

Galvani, Luigi op. cit.

Gelin, L.E., 'Rheologic disturbances and the use of low viscosity dextran in surgery', in *Review of Surgery*, Vol. 19, 1962

Gerson, Max, op. cit.

Goulart, Francis Sheridan, *Super Healing Foods*, West Nyack, New York, Parker Publishing Co., 1998

Hauschka, Rudolph, op. cit.

Heinerman, John, *Heinerman's Encyclopedia of Fruits, Vegetables and Herbs*, West Nyack, New York, Parker Publishing Co., 1998

Hughes, J.H. & Latner, A.L., 'Chlorophyll and haemoglobin regeneration after haemorrhage', in *Journal of Physiology*, Vol. 86, 1936

Hughes, R.E. & Wilson, H.K., 'Flavonoids: Some physiological and nutritional considerations', in *Progress in Medical Chemistry*, Vol. 14, 1977

Irons, V.E. op. cit.

Jean, V., *Aromatherapie*, Paris, Librairie Maloine SA, 1974

Karstrom, Henning, *Ratt Kost* op. cit.

Katahn, Martin, *The Tri-Colour Diet: A Miracle Breakthrough in Diet and Nutrition for a Longer, Healthier Life*, New York, Norton, 1996

Kelsay, J., 'A review of research on effects of fibre intake on man', in *American Journal of Clinical Nutrition*, Vol. 31, January 1978

Knisely, M.H. et al., 'Sludged Blood' in *Science*, Vol. 106, 1947

Kuhn, Thomas op. cit.

Lai, Chiu-Nan, 'Anti-mutagenic activities of common vegetables and their chlorophyll content', in *Mutation Research*, Vol. 77, 1980

Lai, Chiu-Nan, 'The active factor in wheat sprout extract inhibiting the metabolic activation of carcinogens in vitro', in *Nutrition and Cancer*, Vol. 1 (date unknown)

Lakhovsky, G. op. cit.

Lewis, W.H., Memory, P.F. & Elvin, Lewis, *Medical Botany*, New York, John Wiley, 1977

Lund, E.J. op. cit.

Margen, Sheldon, and the editors of the University of California in Berkeley Wellness Letter, *The Wellness Encyclopedia of Food and Nutrition*, New York, Health Letter Associates, 1982

Morgan, Brian L., *Nutrition Prescription*, New York, Crown Publishers, 1987

Moss, T. op. cit.

Murray, Michael T. MD, *Encyclopedia of Nutritional Supplements: The essential guide for improving your health naturally*, Rocklin, CA, Prima Publishing, 1996

Offenkrantz, W.G. op. cit.

Pardee, A.B. & Ingraham, L.L. op. cit.

Patek, A.J., 'Chlorophyll and the Regeneration of the Blood', Annals of Internal Medicine, Vol. 57, 1936

Pfeiffer, C., *Mental and Elemental Nutrients* op. cit.

Pfeiffer, E. op. cit.

Robbins, R.C., 'Action of flavonoids on blood cells: trimodal action of flavonoids elucidates their inconsistent physiologic effects', in *International Journal of Vitamin and Nutrition Research*, Vol. 44, 1974

Robbins, R.C., 'Effects of vitamin C and flavonoids on blood cell aggregation and capillary resistance', in *Internationale Zeitung Vitaminforschung*, Vol. 36, 1966

Robbins, R.C., 'On bioflavonoids: new findings about a remarkable plant defence against disease and its dietary transfer to man', in *Executive Health*, Vol. 16, 1980

Schrodinger, Erwin op. cit.

Seeger, P.G. op. cit.

Simoneton, A. op. cit.

Spiller, Gene, 'Interaction of dietary fiber with other dietary components: a possible factor in certain cancer etiologies', in *American Journal of Clinical Nutrition*, October 1978

Szent-Gyorgyi, Albert, et al. op. cit.

Thompkins, P. & Bird, C. op. cit.

Warburg, Otto op. cit.

Wattenberg, L.W. et al., 'Induction of increased benzpyrene hydroxylase activity by flavones and related compounds', in *Cancer Research*, Vol. 28. 1968

Williams, R. op. cit.

Winter, Ruth, *A Consumer's Guide to Medicine in Food,* New York, Crown Trade Paperbacks, 1995

Zukav, G. op. cit.

Colour Has Clout

Becker, R.O., *Cross Currents: The Promise of Electromedicine, the Perils of Electropollution* op. cit.

Becker, R.O., 'Electromagnetic forces and life processes' op. cit.

Bircher, '*A Turning Point in Nutritional Science*' op. cit.

Bircher, R., *Way to Positive Health.* (ed.) op. cit.

Bircher-Benner, M., *The Essential Nature and Organization of Food Energy and the Application of the Second Principle of Thermo-Dynamics to Food Value and its Active Force* op. cit.

Bircher-Benner, M., *The Prevention of Incurable Disease,* op. cit.

Blauer, Stephen op. cit.

Bohm, David op. cit.

Bray, H.G. & White, K. op. cit.

Brekhman, I.I. op. cit.

Burr, Harold Saxton, op. cit.

Crile, George, *The Bipolar Theory of Living Processes* op. cit.

Crile, George, *The Phenomena of Life: A Radio-Electrical Interpretation* op. cit.

Dakin, H.S., *High Voltage Photography* op. cit.

Eastwood, M.A., & Mitchell W.D. op. cit.

Eppinger, Hans, *'Die Permeabilitatspathologie als Lehre vom Krank-heits-beginn'* op. cit.

Eppinger, Hans, 'Transmineralisation und vegetarische Kost' op. cit.

Eppinger, Hans, 'Uber Rohkostbehandlung' op. cit.

Ershoff, B.H., 'Antitoxic effects of plant fibre', *American Journal of Clinical Nutrition*, Vol. 27, December 1974

Gabor, M. op. cit.

Galvani, Luigi op. cit.

Gelin, L.E. 'Rheologic disturbances and the use of low viscosity dextran in surgery', *Review of Surgery*, Vol. 19, 1962

Gerson, Max op. cit.

Goulart, Francis Sheridan op. cit.

Hauschka, Rudolph op. cit.

Heinermann, John op. cit.

Hughes, J.H. & Latner, A.L. op. cit.

Hughes, R.E. & Wilson, H.K. op. cit.

Irons, V.E. op. cit.

Jean, V. op. cit.

Karstrom, Henning, *Ratt Kost*, op. cit.

Katahn, Martin op. cit.

Kelsay, J. op. cit.

Knisely, M.H. et al. op. cit.

Kuhn, Thomas op. cit.

Lai, Chiu-Nan, 'Anti-mutagenic activities of common vegetables and their chlorophyll content' op. cit.

Lai, Chiu-Nan, 'The active factor in wheat sprout extract inhibiting the metabolic activation of carcinogens in vitro' op. cit.

Lakhovsky, G. op. cit.

Lewis, W.H., Memory, P.F. & Elvin, Lewis op. cit.

Lund, E.J. op. cit.

Margen, Sheldon et al. op. cit.

Morgan, Brian L. op. cit.

Moss, T. op. cit.

Murray, Michael T., MD op. cit.

Offenkrantz, W.G. op. cit.

Pardee, A.B. & Ingraham, L.L. op. cit.

Patek, A.J. op. cit.

Pfeiffer, C., *Mental and Elemental Nutrients* op. cit.

Pfeiffer, E. op. cit.

Robbins, R.C., 'Action of flavonoids on blood cells: trimodal action of flavonoids elucidates their inconsistent physiologic effects' op. cit.

Robbins, R.C., 'Effects of vitamin C and flavonoids on blood cell aggregation and capillary resistance' op. cit.

Robbins, R.C., 'On bioflavonoids: new findings about a remarkable plant defence against disease and its dietary transfer to man' op. cit.

Schrodinger, Erwin op. cit.

Seeger, P.G. op. cit.

Simoneton, A. op. cit.

Spiller, Gene, op. cit.

Szent-Gyorgyi, Albert et al. op. cit.

Thompkins, P. & Bird, C. op. cit.

Warburg, Otto, op. cit.

Wattenberg, L.W. et al. op. cit.

Williams, R. op. cit.

Winter, Ruth, op. cit.

Zukav, G. op. cit.

Foods That Heal

Becker, R.O., *Cross Currents: The Promise of Electromedicine, the Perils of Electropollution* op. cit.

Becker, R.O., 'Electromagnetic forces and life processes' op. cit.

Bircher, R., 'A Turning Point in Nutritional Science' op. cit.

Bircher, R. (ed.) *Way to Positive Health* op. cit.

Bircher-Benner, M., *The Essential Nature and Organization of Food Energy and the Application of the Second Principle of Thermo-Dynamics to Food Value and its Active Force* op. cit.

Bircher-Benner, M., *The Prevention of Incurable Disease*, op. cit.

Blauer, Stephen op. cit.

Bohm, David op. cit.

Bray, H.G. & White, K. op. cit.

Brekhman, I.I. op. cit.

Burr, Harold Saxton, op. cit.

Crile, George, *The Bipolar Theory of Living Processes* op. cit.

Crile, George, *The Phenomena of Life: A Radio-Electrical Interpretation* op. cit.

Dakin, H.S., *High Voltage Photography* op. cit.

Eastwood, M.A. & Mitchell W.D. op. cit.

Eppinger, Hans, '*Die Permeabilitatspathologie als Lehre vom Krank-heits-beginn*' op. cit.

Eppinger, Hans, 'Transmineralisation und vegetarische Kost' op. cit.

Eppinger, Hans, 'Uber Rohkostbehandlung' op. cit.

Ershoff, B.H. op. cit.

Gabor, M. op. cit.

Galvani, Luigi, op. cit.

Gelin, L.E. op. cit.

Gerson, Max, op. cit.

Goulart, Francis Sheridan, op. cit.

Hauschka, Rudolph, op. cit.

Heinermann, John, op. cit.

Hughes, J.H. & Latner, A.L. op. cit.

Hughes, R.E. & Wilson, H.K. op. cit.

Irons, V.E. op. cit.

Jean, V. op. cit.

Karstrom, Henning, *Ratt Kost* op. cit.

Katahn, Martin, op. cit.

Kelsay, J. op. cit.

Knisely, M.H. et al. op. cit.

Kuhn, Thomas, op. cit.

Lai, Chiu-Nan, 'Anti-mutagenic activities of common vegetables and their chlorophyll content', op. cit.

Lai, Chiu-Nan, 'The active factor in wheat sprout extract inhibiting the metabolic activation of carcinogens in vitro', op. cit.

Lakhovsky, G. op. cit.

Lewis, W.H., Memory, P.F. & Elvin, Lewis, op. cit.

Lund, E.J. op. cit.

Margen, Sheldon et al. op. cit.

Morgan, Brian L. op. cit.

Moss, T. op. cit.

Murray, Michael T. MD, op. cit.

Offenkrantz, W.G. op. cit.

Pardee, A.B. & Ingraham, L.L. op. cit.

Patek, A.J. op. cit.

Pfeiffer, C., *Mental and Elemental Nutrients,* op. cit.

Pfeiffer, E. op. cit.

Robbins, R.C., 'Action of flavonoids on blood cells: trimodal action of flavonoids elucidates their inconsistent physiologic effects', op. cit.

Robbins, R.C., 'Effects of vitamin C and flavonoids on blood cell aggregation and capillary resistance', op. cit.

Robbins, R.C., 'On bioflavonoids: new findings about a remarkable plant defence against disease and its dietary transfer to man', op. cit.

Schrodinger, Erwin, op. cit.

Seeger, P.G. op. cit.

Simoneton, A. op. cit.

Spiller, Gene, op. cit.

Szent-Gyorgyi, Albert et al. op. cit.

Thompkins, P. & Bird, C. op. cit.

Warburg, Otto, op. cit.

Wattenberg, L.W. et al. op. cit.

Williams, R. op. cit.

Winter, Ruth, op. cit.

Zukav, G. op. cit.

Sprout for Life

Airola, Paavo O., *How to Keep Slim With Juice Fasting,* Phoenix, Arizona, Health Publishers, 1971

Applegate, W.V. & Connolly, P. *Price Pottenger Lectures,* 1974

Botman, S.G. & Crombie, W.M., *Journal of Experimental Botany*, Vol. 9, 1958

Cancer Control Journal, September/December, 1970, Los Angeles, California

Curtis, C., *An Account of Diseases of India as they appeared in the English Fleet*, Edinburgh, 1807

Hegazi, S.M., *Zeitschrift für Ernarungswissenschaft*, Vol. 13, 1974

Kakade, M.L. & Evans, R.J., *Journal of Food Science*, Vol. 31, 1966

Kirchner, H.E., *Live Food Juices*, Monrovia, California, H.E. Kirchner Publications, 1957

Kirchner, H.E., *Nature's Healing Grasses*, Riverside, California, H.C. White Publications (date unknown)

Kohler, G., *'Unidentified Factors Relating to Reproduction in Animals' Feedstuffs'*, 8 August 1953

Kulvinskas, V., *Nutritional Evaluation of Sprouts and Grasses*, Weathersfield, Connecticut, Omango D'Press, 1978

Kuppuswamy, S., 'Proteins in Food', *Indian Council of Medical Research*, New Delhi, 1958

Leichti-con Brasch, D. et al., *Bircher-Benner Keep Slim Nutrition Plan*, Los Angeles, Nash Publishing, 1973

Mayer, A.M. & Poljakoff-Mayber, A., *The Germination of Seeds*, Oxford, Pergamon Press, 1966

Price, W. op. cit.

Price-Pottenger Foundation, *The Guide to Living Foods Workbook*, La Mesa, California, 1978

Sellman, Per and Gita, *The Complete Sprouting Book*, Wellingborough, Turnstone Press, 1981

Szekely, E.B., *The Essene Gospel of Peace*, International Biogenic Society, Cartago, Costa Rica, 1978

Tsai, C.Y., Dalby, A. et al., 'Lysine and Tryptophan Increases During Cermination of Maize Seed', in *Cereal Chemistry*, Vol. 52, 1975

Walker, N.W., *Natural Weight Control*, op. cit.

Walker, N.W., *Raw Vegetable Juices*, New York, Jove/Harcourt Brace Jovanovich, 1877

RESOURCES

Leslie Kenton's Website: www.lesliekenton.com Here you will find a mass of helpful tools, techniques, inspiration and resources for practitioners and products as well as links to other websites which Leslie has found valuable. The website is highly active. Information changes frequently including messages from Leslie and news about forthcoming events and workshops she is doing throughout the world.

Most of the foods listed in *The Powerhouse Diet* you will be able to find in good 'health food' stores and, increasingly, in good supermarkets. You may have to look quite hard in out-of-the-way places in supermarkets to find tins of coconut milk and packets of seaweed, but they are there. A good health food store, however, will stock most of the products and ingredients I've mentioned or will be able to tell you where you can get them from.

Below are some addresses which may be helpful if you can't immediately find what you want locally, and a list of some of the products and ingredients I have mentioned which might be less than familiar to you with information on where you can get them.

ORGANIC FOODS

Clearspring
Supply organic foods and natural remedies as well as macrobiotic foods by mail order. They have a good range of herbal teas, organic grains, whole seeds for sprouting, dried fruits, pulses, nut butters, soya and vegetable products, sea vegetables, drinks and Bioforce herb tinctures. Write to them for a catalogue:
Clearspring
Unit 19a, Acton Park Estate
London W3 7QE
UK
Tel: +44 (0) 208 749 1781
Fax: +44 (0) 208 746 2249
You can order by telephone, fax, post or shop online at: www.clearspring.co.uk

Organics Direct
Offers a nationwide home delivery service of fresh vegetables and fruits,

delicious breads, juices, sprouts, fresh soups, ready-made meals, snacks and baby foods. They also sell the state-of-the-art 2001 Champion Juicers and the 2002 Health Smart Juice Extractor for beginners. They even sell organic wines – all shipped to you within 24 hours.
Organics Direct
1-7 Willow Street
London EC2A 4BH
UK
Tel: +44 (0) 207 729 2828
Fax: +44 (0) 207 613 5800
Website: www.organicsdirect.com (You can order online.)

The Soil Association
The Soil Association publishes a regularly updated national directory of farm shops and box schemes called *Where to Buy Organic Foods* that costs £5 including postage from:
The Soil Association
Bristol House
40–56 Victoria Street
Bristol BS1 6BY
UK
Tel: +44 (0) 117 929 0661
Fax: +44 (0) 117 925 2504
E-mail: info@soilassociation.org
Website: www.soilassociation.org.

ORGANIC MEAT

Eastbrook Farms Organic Meat
This is my favourite supplier of all sorts of organic meat because they take such care over every order.
Eastbrook Farms Organic Meats
The Calf House
Cues Lane
Bishopstone
Swindon
Wiltshire SN6 8PL
UK
Mail order: +44 (0) 1793 790 460

Helpline: +44 (0) 1793 790 340
Fax: +44 (0) 1793 791 239
E-mail: info@helenbrowningorganics.co.uk
Website: www.helenbrowningorganics.co.uk

Longwood Farm Organic Meats
Good-quality organic beef, pork, bacon, lamb, chicken, turkey, duck
and geese, a variety of types of sausage, dairy products, vegetables and
organic groceries (2000 lines), are available mail order from:
Longwood Farm Organic Meats
Tuddenham St Mary
Bury St Edmunds
Suffolk IP28 6TB
UK
Tel: +44 (0) 1638 717 120
Fax: +44 (0) 1638 717 120

Organic Butchers
A UK Guide to where to buy organic meat www.organicbutchers.co.uk
Organic Butchers
Crescent Consulting
1 The Crescent
Northampton NN1 4SB
UK
Tel: +44 (0) 1604 459962
Fax: +44 (0) 1604 459963
E-mail: butcher@touchstoneconsultants.co.uk

ADDRESSES TO REMEMBER
If you can't find what you want locally, especially if you are looking
for good quality vitamin and mineral supplements, contact either of the
following places.

The Nutri Centre
7 Park Crescent
London W1B 1PF
UK
Tel: +44 (0) 207 436 5122
E-mail: customerservices@nutricentre.com
Website: www.nutricentre.com

The best suppliers of nutritional supplements and information, unique in the world. The NutriCentre is not only the UK's leading supplier of supplements, it also has one of the finest collections of books on holistic health and nutrition including spiritual and psychological books related to health. This small shop in the basement of The Hale Clinic is always at the cutting edge of what is happening in holistic health. Their products can be ordered easily on line or by telephone. The NutriCentre carries more than 20,000 health and natural beauty care products including those which are available in health food stores as well as those sold only through practitioners. What you order is dispatched within 24 hours throughout the world. They have become Britain's largest supplier of complementary medicine textbooks to British colleges and universities. They print an interesting newsletter on holistic health with extracts printed on line. The center is dedicated to service. No order is too small or too large. Almost all of what you need for natural health and beauty you will find here. I can't recommend them highly enough.

Oliver's Wholefood Store

Another excellent place which offers a full range of supplements and natural remedies with an efficient nation-wide mail order service is Oliver's Wholefood Store. They are winner of 'Organic Community Shop of the Year 99' and 'Health Food Store of the Year 99'. Full organic grocer with off-licence, specialising in excellent quality organic food – vegetables, fish, meat etc. Opening Times Monday – Sunday 9am-7pm. Oliver's organise regular health lectures.
5 Station Approach
Kew Gardens
Richmond
Surrey TW9 3QB
UK
Tel: +44 (0) 208 948 3990
Fax: +44 (0) 208 948 3991
E-mail: info@oliverswholefoods.co.uk

HOW TO FIND

Bee Pollen

NatureBee uses various potentiation processes which unlock the power of pollen. NatureBee Potentiated Bee Pollen is available from:
Topline International
PO Box 5853

Wellesley Street
Auckland
New Zealand
Freephone: (NZ) 0800 506 601 and (AUS) 1800 147 009

Head Office and Showroom:
Shed 24,
Princess Wharf
Auckland
Website: www.naturebee.com

In the UK it is available online from www.wmsluk.com or freephone:
0800 917 6664.

Coconut

Coconut oil or fat can be bought in health food stores, many of the major supermarkets, and in Indian and Malaysian stores. Coconut milk, dried coconut, and creamed coconut are available in any supermarket, but make sure that what you buy is pure coconut and contains no sugar or additives.

Flaxseed Oil (Linseed oil)

Organic Flaxseed Oil is available from:
Savant Distribution Ltd
FREEPOST NEA 12027
Leeds LS16 6YY
UK
Order line (UK): 08450 606070
Fax: +44 (0) 113 388 5248
E-mail: info@savant-health.com
Website: www.savant-health.com

Flaxseeds (Linseeds)

Vacuum-packed whole flaxseeds (linseeds) are available in most health-food stores. I use Linusit Gold as they are well packed and fresh. They are available from The Nutri Centre (see above). Keep them refrigerated.

Herbs

Phyto Products Ltd are an excellent company originally set up to supply herbalists with high-quality herbs and plant products. Every plant and herb they sell states the source of origin. All Phyto Products' plants are purchased only from recognisable sources. They do a full range of tinctures, herbal skin creams (including Calendula Cream, Comfrey Cream, Arnica Ointment and St John's Wort Oil), fluid extracts, herbs and the Schoenenberger plant juices. They do not supply herbs in capsules but they now do some herbs in tablet form. Write to them for their price list. They have a minimum order of £20 (before VAT) plus carriage.

Phyto Products Ltd
Park Works
Park House
Mansfield Woodhouse
Mansfield
Nottinghamshire NG19 8EF
UK
Tel: +44 (0) 1623 644 334
Fax: +44 (0) 1623 657 232

Solgar Vitamin & Herb are an American company founded in 1947 which produces good quality nutritional supplements and standardised single herbs and formulas under strict pharmaceutical standards of manufacture – in many cases stricter than USA government requirements. These include standardised full potency Herbal Female Complex (containing soy isoflavones), Feverfew Willow Complex, Milk Thistle Dandelion Complex, Ginger Fennel Complex, Olive Leaf Echinacea Complex, and Herbal Male Complex. Solgar products are available from top health-food stores, some chemists, and the Nutri Centre.

Solgar Vitamins Ltd.
Beggar's Lane
Aldbury
Tring
Herts HP23 5PT
UK
Tel: +44 (0) 1442 890 355
Fax: +44 (0) 1442 890 366
E-mail: solgarinfor@solgar.com
Website: www.solgar.com

Herb Teas
Some of my favourite blends include Cinnamon Rose, Orange Zinger and Emperors Choice by Celestial Seasonings: Warm & Spicy by Symmingtons and Creamy Carob French Vanilla. Yogi Tea by Golden

Temple Products is a strong spicy blend, perfect as a coffee replacement. Green tea is available from health food stores and Oriental supermarkets.

Juicers

Veteran juicers wax lyrical about the virtues of The Champion masticating juicer: an indestructible American juicer that some people claim makes better juice than any centrifugal extractor can. The Champion is basically a rotating cutter on a shaft, which expels dry pulp from it spout at one end as the juice is drained through a nozzle underneath. There are many UK suppliers, including Savant-Health (see Flaxseed Oil)

Another favourite juicer is The Vita-Mix Total Nutrition Centre: basically a turbo charged, super-efficient blender with an indestructible stainless steel blades and an extremely powerful motor, the TNC is dynamic. It's the only machine that is properly able to make the fibre-rich juices – the kind of molecular – or total – juicing. It is also effective for making cereal grass juices, which must be strained before use.
Contact:
Country Life Natural Food Shop Ltd
3-4 Warwick Street
London W1B 5LS
UK
Tel: +44 (0) 207 434 2922
Fax: +44 (0) 207 434 2838

Maldon Salt Flakes and Celtic Salt: Available from good health food stores and some supermarkets. These are the best tasting salts I have found.

Manuka Honcy

Manuka honey should be easy to find in your local health food store. One of my favourites is "Active" Manuka Honey from NatureBee. See above.

Comvita Manuka Honey is available from Xynergy Health Products (see Super Green Foods).

The Garvin Honey Company has a good selection of set and clear honeys form all over the world.
The Garvin Honey Co.
Avenue Three

Station Lane
Witney
Oxon OX28 4HZ
UK
Tel: +44 (0) 1993 775 423
Fax: +44 (0) 1993 774 227
E-mail: Sales@honeyonline.co.uk
Website: www.honeyonline.co.uk

Marigold Swiss Vegetable Bouillonn Powder: This instant broth made from vegetables and sea salt comes in regular, low-salt, vegan and organic varieties. It is available from health food stores or direct from:
Marigold Foods
102 Camley Street
London NW1 OPF
UK
Tel: +44 (0) 207 388 4515
Fax: +44 (0) 207 388 4516

Microfiltered Whey Protein
Solgar produce Whey To Go Protein Powder in vanilla, chocolate, honey nut and mixed berry flavours, I prefer the vanilla and chocolate (although the chocolate contains artificial sweetener).
Solgar Vitamin & Herb
Beggar's Lane
Aldbury
Tring
Herts HP23 5PT
UK
Tel: +44 (0) 1442 890 355
Fax: + 44 (0) 1442 890 366
E-mail: solgarinfo@solgar.com
Website: www.solgar.com

BioPure Pure Protein by Metagenics or Twinlab Super Whey Powder are also good sources of microfiltered whey protein. Whey To Go and BioPure can be purchased from the Nutri Centre (see above).

MSM Max
These MSM tablets are the purest and most potent form of MSM available – fast-acting and 100% pure with no additives or binders.

PO Box 33830
Portland
OR 97292
USA
Tel: ++1 (503) 761 7450
Fax: ++1 (503) 761 5383
Website: www.richdistributing.com

Also available from:
The Naturally Curious Company
P O Box 46
Pukekohe
Auckland 1800
New Zealand
Tel: +64 (9) 239 0496.
Fax: +64 (9) 239 0936
Website: www.naturalchoices.co.nz

Sea plants/Seaweed
You can buy seaweed and sea plants in good health food stores, Japanese supermarkets, and an increasing number of supermarkets. The range available in supermarkets is often pretty limited so for the best choice find your nearest Japanese supermarket. Or contact Olivers Wholefood Store (see above).

Soya Milk
The best soya milk I have come across is called Bonsoy. It is particularly good soya milk, unusual in that it is not packed in aluminium. It is organic and available from good health food stores. Try:
Fresh and Wild
196 Old Street
London EC1V 9FR.
UK
Tel: +44 (0) 207 250 1708

or Wild Oats
210 Westbourne Grove
London W11 2RH
UK
Tel: +44 (0) 207 229 0468

Stevia

In most countries stevia is readily available in health food stores in many forms. Not in the UK, alas. It comes as clear liquid extract in distilled water, powdered stevia leaf, as full strength (very sweet) stevioside extract. You can sprinkle stevia like sugar on foods and in drinks. It even comes in tiny single serving packets which you can carry around with you in your pocket or handbag. You may find you can order stevia direct from abroad over the internet. Or asking a friend who lives in the US to send you some. Stevia is unquestionably the best form of sweetener in the world. Far from doing harm it actually has many beneficial properties. Keep an eye on my website as the friends of the website often post updates on how to order stevia from abroad if you live in the UK or EU.

Super Green Foods

Xynergy Health Products specialise in selling the finest green nutritional products – such as spirulina and cereal grasses – you can buy. They also sell the only fully natural multiple vitamin and mineral formula derived from plants, called Pure Synergy ™ . Xynergy products are available in sophisticated health food stores or can be ordered by post direct from them.

Xynergy Health Products
Elsted
Midhurst
West Sussex GU29 0JT
UK
Tel: +44 (0) 1730 813 642
Fax: +44 (0) 1730 815 109
E-mail: naturally@xynergy.co.uk
Website: www.xynergy.co.uk

Water

Getting pure water can be difficult. One in ten of us drink water which is contaminated with poisons above international standards. I have finally found a water purifier which I think is good – the Fresh Water 1000 Water Filter System. It removes more than 90 percent of heavy metals, pesticides and hydrocarbons such as benzene, trihalmethanes, chlorine, oestrogen and bacteria without removing essential minerals like calcium. Available from:

The Fresh Water Filter Company Ltd
Gem House

895 High Road
Chadwell Heath
Essex RM6 4HL
UK
Tel: +44 (0) 208 597 3223
Fax: +44 (0) 870 056 7264
E-mail: mail@freshwaterfilter.com
Website: www.freshwaterfilter.com

FOR FURTHER INFORMATION

Bio Dynamic Agricultural Association
Painswick Inn
Stroud
Gloucester
UK
Tel/Fax: +44 (0) 1453 759 501
E-mail: office@biodynamic.org.uk
Website: www.anth.org.uk/biodynamic

Advice, information, bio-dynamic preparations, regional groups, journal.

Henry Doubleday Research Association (HDRA)
Ryton Organic Gardens
Coventry
Warwickshire CV8 3LG
UK
Tel: +44 (0) 247 630 3517
Fax: +44 (0) 247 663 9229
Website: www.hdra.org.uk

Advice, information, quarterly magazine, courses, beautiful demonstrations of organic growing techniques

The Weston A Price Foundation
Website: www.westonaprice.org

INDEX